Interventional Cardiology

Self–Assessment & Review

Martin B. Leon, MD

Director, Cardiology Research Foundation
Washington Hospital Center
Washington, D.C.

Robert D. Safian, MD

Director, Interventional Cardiology
William Beaumont Hospital
Royal Oak, Michigan

Mark Freed, MD

Division of Cardiology
William Beaumont Hospital
Royal Oak, Michigan

**PHYSICIANS'
PRESS**

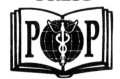

Birmingham, Michigan

ABOUT PHYSICIANS' PRESS

Physicians' Press is a unique entry into the medical publishing industry. Owned and operated by physicians, Physicians' Press specializes in innovative and user-friendly manuals, textbooks, and newsletters in the fields of Interventional Cardiology, Clinical Cardiology, and Internal Medicine. Physicians' Press stands apart from all other medical publishers in being able to produce <u>completely current publications</u>; literature references are *less than 2 weeks old* at the time of book release, compared to 18 months old for most other texts. We frequently receive comments such as "I am astounded at how current your information is," and, "The only books I bother reading are yours, the rest are outdated." Physicians' Press is committed to providing its readers with the most current, practical, and user-friendly information, as we continue to distinguish ourselves as the new gold-standard in medical publishing.

Be sure to visit us on the internet at **www.physicianspress.com**, where you'll find interventional cases, self-assessment questions and answers, information about upcoming meetings, and more.

If you are looking for a publisher or have comments and suggestions, please contact us at:

Physicians' Press
555 South Woodward Ave., Suite 1409
Birmingham, Michigan 48009
Tel: (248) 645-6443
Fax: (248) 642-4949
http://www.physicianspress.com

Printed in the United States of America   ISBN 1-890114-04-9

DEDICATION

To my wife, Linda, and my children, Yelena and Ari, who make all things in life possible.

— Martin B. Leon

To my wife, Maureen, and to my sons, Ryan and Luke: The more you learn, the more you want to know.

— Robert D. Safian

To those who dedicate their lives to the pursuit of scientific investigation, and to my wonderfully dear and loving family.

— Mark Freed

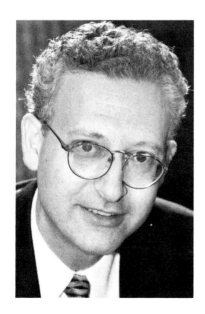 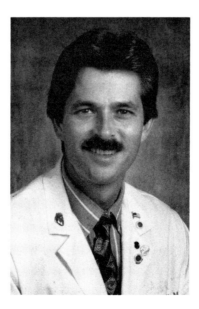 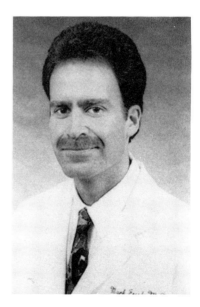

Martin B. Leon, MD   Robert D. Safian, MD   Mark Freed, MD

PREFACE

In the near future, organizations such as the American College of Cardiology (ACC) and the Society for Cardiac Angiography and Interventions (SCAI) will put forth two important proposals to improve the practice of interventional cardiology: Implementation of a national board examination, and development of specific criteria for certification. There is no doubt that within the next few years, physicians who wish to practice interventional cardiology will be required by hospital credentialing committees to meet all the requirements for certification, including passing the interventional cardiology board examination.

Interventional Cardiology: Self-Assessment and Review has been developed in anticipation of the requirement for formal certification in interventional cardiology. This unique reference, the first of its kind in interventional cardiology, also serves as a powerful teaching aid for physicians and other medical professionals who wish to test and supplement their knowledge of the field. Over 500 multiple choice and matching questions span the entire breadth of interventional cardiology, including simple and complex angioplasty; stents, atherectomy, and lasers; adjunctive imaging and pharmacotherapy; intraprocedural complications; recent clinical trials; peripheral vascular intervention; and balloon valvuloplasty. Answers and explanations are supplemented by completely current references from journals and international meetings.

Additional self-assessment questions and answers, along with interventional cases and a listing of meetings and conferences can be found on the Physicians' Press web site at **www.physicianspress.com**

We hope you enjoy the challenge of **Interventional Cardiology: Self-Assessment and Review**, as Physicians' Press continues to distinguish itself by producing the most practical, easy-to-read, comprehensive, and completely up-to-date publications for the interventional cardiologist.

Martin B. Leon, MD
Robert D. Safian, MD
Mark Freed, MD

ACKNOWLEDGMENTS

We would like to acknowledge the dedicated and tireless efforts of Dianna Frye in preparing this manuscript for publication, Norm Lyle of *The Lyle Group* for cover design, Steven Kronenberg of *Imprint Graphic Design* for graphic arts, and Dickinson Press for their printing expertise.

Martin B. Leon, MD
Robert D. Safian, MD
Mark Freed, MD

NOTICE

The explosive growth of new equipment and drug therapy has resulted in the rapid evolution and acceptance of practice patterns often based on retrospective nonrandomized data and personal experience. Their ultimate role will require close inspection of prospective randomized trials. The clinical recommendations set forth in this book are those of the authors; they are offered as *general guidelines only and are not to be construed as absolute indications.* In addition, not all equipment or medications have been accepted by the U.S. Food and Drug Administration (USFDA) for usages described in this manual. The use of any device or drug should be preceded by a careful review of the package insert, which provides indications (and dosages) as approved by the USFDA. The reader is advised to consult the package insert before using any therapeutic agent. The authors and publisher disclaim responsibility for adverse effects resulting from omissions or undetected errors.

Interventional Cardiology

- Questions -

1. Which medical conditions require postponement of elective coronary intervention:

   a. Aspirin allergy
   b. Compensated left ventricular dysfunction
   b. Mobitz Type I second-degree AV block
   d. Mobitz Type II second-degree AV block
   e. Compensated chronic obstructive pulmonary disease
   f. Uncontrolled diabetes
   g. Potassium = 2.7 mEq/L
   h. Active GI bleeding
   i. Platelet count = 60,000/μl
   j. Prothrombin time > 16 seconds
   k. Unexplained or progressive renal insufficiency
   l. Unexplained fever
   m. Unexplained leukocytosis

2. Aspirin has been shown to reduce the incidence of acute occlusion after PTCA by 50-75% and is considered essential therapy prior to non-emergent interventions:

   a. True
   b. False

3. Which of the following statements about aspirin-induced asthma and rhinosinusitis are true:

   a. Over 10% of adults with asthma and 30% of those with asthma and rhinosinusitis develop aspirin sensitivity
   b. The absence of a prior adverse reaction predicts continued tolerance
   c. Most aspirin allergic patients have nasal polyps, eosinophils and mast cells on nasal smear, and abnormal sinus radiographs
   d. Aspirin desensitization is safe but unreliable
   e. Patients with aspirin allergies requiring desensitization should be referred to a center experienced in this technique

4. Which of the following statements about aspirin-induced cutaneous reactions are true?

   a. Desensitization of individuals with aspirin-induced angioedema and/or urticaria is unreliable and these patients should not undergo desensitization
   b. A previous cutaneous reaction to aspirin places the individual at increased risk for anaphylaxis upon readministration of the drug
   c. H$_1$ and H$_2$ and antagonists can usually control cutaneous symptoms during the peri-procedural period

5. Desensitization is recommended for individuals who have had an anaphylactic reaction to aspirin:

   a. True
   b. False

6. Reasonable approaches to the management of patients with aspirin-induced anaphylaxis who require percutaneous intervention include:

   a. Aspirin desensitization
   b. Ticlopidine
   c. ReoPro
   d. Dextran
   e. IV heparin alone without antiplatelet agents

7. Clinical factors that increase the risk of complications and/or decrease the rate of success during PTCA include:

   a. Advanced age
   b. Mitral stenosis
   c. Aortic stenosis
   d. Pulmonary hypertension
   e. Ejection fraction < 40%
   f. Diabetes mellitus
   g. Silent ischemia
   h. Atrial fibrillation
   i. Previous CABG
   j. Peripheral vascular disease
   k. Acute myocardial infarction

8. All of the following angiographic factors increase the risk of complications and/or decrease the rate of successful during PTCA except:

    a. Multivessel disease
    b. Single patent vessel
    c. Bend point of 30°
    d. Bifurcation lesion
    e. Thrombus
    f. Severe proximal vessel tortuosity
    g. Calcification
    h. Ostial lesion
    I. Degenerated vein graft

9. An activated clotting time ___ seconds is recommended before PTCA hardware is advanced into the coronary artery:

    a. 200
    b. 200-250
    c. 250-300
    d. 300-400
    e. > 400

10. Patients receiving continuous heparin prior to PTCA may be resistant to heparin during the procedure:

    a. True
    b. False

11. When sizing the PTCA balloon, the diameter of the final balloon should be:

    a. 10% less than the normal reference diameter adjacent to the lesion
    b. Equal to the normal reference diameter adjacent to the lesion
    c. Equal to the diameter of the target vessel at its ostium
    d. 10% larger than the normal reference diameter adjacent to the lesion

12. Balloon/artery ratios < 0.9 frequently result in significant residual stenosis, while balloon/artery ratios ≥ 1.2 increase the risk of emergency bypass surgery and myocardial infarction:

    a. True
    b. False

13. Which of the following angiographic views best show region-3 on the figure below:

    a. 30° LAO, 20° cranial
    b. 90° LAO
    c. 20° RAO

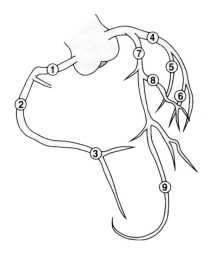

14. If buckling occurs during attempts to cross a lesion with the guidewire, the wire should be:

    a. Forcefully prolapsed beyond the lesion
    b. Retracted and readvanced
    c. Retracted and the case terminated

15. Match each of the procedures below to their recommended vascular sheath size:

    a. PTCA   1. 8-11 French
    b. Atherectomy   2. 18-22 French
    c. Aortic Valvuloplasty   3. 12-14 French
    d. Percutaneous cardiopulmonary bypass   4. 6-8 French

16. Which of the following statements about PTCA of the LAD are true:

    a. The LAD normally arises in an anterior and superior position
    b. A Judkins Left 4.0 is the guide catheter of choice in the majority of cases
    c. If the ostium of the left main is high or the aortic root is small, a JL 4.5 catheter may be preferred
    d. Once in the left main, gentle clockwise rotation of the guiding catheter will frequently direct it anteriorly

17. Which of the following statements about PTCA of the left circumflex are true:

    a. Left circumflex angioplasty is often associated with difficulties in guidewire passage and balloon tracking
    b. Stable coaxial alignment of the guide catheter may be facilitated by gentle counterclockwise rotation of a JL4 guiding catheter once in the left main
    c. An Amplatz left guiding catheter should be considered for sharply angulated or an inferiorly positioned circumflex origin

18. Which of the following statements about use of an Amplatz guide catheter are true:

    a. Amplatz guides should be withdrawn from the vessel in a manner similar to a Judkins guide
    b. Deeply engaged Amplatz guides should be partially withdrawn over an extended balloon
    c. Proper disengagement may require slight advancement until the tip prolapses out of the artery, followed by rotation away from the ostium prior to withdrawal
    d. The Amplatz guide catheter derives its support from the opposite wall of the aorta

19. Which of the following statements about PTCA of the right coronary artery are true:

    a. Compared to the left coronary artery, guide engagement of the right coronary artery more often results in dampened arterial pressure tracings
    b. A "Shepherd Crook" RCA should not be engaged with a hockey stick guide because of the risk of dissection
    c. For marked inferior orientations, multipurpose and Amplatz guides should be avoided

20. Which of the following statements about damping of the arterial pressure tracing are true:

    a. Causes include the presence of a diseased ostium, coronary spasm, non-coaxial alignment of the guide and vessel wall, and mismatch between the vessel diameter and diameter of the guide
    b. Forceful contrast injections increase the risk of coronary dissection
    c. Consider the use of a smaller guide catheter, guide catheter with a different tip configuration, or a side-hole catheter

21. Potential problems with sidehole catheters include all of the following except:

    a. Suboptimal opacification of the target vessel
    b. Increased risk of ostial trauma during engagement
    c. Decreased back-up support
    d. Kinking of the guide catheter at the sideholes

22. Which of the pressure tracings below is:

    a. Damped
    b. Normal
    c. Ventricularized

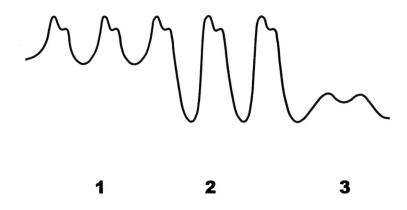

1   **2**   **3**

23. All the following statements about PTCA guidewires are true except:

    a. Wires with increased flexibility have decreased steerability
    b. Wires with increased torque-control have decreased flexibility
    c. Larger wires have decreased steerability, resulting in greater straightening of tortuous segments and providing more support for balloon catheter advancement

24. Which of the following characteristics about balloon catheters are true:

    a. Balloon "compliance" is defined as the change in balloon diameter per atmosphere of inflation pressure and is an index of the stretchability of a balloon
    b. Balloon "creep" refers to the tendency of a balloon to enlarge after serial inflations at the same pressure
    c. Less compliant balloons are generally associated with more creep
    d. Data clearly demonstrate clinical superiority of compliant over non-compliant balloons
    e. Rated burst pressure is defined as the pressure below which 99.9% of balloons will not rupture
    f. Mean burst pressure is defined as the pressure at which 50% of balloons will rupture and is higher than rated burst pressure

25. Femoral sheaths can be removed after discontinuing heparin when the:

    a. ACT is less than 190 seconds
    b. ACT is less than 150 seconds
    c. PTT is less than 50 seconds
    d. Fibrinogen level is less than 100 mg/dl if lytics have been given
    e. Fibrinogen level is between 100-150 mg/dl if lytics have been given
    f. Fibrinogen level exceeds 150 mg/dl if lytics have been given

BRACHIAL AND RADIAL APPROACH

26. Compared to the femoral approach, the brachial approach to coronary intervention is associated with:

    a. More difficult catheter manipulation
    b. Less radiation exposure
    c. Easier superselective coronary intubation

    d. More local bleeding

    e. Increased loss of pulse

    f. Less transfusion requirements

27. Clinical situations favoring brachial and/or radial approaches over the femoral approach include:

    a. Peripheral vascular disease

    b. Need for uninterrupted anticoagulation

    c. Difficult internal mammary artery cannulation

    d. Degenerated saphenous vein graft disease

    e. Severe coronary artery tortuosity

    f. Poor left ventricular dysfunction

28. The incidence of brachial artery occlusion and significant hematoma following the brachial approach to coronary intervention are:

    a. 1% and 1%

    b. 0.1% and 0.1%

    c. 0.1% and 1%

    d. 1% and 0.1%

MULTIVESSEL AND HIGH-RISK INTERVENTION

29. Which of the following statements are true about the randomized PTCA versus CABG trials for multivessel disease (RITA, ERACI, GABI, CABRI, EAST, BARI):

    a. 50% of patients with multivessel disease met the inclusion criteria

    b. Less than 10% of patients screened were actually randomized

    c. Most patients had two-vessel disease and normal LV function

    d. Complete revascularization varied between trials

    e. Patients with total occlusions were excluded from all trials

    f. Use of new devices and internal mammary artery grafting were not allowed

Questions

30. Which of the following statements about **in-hospital** results of the randomized PTCA versus CABG trials are true:

    a. In-hospital mortality was similar between PTCA and CABG groups
    b. In-hospital MI rate was higher in the PTCA group
    c. Emergency CABG for failed PTCA was required in 1.5-10%
    d. Length of hospital stay was 2-3 fold higher in the CABG group

31. Which of the following statements about **late outcome** of patients randomized to the PTCA versus CABG trials are true:

    a. Infarct-free survival at 1 year was similar
    b. Diabetics treated with PTCA had higher late mortality
    c. PTCA resulted in equal degrees of angina, need for anti-anginal therapy, and repeat revascularization
    d. Approximately 20% of PTCA patients required CABG at 1-3 years

32. Which of the following statements about multivessel angioplasty in patients with LV dysfunction are true:

    a. LV dysfunction adversely impacts long-term outcome after multivessel PTCA
    b. Complete anatomical revascularization may be more important in patients with LV dysfunction compared to those with normal LV function
    c. CABG may be preferred if PTCA cannot achieve complete revascularization, particularly in patients with diabetes, unstable angina, high-risk lesion morphology, and/or proximal LAD disease

33. Indications for staging procedures in patients with multivessel disease include all of the following except:

    a. Thrombus after PTCA of first lesion
    b. Severe dissection after intervention on first lesion
    c. Procedure duration > 3 hours
    d. Contrast volume of 250 cc
    e. Second lesion has a 50-70% stenosis without objective evidence for ischemia
    f. PTCA for acute MI

34. Preprocedural considerations aimed at risk reduction in patients undergoing high-risk angioplasty include:

    a. Referral to an interventional center experienced with the use of new devices and support strategies
    b. Insertion of a pulmonary artery catheter in patients with labile hemodynamics or heart failure
    c. Maintenance of urine output > 40cc per hour with IV crystalloids in patients with pre-existing renal insufficiency or a history of renal dysfunction after contrast exposure

35. Post-procedural recommendations after high-risk angioplasty include:

    a. Transfer to a monitored medical bed
    b. Immediate return to the cath lab to exclude abrupt closure for recurrent chest pain with ECG changes or hemodynamic instability
    c. Abrupt discontinuation of heparin 12-24 hours post PTCA for procedures complicated by slow-flow or thrombus

36. Asymptomatic hypotension may be caused by:

    a. Medications (sedatives, nitrates, calcium-channel blockers, beta-blockers)
    b. Hypovolemia
    c. Cardiac tamponade
    d. Retroperitoneal bleeding
    e. Sepsis

37. Which of the following statements about left main disease are true:

    a. Left main disease occurs in 7% of patients with stable angina and 15% of patients with unstable angina
    b. Bypass surgery has been shown to prolong survival in patients with left main stenoses of 40-50% and normal left ventricular function
    c. PTCA can be performed with success rates exceeding 90%
    d. In-hospital and 3-year mortality rates following PTCA approach 10% and 60%, respectively
    e. Left main coronary disease can be treated equally well with bypass surgery or stents

UNSTABLE ISCHEMIC SYNDROMES

38. Only _____ % of acute MI patients receive thrombolytic therapy:

    a. 10%
    b. 33%
    c. 50%
    d. 60%

39. Following IV thrombolytic therapy for acute MI, _____ % of vessels remain occluded and _____ % have impaired (TIMI ≤ 2) flow:

    a. 10% and 20%
    b. 45% and 20%
    c. 20% and 45%
    d. 45% and 55%

40. Following IV thrombolytic therapy for acute MI, recurrent ischemia occurs in _____ % and intracranial bleeding in _____ %:

    a. 15-30% and 3-5%
    b. 30-45% and 0.5-1.5%
    c. 15-30% and 0.5-1.5%
    d. 30-45% and 2-5%

41. Compared to IV thrombolysis for acute MI, primary (direct) PTCA:

    a. Allows immediate definition of coronary anatomy
    b. Results in similar rates of acute vessel patency and similar rates of TIMI-3 flow
    c. Results in less reocclusion, recurrent ischemia, and reinfarction
    d. Results in better survival in high-risk patients
    e. Results in more reperfusion injury and myocardial rupture
    f. Is associated with a similar risk of intracranial hemorrhage
    g. Results in a shorter length of hospital stay

42. Procedure-related mortality is higher when primary PTCA is performed on lytic-ineligible patients compared to lytic-eligible patients:

    a. True
    b. False

43. Patient groups especially well-suited for primary PTCA include:

    a. The elderly
    b. Patients who present late after symptom onset
    c. Patients with acute vein graft occlusion
    d. Patients without ST elevation

44. Survival rates in patients presenting with acute MI and cardiogenic shock are ____ % after PTCA, ____ % after lytic therapy, and ____ % after medical therapy.

    a. 50-80% and 30% and 10%
    b. 30-50% and 10% and 2%
    c. 50-80% and 50% and 20%

45. Rescue PTCA of a persistent occlusion following lytics is not recommended due to significant morbidity and mortality associated with this interventional strategy:

    a. True
    b. False

46. Which of the following statements about rescue (salvage) PTCA for failed thrombolysis are true:

    a. Rescue PTCA often improves regional wall motion and LV function, and reduces the risk of heart failure, shock, and death in patients with large infarctions
    b. The prognosis of patients after successful rescue PTCA is similar to that after successful thrombolysis
    c. Patients requiring rescue PTCA are at no higher risk for reocclusion than patients treated with primary PTCA or successful thrombolytic therapy
    d. Early mortality is high if rescue PTCA is unsuccessful

47. Immediate PTCA of a high-grade residual stenosis after thrombolysis for acute MI is routinely recommended for asymptomatic patients with TIMI 3 flow:

    a. True
    b. False

48. Randomized trials have shown that after successful thrombolysis, a strategy of routine PTCA before discharge in asymptomatic patients results in higher survival, less infarction, and better ejection fraction compared to a conservative approach of PTCA for spontaneous or inducible ischemia:

    a. True
    b. False

49. Which of the following statements about direct PTCA for acute MI are true:

    a. Profound hypotension and bradycardia due to the Bezold-Jarisch reflex occur more commonly after PTCA of the right coronary artery (compared to left coronary artery)
    b. In-hospital recurrent ischemia occurs in 10-15%
    c. The need for blood transfusion after primary PTCA has been associated with thrombolytic agents, bypass surgery, prolonged anticoagulation, and indwelling sheaths

50. In-hospital rate of re-infarction following primary PTCA for acute MI is ____%:

    a. 8%
    b. 10%
    c. 0.5%
    d. 2%

51. Vessel reocclusion after primary PTCA occurs in ____ % of patients prior to discharge:

    a. 5%
    b. 10%
    c. 15%
    d. > 20%

52. Vessel reocclusion after successful rescue PTCA occurs in _____ % of patients prior to discharge:

    a. 5%
    b. 10%
    c. 15%
    d. > 20%

53. By 6-months after successful primary PTCA for acute MI, reocclusion occurs in _____ % and restenosis in _____ %:

    a. 30% and 60%
    b. 30% and 20%
    c. 15% and 40%
    d. 15% and 20%

54. Medical therapy for unstable angina is associated with in-hospital mortality in _____ % and myocardial infarction in _____ %:

    a. 1% and 10%
    b. 1% and 20%
    c. 5% and 10%
    d. 5% and 20%

55. Patients presenting with unstable angina and a history of antecedent angina are more likely to have multivessel disease compared to patients with new onset unstable angina:

    a. True
    b. False

56. Which of the following statements about PTCA for unstable angina are true:

    a. Technical success rates for unstable angina are similar to those for stable angina
    b. Periprocedural complications of PTCA for unstable angina are similar to PTCA for stable angina

c. Compared to an initial strategy of medical therapy, PTCA reduces the incidence of death and MI

57. Which of the following statements about the use of devices for MI or unstable angina are true:

a. The routine use of IABPs to reduce reinfarction and reocclusion after primary PTCA is controversial
b. In the CAVEAT trial, DCA was associated with more non-Q-wave MI than PTCA
c. Rotablator atherectomy is not recommended in acute MI
d. Preliminary experience does not support the feasibility and safety of stenting in the setting of recent or acute MI

58. Which of the following statements about drugs for MI or unstable angina are true:

a. Aspirin reduces the incidence of acute closure by 30-50%
b. Ticlopidine is not useful for percutaneous intervention
c. ReoPro reduces the rate of MI following PTCA for unstable or post-MI angina
d. Intraprocedural heparin doses and "ideal" ACT levels may be higher in patients with acute ischemic syndromes than with stable angina
e. Compared to heparinized patients undergoing primary PTCA, hirudin reduces late cardiac events
f. Routine intracoronary thrombolytic therapy should be avoided in patients undergoing PTCA for unstable angina

LV DYSFUNCTION

59. Potential indications for supported angioplasty conclude:

a. Target vessel supplies the majority of viable myocardium
b. Ejection fraction < 30%
c. Triple vessel disease with LV ejection fraction ≥ 40%
d. Jeopardy score ≥ 3
e. Cardiogenic shock and multivessel disease

60. Which of the following statements about intra-aortic balloon pumping (IABP) are true:

    a. IABP decreases myocardial oxygen demand, increases coronary perfusion pressure, and increases cardiac output by 20-40%
    b. The incidence of vascular complications, including AV fistula, pseudoaneurysm, iliofemoral thrombosis, and local bleeding is about 50%
    c. Complications are more common in patients with pre-existing vascular disease, diabetics, and males
    d. Effective diastolic augmentation requires a stable cardiac rhythm
    e. Significant hemolysis and platelet counts below 50,000 are usual

61. When percutaneous cardiopulmonary support is used, intravenous heparin should be dosed to maintain the ACT at _____ seconds:

    a. 200-250
    b. 250-300
    c. 300-350
    d. 350-400
    e. > 400

62. Hypotension is common within the first few minutes of CPS and usually responds to a bolus of normal saline rather than increasing the flow rate:

    a. True
    b. False

63. Which of the following statements about percutaneous CPS are true:

    a. CPS provides excellent systemic perfusion independent of ventricular function and intrinsic cardiac rhythm
    b. The perception of ischemic chest pain during PTCA is reduced in CPS-supported patients
    c. Myocardial ischemia, regional wall motion abnormalities, and anaerobic metebalism do not occur during balloon inflation
    d. CPS can be continued up to 12 hours after its initiation

64. Only 5-10% of patients with standby CPS (contralateral arterial and venous access obtained; cannulas placed only if needed) will actually require initiation of CPS:

a. True
b. False

65. All of the following statements about autoperfusion catheters are true except:

    a. They are more difficult to place in tortuous vessels and distal coronary segments because their profile and trackablity are inferior to nonperfusion catheters
    b. Balloon inflation pressures greater than 6 atmospheres may impair perfusion
    c. Intermittent flushing of the central lumen with heparinized saline is recommended to prevent thrombosis
    d. Flow rates as high as 40-60cc per minute may be achieved independent of systemic blood pressure
    e. When used as a bailout catheter for failed PTCA prior to emergency bypass surgery, successful placement results in a lower incidence of Q-wave MI, less ST segment elevation, and greater use of internal mammary grafts

PATIENT CHARACTERISTICS

66. Which of the following statements about the impact of age on coronary revascularization are true:

    a. Compared to older patients, patients < 40 years of age typically have more cardiac risk factors and less extensive disease
    b. PTCA success rates among elderly patients (65-75 years) exceed 90%; however, there is increased risk of death after acute closure and a 2-3 fold increase in peripheral vascular complications and blood transfusion
    c. CABG and PTCA achieve similar long-term survival rates for patients between the ages of 65-75 years
    d. Compared to younger patients, octogenarians have more acute complications and late cardiac death after PTCA

67. After accounting for differences in the prevalence of diabetes mellitus, hypertension, unstable angina, and prior MI, gender still has a significant independent effect on PTCA outcome:

    a. True
    b. False

68. Most studies indicate that PTCA outcome is independent of race:

    a. True
    b. False

69. Which of the following statements about diabetics are true:

    a. Compared to non-diabetics, patients with diabetes have a 2-3 fold higher rate of coronary disease, and are at increased risk of myocardial infarction, congestive heart failure, and death
    b. Compared to non-diabetics undergoing bypass surgery, diabetics have similar in-hospital stroke and long-term survival, but more late MI and repeat revascularization
    c. Acute procedural successful rates for PTCA are similar between diabetics and non-diabetics
    d. In the Bypass Angioplasty Revascularization Investigation (BARI), 5-year mortality rates for diabetics with multivessel disease were independent of the mode of initial revascularization

70. PTCA patients on chronic dialysis have more ischemic and vascular complications, late cardiac events, and restenosis than PTCA patients not on dialysis:

    a. True
    b. False

71. All of the following statements about cardiac transplantation patients are true except:

    a. Coronary artery disease is the leading cause of death among patients who survive more than 1-year after cardiac transplantation
    b. Angina pectoris is a common manifestation of coronary disease
    c. Diltiazem and lipid lowering agents may reduce the progression of allograft vasculopathy
    d. PTCA can be performed with acceptable success and complication rates

72. Elective PTCA for patients with silent ischemia is safe, relieves objective evidence of ischemia, and improves 1-year survival:

    a. True
    b. False

INTRACORONARY THROMBUS

73. What percentage of patients undergoing PTCA for medically refractory unstable ischemic syndromes demonstrate thrombus by angioscopy:

    a. 30%
    b. 50%
    c. 75%
    d. 90%

74. Which of the following statements about the sensitivity and specificity of angiography for the detection of intracoronary thrombus are correct:

    a. Sensitivity and specificity are low
    b. Sensitivity and specificity are high
    c. Sensitivity is low and specificity is high
    d. Sensitivity is high and specificity is low

75. The most accurate means of detecting intracoronary thrombus is:

    a. Angiography
    b. Ultrafast CT scan
    c. Angioscopy
    d. Intravascular ultrasound

76. Compared to PTCA of nonthrombotic lesions, PTCA of thrombotic lesions is associated with a similar incidence of acute closure but more distal embolization and no-reflow:

    a. True
    b. False

77. All laser, atherectomy, and stent devices are associated with an increase risk of complications when thrombus is present:

    a. True

b. False

78. Which of the following statements about pharmacologic therapy of pre-existing thrombus are true:

a. Pretreatment with a 2-14 day course of heparin and aspirin may reduce the risk of PTCA
b. High-dose intravenous heparin (ACT > 350 seconds) may be associated with lower rates of abrupt closure
c. Systemic thrombolytic therapy has consistently been shown to improve outcome in patients with unstable angina

79. In the TAUSA study, patients with ischemic rest pain treated with intracoronary urokinase prior to PTCA had a higher incidence of acute vessel occlusion, even in lesions that were complex or contained filling defect suggestive of thrombus:

a. True
b. False

BIFURCATION LESIONS

80. Which of the following statements about sidebranch closure are true:

a. Branch vessels that do not originate from the parent vessel stenosis but may be transiently covered by the inflated balloon have a 5-10% likelihood of persistent occlusion
b. Sidebranches that originate from the parent vessel stenosis but are themselves normal have < 1% chance of occlusion
c. The risk of sidebranch occlusion is highest when both the parent vessel and ostium of the branch contain diameter stenoses > 50%

81. Sidebranch protection is recommended for which of the following types of bifurcation lesion (see figure, next page):

a. Type 1A   b. Type 1B   c. Type 2A
d. Type 2B   e. Type 3A
f. Type 3B   g. Type 4

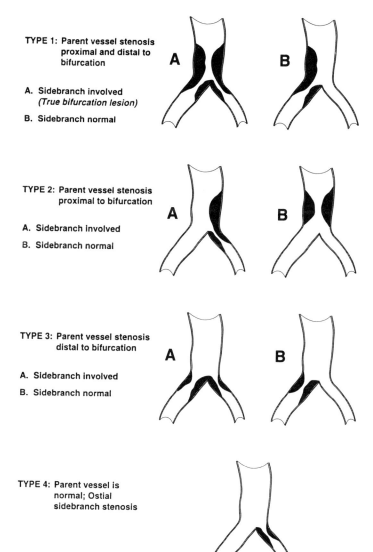

TYPE 1: Parent vessel stenosis proximal and distal to bifurcation

A. Sidebranch involved (True bifurcation lesion)

B. Sidebranch normal

TYPE 2: Parent vessel stenosis proximal to bifurcation

A. Sidebranch involved

B. Sidebranch normal

TYPE 3: Parent vessel stenosis distal to bifurcation

A. Sidebranch involved

B. Sidebranch normal

TYPE 4: Parent vessel is normal; Ostial sidebranch stenosis

82. Bifurcation angioplasty is associated with the usual risks of PTCA and the additional risks of:

   a. Sidebranch occlusion

   b. Incomplete dilation due to the snow-plow effect

   c. Aneurysm formation

   d. Retrograde propagation of dissection from sidebranch to parent vessel

83. All the following are causes of sidebranch occlusion except:

    a. Snow-plow injury
    b. Spasm
    c. No-reflow
    d. Dissection
    e. Thrombus

84. In the CAVEAT-I trial, compared to PTCA of bifurcation lesions, DCA resulted in higher success, less restenosis, and similar ischemic complications:

    a. True
    b. False

85. The presence of a true bifurcation lesion is a contraindication to stenting:

    a. True
    b. False

86. Which of the following statements about retrieval of occluded sidebranches after bifurcation intervention are true:

    a. Acutely occluded sidebranches without ostial stenoses can be reopened in > 75%
    b. Acutely occluded sidebranches with ostial stenosis can be reopened in > 50%
    c. It is imperative to protect the parent vessel with a guidewire during attempted salvage of a sidebranch

87. Following sidebranch occlusion:

    a. Parent vessel closure is uncommon
    b. Myocardial infarction occurs in > 50% of patients
    c. In-hospital mortality is < 1%

TORTUOSITY AND ANGULATED LESIONS

88. Balloon angioplasty of vessels with proximal tortuosity is associated with:

    a. Increase incidence of procedural failure due to inability to cross the lesion with a guidewire
    b. Increase incidence of procedural failure due to inadequate guiding catheter support
    c. Increase incidence of acute complications

89. The most flexible atherectomy device is the:

    a. Rotablator
    b. Directional Atherocath
    c. TEC catheter

90. PTCA of angulated (> 45-60°) stenoses is associated with:

    a. Increased incidence of procedural failure
    b. Increased incidence of major ischemic complications
    c. Lower incidence of restenosis
    d. Increased incidence of no-reflow

91. Severe angulation is a strong predictor of laser and atherectomy failure and may lead to suboptimal stenting due to prolapse of atheroma through stent coils or the articulation site:

    a. True
    b. False

92. Revascularization of angulated lesions using laser or atherectomy devices is safer when plaque is on the inner curve rather than when plaque is on the outer curve:

    a. True
    b. False

93. Angiography is very sensitive for detecting mild-to-moderate lesion calcium:

    a. True
    b. False

94. Up to 10% of lesions with angiographic calcium fail to show calcium by intravascular ultrasound (i.e., false positive):

    a. True
    b. False

95. Coronary dissection is more common after PTCA of calcified lesions than non-calcified lesions:

    a. True
    b. False

96. Lesion calcium is a risk factor for restenosis:

    a. True
    b. False

97. Acceptable interventional techniques for undilatable calcified lesions include:

    a. Force-focused angioplasty
    b. TEC atherectomy
    c. Excimer laser
    d. Rotablator
    e. PTCA using oversized balloons

98. The device of choice for the treatment of calcified lesions is:

    a. High-pressure PTCA
    b. Directional atherectomy
    c. Rotablator
    d. TEC atherectomy
    e. Excimer laser
    f. Stent

99. Both directional atherectomy and TEC atherectomy are reasonable modalities for moderately calcified lesions:

    a. True
    b. False

100. When a balloon cannot be fully expanded in a calcified lesion, immediate stent placement can still be performed with good acute and long-term results:

    a. True
    b. False

101. ELCA techniques for mildly calcified lesions include all except:

    a. Small initial fibers
    b. Long laser trains (> 5 seconds)
    c. High fluence (50-60 mJ/mm^2)
    d. Saline infusion technique

102. Techniques to minimize no-reflow after Rotablator atherectomy of calcified lesions include:

    a. Small initial burr
    b. Large single burr
    c. 20% decrease in initial platform speed
    d. Ablation runs < 30 seconds
    e. Rotaflush "cocktail" of a nitrate, calcium channel blocker, and heparin

103. All of the following statements about lesions with deep calcium (i.e., at or near the medial-adventitial border) are true except:

    a. Deep calcium does not usually interfere with PTCA, DCA, or stenting
    b. Initial use of Rotablator or ELCA is not generally required
    c. Results in a greater incidence of procedural failure and acute complications
    d. Device selection can be based on associated lesion morphologies

ECCENTRIC LESIONS

104. Contrast angiography has good predictive value for detecting eccentric plaque morphology:

    a. True
    b. False

105. Compared to concentric lesions, PTCA of eccentric lesions may be associated with:

    a. More elastic recoil
    b. Less effective plaque compression
    c. Increased risk of acute closure
    d. More vasospasm
    e. Suboptimal lumen enlargement

106. Match each of the following lesion morphologies with the most appropriate device.

Lesion Type	Device
a. Extreme eccentricity in a large vessel	1. TEC atherectomy
b. Eccentric stenosis with extensive calcification	2. Rotablator
c. Vein graft with thrombus	3. Directional atherectomy

107. Virtually all stent designs are capable of treating eccentric lesions:

    a. True
    b. False

OSTIAL LESIONS

108. Of all lesions considered for PTCA, ostial lesions are the most likely be associated with suboptimal lumen enlargement due to lesion rigidity and elastic recoil:

    a. True
    b. False

109. When PTCA of ostial lesions is attempted:

    a. Coaxial guiding catheter alignment is crucial
    b. Aggressive vessel intubation is recommended
    c. Sidehole catheters are useful to minimize pressure damping
    d. Long balloons are often useful to prevent "watermelon seeding"
    e. Once the balloon is properly positioned, the guiding catheter should be gently retracted 1-2 cm into the aorta
    f. A portion of the balloon should remain inside the guiding catheter during inflation

110. To ensure that an ostial stenosis is not due to transient spasm it is helpful to:

    a. Administer intracoronary nitroglycerin
    b. Perform a subselective injection in the Sinus of Valsalva
    c. Administer ergonovine
    d. Perform IVUS

111. Which of the following statements about new device intervention for ostial lesions are true:

    a. DCA is well suited for calcified ostial stenoses in vessels ≥ 3 mm in diameter
    b. TEC may be useful for ostial vein graft lesions with thrombus, but is contraindicated in the presence of significant calcification, extreme angulation, or dissection
    c. Rotablator may be useful to treat ostial lesions with calcification and thrombus
    d. ELCA may be used for noncalcified ostial lesions, particularly with long (> 30 mm) segments of disease
    e. Directional ELCA may be useful for eccentric ostial lesions
    f. Stents can be used for ostial lesions that can be fully expanded with a balloon, particularly for vessels ≥ 3 mm in diameter

LONG LESIONS

112. Which of the following statements about balloon angioplasty of long lesions are true:

    a. Angioplasty success decreases as lesion length increases
    b. Intravascular ultrasound has shown that residual stenosis is underestimated by contrast angiography, since the "normal" reference segment is often diseased
    c. The relationship between lesion length and restenosis is controversial
    d. Long (30-40 mm) balloons offer no advantage over 20 mm balloons

113. Which of the following statements about Rotablator atherectomy of long lesions are true:

    a. Success and complication rates are independent of lesion length
    b. Rotablator is the preferred method of revascularizing long lesions with deep calcium
    c. When Rotablator is performed on such lesions, it is important to use slow passes and a small burr to minimize slow-flow and ischemic complications

114. Compared to DCA of focal lesions, DCA of long lesions is associated with lower success, more ischemic complications, and higher restenosis rates:

    a. True
    b. False

115. Which of the following statements about excimer laser coronary angioplasty (ELCA) of long lesions are true:

    a. Procedural success is independent of lesion length
    b. Dissections are more common in long lesions
    c. In the Amstrodam-Rotterdam (AMRO) trial, ELCA resulted in higher procedural success, and less restenosis than PTCA
    d. In the Excimer Laser Rotablator Balloon Angioplasty for C-Lesions (ERBAC) trial, there was no difference in restenosis between ELCA, Rotablator, and PTCA at 6-months

116. Lesion length > 20 mm is a contraindication to stenting due to the increased risk of subacute thrombosis:

    a. True
    b. False

CHRONIC TOTAL OCCLUSION

117. Which of the following statements about chronic total coronary occlusion are true:

    a. Patients often present with a change in exertional angina due to collateral insufficiency
    b. Histopathology usually demonstrates a ruptured fibrous cap overlying soft atheroma with fresh occlusive thrombus
    c. Spontaneous recanalization is rare
    d. Intercoronary collaterals are rare
    e. Myocardial viability is uncommon in the distribution of the totally occluded vessel

118. When PTCA is used to treat chronic total occlusions, the most common cause of procedural failure is:

    a. Failure to cross the occlusion with a balloon
    b. Failure to cross the occlusion with a guidewire
    c. Inability to dilate the stenosis

119. Case selection is the most important predictor of PTCA success for chronic total occlusions:

    a. True
    b. False

120. Factors favoring success for PTCA of chronic total occlusions include:

    a. Functional occlusion
    b. Occlusion age > 12 weeks
    c. Length of occlusion > 15 mm

    d.   Tapered stump

    e.   Sidebranch present at point of occlusion

    f.   Extensive bridging collaterals

121. Percutaneous revascularization should not be attempted when the chronic total occlusion is 6 months old or shows extensive bridging collaterals ("Caput Medusa"):

    a.   True

    b.   False

122. The risk of major complications is similar for PTCA of total and nontotal occlusions:

    a.   True

    b.   False

123. Which of the following features favor successful revascularization of a chronic total occlusion:

    a.   Tapered stump

    b.   Functional occlusion

    c.   Bridging collaterals

    d.   Flush occlusion at a sidebranch

124. Which of the following statements about late outcome after PTCA of chronic total occlusions are true:

    a.   More than 60% of patients with successful PTCA are asymptomatic at follow-up

    b.   The absence of symptoms excludes restenosis

    c.   Successful recanalization reduces the need for CABG by 50-75%

    d.   Successful PTCA appears to improve survival and reduce the incidence of late myocardial infarction

125. Potentially useful equipment for chronic total occlusions which cannot be crossed with a PTCA guidewire include:

    a.   Glidewire

b. Magnum wire

c. Laserwire

d. Vibrational angioplasty

e. ROTACS

126. Prolonged intracoronary thrombolytic infusions have not been shown to improve the recanalization rate of chronic total coronary occlusions:

a. True

b. False

CORONARY ARTERY BYPASS GRAFTS

127. Which of the following statements about saphenous vein graft occlusion are true:

a. Approximately 10% and 50% of saphenous vein bypass grafts will be occluded 1 year and 10 years after operation, respectively

b. 40% of patients will require reoperation within 10 years

c. Repeat CABG is technically more difficult and associated with increased morbidity and mortality than initial CABG

d. Vein graft occlusion within the first month of operation is almost always due to graft thrombosis from poor surgical technique or poor distal runoff

e. Between 1 and 12 months, graft atherosclerosis is the most common cause of vein graft occlusion

f. After 1 year, occlusion is most often caused by intimal hyperplasia, which is indistinguishable from restenosis

128. Following PTCA of a chronically occluded saphenous vein graft, there is a:

a. High incidence (10%) of distal embolization

b. High incidence of late cardiac events (event-free survival of 30% at 3 years)

c. High incidence (40-50%) of late graft occlusion

129. Despite the ability of coronary artery bypass surgery to relieve angina:

    a. Ischemia recurs in 20% and 60% of patients at 1- and 10-years, respectively
    b. The rate of vein graft failure is about 10% at 1-year, 40% at 5-years, and 75% at 10-years
    c. In asymptomatic patients, silent occlusion occurs in 30% of vein grafts at 1-3 years
    d. Repeat CABG or PTCA is required in 20% of patients at 10 years

130. Which of the following statements about repeat CABG and PTCA for vein graft disease are true:

    a. The risks of repeat CABG are 2-4 fold higher than initial CABG, with periprocedural death and MI in 2-5% and 2-8% of patients, respectively
    b. Preliminary data suggests that c7E3 (ReoPro) may lead to significant reduction in distal embolization and non-Q-wave MI during vein graft PTCA
    c. The incidence of no-reflow following vein graft PTCA is 5-15% and is more frequent in old (> 3 years) degenerated grafts
    d. Abrupt closure complicates 5-15% vein graft interventions, which is higher than the 2-10% incidence following native vessel intervention
    e. Perforation occurs with similar frequency among vein graft and native coronary artery interventions
    f. Cardiac tamponade is unusual after vein graft perforation

131. Match the angiographic complication with the most appropriate therapy:

    <u>Complication</u>
    a. Distal embolization leading to abrupt cut-off of a distal branch
    b. No-reflow
    c. Abrupt closure
    d. Perforation

    <u>Therapy</u>
    1. Prolonged balloon inflation, pericardiocentesis, emergency surgery for refractory cases
    2. Intracoronary calcium-channel blockers
    3. Prolonged balloon inflations or stent
    4. Gentle guidewire manipulation, repeat PTCA, infusion of thrombolytic drugs

132. Graft age is the most important determinant of procedural success after percutaneous intervention:

    a. True
    b. False

133. PTCA of lesions in the proximal portion of the vein graft or the aorto-ostial position have lower success rates and higher restenosis rates than PTCA of other vein graft sites:

    a. True
    b. False

134. Acute myocardial infarction from saphenous vein graft occlusion is:

    a. Generally associated with more intraluminal clot than acute occlusion of a native vessel
    b. Commonly refractory to intravenous thrombolytic therapy
    c. More effectively treated with mechanical techniques

135. Which of the following statements about the internal mammary artery are true:

    a. Compared to saphenous veins grafts, IMAs demonstrate better flow, less atherosclerosis, and higher 10-year patency rates
    b. PTCA failure is largely due to elastic recoil
    c. Restenosis rates after PTCA are 30-50%
    d. Restenosis rates are lower for lesions at the distal anastomosis than in the body of the IMA graft

136. Which of the following statements about coronary fistulae are true:

    a. They are the most common hemodynamically-significant coronary anomaly
    b. Most drain into the arterial circulation (left ventricle, left atrium, aorta)
    c. The majority of patients develop angina in the second or third decade
    d. Indications for closure include a significant left-to-right shunt, heart failure, or ischemia
    e. Selected coronary fistulae can be closed percutaneously

CORONARY ARTERY SPASM

137. Match the clinical features to the type of coronary artery spasm:

Features:
a. Occurs in 1-5% of PTCA procedures and can usually be treated by intracoronary nitrates, calcium channel blockers, or repeat PTCA at low inflation pressure
b. Rarely responds to nitrates
c. Very common after PTCA and all percutaneous devices.

Spasm Type:
1. Spasm of the distal epicardial vessel (distal to the treatment site)
2. Intralesional spasm (at the treatment site)
3. Distal microvascular spasm

138. The treatment site remains susceptible to spasm for several months after PTCA:

a. True
b. False

139. Coronary artery spasm may occur with:

a. PTCA
b. Rotablator
c. TEC atherectomy
d. Excimer laser
e. Directional atherectomy
f. Stents

140. The usual dose of intracoronary nitroglycerin for the treatment of coronary artery spasm is:

a. 50-100 mcg repeated at 50 mcg increments as needed up to a total of 300 mcg
b. 100-300 mcg repeated as needed up to a total of 1-2 mg
c. 1-2 mg repeated as needed up to 5-10 mg

141. If spasm occurs at the treatment site, the guidewire should be partially or completely removed:

    a. True
    b. False

142. Intracoronary calcium channel blockers may reverse nitrate- resistant coronary artery spasm:

    a. True
    b. False

143. A temporary transvenous pacemaker should be inserted prior to the administration of intracoronary verapamil or diltiazem when used to treat coronary spasm, due to the risk AV block, bradycardia, and significant hypotension:

    a. True
    b. False

144. Doses of calcium channel blockers recommended to treat coronary artery spasm include:

    a. Verapamil: 0.1-0.2 mg IC repeated every 1-5 min as needed up to a maximum of 1.0-1.5 mg
    b. Verapamil: 0.1-0.2 mg IV repeated every 1-5 min as needed up to a maximum of 1.0-1.5 mg
    c. Verapamil: 1-2 mg IC repeated every 1-5 min as needed up to a maximum of 10-15 mg
    d. Diltiazem: 0.5-2.5 mg IC over 1 min up to 5-10 mg as needed
    e. Diltiazem: 0.5-2.5 mg IV over 1 min up to 5-10 mg as needed
    f. Diltiazem: 5-25 mg IC over 1 min up to 50-100 mg as needed

145. A prolonged low-pressure inflation using a balloon matched to the reference segment is often successful at treating intralesional spasm:

    a. True
    b. False

146. Intracoronary stenting may successfully treat refractory spasm, but should only be considered after other non-operative alternatives have failed:

    a. True
    b. False

147. Emergency bypass surgery is rarely necessary to treat coronary artery spasm:

    a. True
    b. False

148. Which of the following statements about PTCA of organic stenoses in patients with variant angina are true:

    a. A high technical success rate can be achieved
    b. Procedural complications occur more often in patients with variant angina
    c. Restenosis rates exceed 70%

DISSECTION AND ABRUPT CLOSURE

149. Which of the following statements about the incidence and timing of abrupt closure are true:

    a. Acute closure occurs in 2-11% of elective PTCA cases
    b. Most episodes occur after the patient has left the catheterization laboratory
    c. Episodes developing outside the angioplasty suite usually occur within the first 6 hours and are rare after 24 hours
    d. The incidence of acute closure has been reduced by directional atherectomy
    e. The lowest incidence of acute closure occurs after intracoronary stenting

150. The most common cause of acute closure is thrombus formation:

    a. True
    b. False

Questions

151. Following "routine" PTCA, coronary dissection is detected by angiography in 20-40% of cases, and by intravascular ultrasound or angioscopy in 60-80% of cases:

   a. True
   b. False

152. Situations that may give rise to a false impression of coronary dissection by angiography include:

   a. Weak contrast injections
   b. Deep guide catheter intubation that deforms the proximal vessel
   c. Straightening and invagination of the vessel wall by extra-support guidewires

153. Angiographic dissections occur with equal frequency after PTCA, atherectomy, and stents:

   a. True
   b. False

154. The saline infusion technique has reduced the incidence of dissection after:

   a. Rotablator
   b. ELCA
   c. DCA
   d. PTCA
   e. TEC atherectomy
   f. Stents

155. Which NHLBI dissections types, if left untreated, increase the risk of myocardial infarction, emergency CABG, or death:

   a. Type A
   b. Type B
   c. Type C
   d. Type D
   e. Type E
   f. Type F

156. Dissection characteristics associated with an increased risk of ischemic complications include:

    a. Length > 10 mm
    b. Impaired flow
    c. Residual stenosis > 50%

157. Which of the following statements about the pathophysiology of dissection are true:

    a. Complex dissections associated with an increased incidence of ischemic complications demonstrate intimal splitting without medial dissection
    b. Dissections frequently occur at the junction between calcified and noncalcified plaque
    c. Laser-induced dissection is most often caused by acoustic shock waves generated from absorption of excimer laser energy

158. Risk factors for major ischemic events in the presence of a dissection include all of the following except:

    a. Dissection length > 15 mm
    b. NHLBI dissection types C-F
    c. Residual diameter stenosis > 30%
    d. Residual cross sectional area > 2 mm^2
    e. Unstable angina
    f. Chronic total occlusion.

159. Which of the following factors increase the risk of coronary dissection:

    a. Use of compliant balloon material
    b. Use of oversized balloons (balloon: artery > 1.2:1)
    c. Slow deflation speed
    d. Long balloons for long lesions

160. Which of the following statements about prognosis after coronary dissection are true:

    a. Severe dissection increases the risk of ischemic complications 5-fold
    b. The majority of dissections not resulting in acute ischemic complications disappear with time

c. Dissections not resulting in acute ischemic complications are associated with a lower incidence of restenosis

161. The most powerful predictor of acute closure is:

a. Unstable angina
b. Inadequate antiplatelet therapy
c. Bend > 45°
d. Long lesion
e. Complex dissection

162. The most powerful predictor of cardiac death after acute closure is:

a. Female gender
b. Collaterals originating from the target vessel
c. Jeopardy score
d. PTCA of a proximal LAD

163. Preprocedural aspirin reduces the risk of coronary occlusion by 50-75%:

a. True
b. False

164. In the EPIC trial, ReoPro reduced the incidence of major ischemic complications at 30 days and angiographic restenosis at 6 months:

a. True
b. False

165. In the EPILOG trial, the combined endpoint of death or MI (CPK $\geq$ 3 x normal) at 30 days was lower in patients receiving ReoPro plus low-dose heparin compared to those receiving standard-dose heparin without ReoPro:

a. True
b. False

166. Conventional bolus dosing of 10,000 units of heparin results in optimal prolongation of the activated clotting time (ACT) in > 95% of patients with stable and unstable angina:

    a. True
    b. False

167. Lytic therapy is routinely recommended for abrupt closure caused by dissection:

    a. True
    b. False

168. Prolonged perfusion balloon inflations and stenting have proven to be equally efficacious in the treatment of flow-limiting dissection:

    a. True
    b. False

169. When directional atherectomy is used to excise focal flow-limiting dissections, the risk of perforation can be minimized by:

    a. Use of a slightly undersized AtheroCath
    b. Low inflation pressure
    c. Orientation of the AtheroCath toward the angiographically normal vessel wall

170. Directional atherectomy should not be used to excise dissections that:

    a. Are more than 10 mm in length
    b. Are located in vessels with diameters > 3 mm
    c. Are located in vessels with moderate-to-severe tortuosity or heavy calcification
    d. Have periadventitial dye staining
    e. Have a large amount of untreated clot

171. The majority of small intimal dissections (residual stenosis < 30%, length < 10 mm, normal flow) may not require further mechanical or drug therapy:

a. True
b. False

172. Stenting has clearly been shown to confer a clinical benefit over conventional therapy for non-flow-limiting dissection with high-risk features such as residual stenosis ≥ 30% or dissection length > 15 mm:

a. True
b. False

173. Primary thrombosis and vessel dissection are equally common causes of abrupt closure after PTCA:

a. True
b. False

174. Primary thrombosis and vessel dissection are equally common causes of abrupt closure after directional atherectomy:

a. True
b. False

175. Potentially useful treatment modalities for thrombotic acute closure include:

a. TEC atherectomy
b. Rotablator
c. Hydrolyser
d. AngioJet
e. Overnight superselective infusion of urokinase
f. ReoPro

176. No-reflow can be diagnosed when dissection is present at the treatment site:

a. True
b. False

NO-REFLOW

177. Risk factors for no-reflow include:

    a. Thrombus-containing lesions
    b. Angulated lesions
    c. Degenerated vein grafts
    d. Rotablator atherectomy

178. No-reflow does not usually cause ECG changes or symptoms:

    a. True
    b. False

179. No-reflow increases the risk of death and myocardial infarction after percutaneous revascularization:

    a. True
    b. False

180. Techniques to minimize the risk of no-reflow after Rotablator atherectomy of calcified lesions include:

    a. Small initial burr
    b. Large single burr
    c. Reduction in platform speed by 20%
    d. Ablation runs < 30 seconds

181. Potentially useful therapies for no-reflow include:

    a. Intracoronary calcium channel blockers
    b. Intracoronary nitrates
    c. Intracoronary beta blockers
    d. Coronary artery bypass surgery

182. No-reflow resulting in hypotension is a contraindication to intracoronary calcium channel blockers:

    a. True
    b. False

CORONARY ARTERY PERFORATION

183. Coronary artery perforation has been reported in ___% of lesions treated with PTCA and ___% of lesions treated with Rotablator, DCA, TEC, or ELCA:

    a. 1% and 5-10%
    b. 0.1% and 0.5-3%
    c. 0.5-3% and 0.1%
    d. 1% and 0.5-3.0%

184. Mechanisms of PTCA-induced perforation include:

    a. Guidewire advancement
    b. Forceful contrast injection
    c. Balloon advancement
    d. Balloon inflation
    e. Balloon rupture

185. Factors that may increase the risk of coronary perforation include:

    a. Use of oversized balloons (balloon-to-artery ratio > 1.2)
    b. Use of extra-support wires
    c. Complex lesion morphology (chronic total occlusion, vessel bifurcation, severe tortuosity or angulation)
    d. Unstable angina
    e. Females
    f. Elderly patients
    g. Atherectomy and laser devices

186. Some perforations are angiographically inapparent and may go undetected during the interventional procedure, only to manifest 8-24 hours later with the sudden appearance of cardiac tamponade:

a. True
b. False

187. Cardiac tamponade is uncommon following PTCA-induced perforation of saphenous vein grafts:

a. True
b. False

188. When ELCA, Rotablator or TEC is being used to treat lesion morphologies at high risk for perforation (i.e., bifurcations, angulated stenoses, total occlusion) initial device-to-artery ratios of 0.7-0.8 are recommended:

a. True
b. False

189. Most guidewire perforations have adverse clinical and hemodynamic effects:

a. True
b. False

190. All of the following statements about the non-operative management of free coronary perforation are true except:

a. A balloon should be immediately positioned at the site of contrast extravasation and inflated to 2-6 ATM for at least 10 minutes
b. If sealing is incomplete after PTCA, a second low-pressure inflation should be performed for 15-45 minutes using a perfusion balloon catheter wherever possible
c. If pericardial hemorrhage is present, a pericardiocentesis needle should be exchanged for a multiple sidehole catheter while non-operative measures to treat the perforation proceed
d. Under no circumstances should protamine be administered
e. Emergency surgery is recommended for all refractory perforations

191. Prolonged balloon inflations successfully seal 20-30% of coronary artery perforations:

    a. True
    b. False

192. Indications for emergency cardiac surgery following coronary intervention include all except:

    a. Acute occlusion of a major coronary artery that is not amenable to percutaneous revascularization
    b. Severe dissection with refractory myocardial ischemia
    c. No reflow of a major coronary artery
    d. Coronary artery perforation with refractory pericardial tamponade
    e. Occlusion of the left main coronary artery

RESTENOSIS

193. Restenosis rates vary widely, depending on which definition of restenosis is used:

    a. True
    b. False

194. Match the following parameters to their definitions:

    Parameter
    a. Acute gain
    b. Late loss
    c. Loss index

    Definition
    1. Difference in lumen diameter immediately after intervention and at follow-up
    2. Acute gain divided by late loss
    3. Late loss divided by acute gain
    4. Difference in lumen diameter before and immediately after intervention

195. Which of the following statements about acute gain, late loss, and loss index are true:

    a. Acute gain is to due to plaque removal, not arterial expansion
    b. Late loss reflects the net effects of intimal hyperplasia, elastic recoil, and vascular remodeling
    c. A typical loss index is 0.5

196. Which of the following statements about the mechanisms of restenosis are true:

    a. Most elastic recoil occurs within 30 minutes after balloon deflation
    b. Elastic recoil is greatest after DCA, intermediate after PTCA, and lowest after stenting
    c. Atherectomy specimens from restenotic lesions show intimal hyperplasia
    d. Late arterial remodeling is an important mechanism of restenosis after stenting

197. Restenosis is common in the first month, plateaus at 3-6 months, and is unusual after 12 months:

    a. True
    b. False

198. The time course of restenosis after atherectomy, laser, and stenting differs substantially from PTCA:

    a. True
    b. False

199. Predictors of restenosis include:

    a. Post-procedure lumen diameter
    b. Dissection
    c. Deep wall excision after directional atherectomy

200. Risk factors for restenosis include:

    a. Unstable angina
    b. Dissection
    c. Chronic total occlusion
    d. Proximal lesion location

e. Residual stenosis > 30%

201. Factors shown to decrease angiographic restenosis include:

   a. ACE inhibitors
   b. ReoPro
   c. ELCA
   d. Stents
   e. Aspirin
   f. Rotablator

202. Which of the following statements about restenosis are true:

   a. Recurrent symptoms have a low positive predictive value for restenosis
   b. Absence of symptoms in previously symptomatic patients has a high predictive value for the absence of restenosis
   c. Exercise testing using thallium-201 scintigraphy, exercise radionuclide angiography, and dobutamine echocardiography have better sensitivity for detecting restenosis than exercise testing without perfusion imaging
   d. Functional testing performed within four weeks of PTCA is frequently associated with false positives

203. Routine non-invasive testing is recommended for all patients following percutaneous revascularization within the first 6 months:

   a. True
   b. False

204. PTCA of a restenotic lesion is associated with fewer complications than initial PTCA:

   a. True
   b. False

MEDICAL & PERIPHERAL COMPLICATIONS

205. Which of the following statements about periprocedural renal insufficiency are true:

    a. The most common manifestations include decreasing urine output and a rising serum creatinine in the first few days after PTCA

    b. The most common cause of renal insufficiency in the post-PTCA patient is prerenal azotemia from intraprocedural myocardial ischemia and LV dysfunction

    c. Dye-induced renal dysfunction occurs in < 1% of PTCA patients with normal renal function

206. Risk factors for dye-induced nephrotoxicity include all of the following except:

    a. Pre-existing renal insufficiency
    b. Diabetic nephropathy
    c. Large contrast load
    d. Female patients
    e. Hypertensive patients
    f. Baseline hypovolemia
    g. Impaired left ventricular function

207. Once dye-induced renal dysfunction develops, creatinine levels generally peak at ___ days and remain elevated for ___ days:

    a. 1 and 7-14
    b. 3-5 and 7-14
    c. 7 and 14-21
    d. 1 and 7-14

208. Non-ionic contrast agents reduce the risk of contrast nephropathy:

    a. True
    b. False

209. Which of the following statements about the management of PTCA-induced renal insufficiency/failure are true:

    a. Retroperitoneal bleeding or bladder obstruction may first manifest as diminished urine output and should be excluded
    b. A useful "rule of thumb" is to match urine output with IV fluids during the first 8-10 hours post-procedure
    c. If the patient is felt to have adequate intravascular volume and renal insufficiency, hydrochlorothiazide will frequently relieve the prerenal state
    d. Right heart catheterization and hemodynamic monitoring should be considered in all cases of oliguria and anuria when volume status is in question

210. Which statements about contrast agents are true:

    a. Patients with a previous history of an adverse dye reaction are at highest risk for a subsequent severe reaction
    b. Transient ventricular dysfunction and hypotension are equally common with high and low osmolar agents
    c. Low osmolar agents cause fewer minor reactions (nausea, urticaria, itching, heat sensation, vomiting) than high osmolar agents
    d. Compared to ionic contrast, nonionic agents have greater anticoagulant and antiplatelet activities

211. When using corticosteroids to reduce the risk of contrast reactions, it is important to begin pretreatment at least 12 hours before exposure:

    a. True
    b. False

212. Which statements about contrast reactions are true:

    a. Minor reactions (i.e., nausea, burning sensation, flushing, mild urticaria without hives, mild bradycardia) usually occur within minutes of contrast exposure and do not require treatment with steroids or epinephrine
    b. Moderate contrast reactions (i.e., persistent nausea and vomiting, persistent bradycardia or vasovagal episodes with hypotension) usually occur within minutes to hours of contrast exposure and require intravenous steroids and epinephrine

c. Anaphylactoid reactions (urticaria with hives and tongue swelling) can occur within minutes to hours of contrast exposure and should be treated with epinephrine

d. Anaphylaxis (bronchospasm, laryngeal edema, and/or profound hypotension(may occur immediately after a single contrast injection and requires intravenous steroids and epinephrine

213. What initial epinephrine dose is recommended for the treatment of contrast-induced urticaria and tongue swelling:

a. 0.1 - 0.5 cc of a 1:10,000 dilution subcutaneously
b. 0.1 - 0.5 cc of a 1:1,000 dilution subcutaneously
c. 0.1 - 0.5 cc of a 1:1,000 dilution subcutaneously

214. What initial epinephrine dose is recommended for contrast-induced anaphylaxis (i.e., severe bronchospasm, laryngeal edema, and/or profound hypotension):

a. 0.1 - 0.5 cc of a 1:10,000 dilution subcutaneously
b. 0.1 - 0.5 cc of a 1:1,000 dilution subcutaneously
c. 0.1 - 0.5 cc of a 1:1,000 dilution intravenously
d. 0.1 - 0.5 cc of a 1:10,000 dilution intravenously

215. Which statements about peripheral vascular complications after coronary intervention are true:

a. All AV fistulas should be repaired surgically or by ultrasound-guided compression
b. All pseudoaneurysms should be repaired surgically by ultrasound-guided compression
c. Arterial thrombosis should be managed with heparinization and urgent thrombectomy
d. Most guidewire-induced peripheral arterial perforations are benign and rarely require surgical treatment
e. The majority of retroperitoneal bleeds stop spontaneously
f. Blue-toe syndrome and livedo reticularis are often manifestations of cholesterol embolization

ADJUNCTIVE PHARMACOTHERAPY

216. Demerol is a contraindicated in patients who have received a monoamine oxidase inhibitor within 14 days:

a. True
b. False

217. Aspirin does not prevent platelet aggregation caused by thrombin, ADP, catecholamines, or shear-stress:

a. True
b. False

218. Which statements about ticlopidine are true:

a. In contrast to aspirin, ticlopidine can inhibit platelet aggregation to thrombin and shear-stress
b. Ticlopidine (250 mg PO BID) should be administered for at least 3 days prior to the procedure to maximize antiplatelet effects
c. The most serious side effect of ticlopidine is thrombocytopenia, which occurs in 1-2% of patients after 4 weeks of use

219. Which statements about ReoPro are true:

a. It binds to and inhibits platelet glycoprotein IIb/IIIa receptors
b. In the EPIC trial, ReoPro reduced ischemic endpoints at 30 days and 6 months, and reduced the need for repeat target vessel revascularization at 6 months
c. In the EPILOG trial, patients receiving ReoPro prior to elective PTCA had a lower incidence of death or MI (CPK 3x normal) at 30 days compared to placebo
d. In the CAPTURE trial, patients treated with ReoPro for 18-24 hours prior to PTCA had a reduction in the 30-day combined endpoint of death, MI, or urgent revascularization compared to those treated with conventional medical therap

220. For the same heparin concentration, a higher ACT value is expected using the HemoChron compared to the HemoTec system:

a. True
b. False

221. Heparin's anticoagulant effect is limited by:

    a. Inability to inactivate clot-bound thrombin
    b. Neutralization by platelet factor 4 (from platelet-rich thrombi)
    c. Inactivation by fibrin-II monomers, which are formed by the action of thrombin on fibrinogen

222. Which statements about heparin-induced thrombocytopenia (HIT) are true:

    a. Type I HIT is due to heparin's direct platelet aggregating effect and is associated with platelet counts of 50,000 to 150,000/mm^2
    b. Type II HIT (heparin-associated thrombotic thrombocytopenia; HATT) is due to an autoantibody directed against the platelet factor IV-heparin complex and is typically associated with platelet counts < 50,000/mm^2
    c. Type I HIT is more common than HATT, has a benign clinical course, and often improves even if heparin is continued
    d. HATT can be associated with fatal venous and arterial thromboses
    e. HATT requires discontinuation of all heparin

223. Which statements about hirudin are true:

    a. Unlike heparin, hirudin does not require antithrombin III for its anticoagulant effect
    b. Hirudin forms a highly stable noncovalent complex with circulating <u>and</u> clot-bound thrombin
    c. Hirudin is inhibited by platelet factor IV from platelet-rich thrombi

CORONARY STENTS

224. Important features of the coronary Wallstent include all of the following except:

    a. Stainless steel wire construction
    b. Stent shortening by only 5% after deployment
    c. Impregnation with tantalum to enhance radiopacity
    d. Expansion of the stent until an equilibrium is achieved between the stent and the vessel wall
    e. Wallstents are selected to achieve diameters 0.5 mm larger than the adjacent reference segment

225. All of the following stents are mounted on a balloon and deployed by balloon expansion except:

    a. The Gianturco-Roubin stent
    b. The Palmaz-Schatz stent
    c. The Multilink stent
    d. The Radius stent
    e. The Micro stent
    f. The NIR stent

226. Important characteristics of stents constructed of tantalum include all of the following except:

    a. Excellent flexibility
    b. Excellent radiopacity
    c. Low profile
    d. Premature expansion at body temperature

227. Match the stent designs with stent types:

    1. Self expanding Wallstent
    2. Palmaz-Schatz stent
    3. Gianturco-Roubin stent
    4. GR-II stent
    5. Microstent
    6. Multi-Link stent

a.

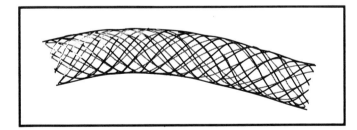

b.

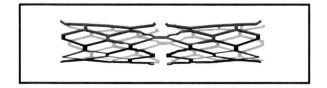

c.

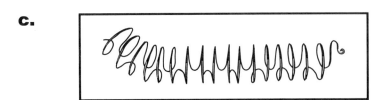

d.

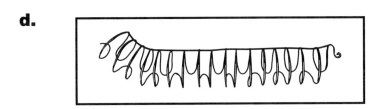

e.

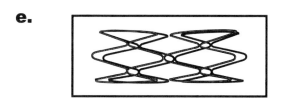

f.

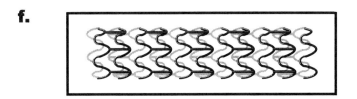

228. Clinical studies have confirmed that tantalum and Nitinol stents are less thrombogenic than stainless steel stents:

    a.   True
    b.   False

229. Newer techniques involving the use of highly polished and ultrapure grades of stainless steel with thrombo-resistant coatings have eliminated the need for antiplatelet medication after stent implantation:

    a.   True
    b.   False

230. Which of the following stents is the least flexible:

    a. Palmaz-Schatz coronary stent
    b. Gianturco-Roubin stent
    c. Microstent
    d. NIR stent
    e. Wiktor stent
    f. Wallstent

231. Newer balloon-expandable stent designs have eliminated the need to visualize the stent to ensure optimal stent placement; visualization of balloon markers is sufficient to reliably deploy these stents:

    a. True
    b. False

232. A potential advantage of tantalum compared to stainless steel is enhanced radiopacity:

    a. True
    b. False

233. Enhanced radiopacity of Palmaz biliary stents compared to Palmaz-Schatz coronary stents is due to special heparin coating:

    a. True
    b. False

234. Balloon expandable coronary stents can be expanded to virtually any diameter in any vessel, depending on the final size of the balloon used to dilate the stent:

    a. True
    b. False

235. Biliary stents can be crimped on virtually any balloon for use in virtually all coronary arteries and vein grafts:

    a. True
    b. False

236. All of the following statements about stent surface area are true except:

    a. The stent surface area ranges from 7-20% for most stents
    b. Stents with extremely low surface areas may be less thrombogenic, but may also have insufficient radial strength
    c. Stent recoil or inadequate coverage of the lesion due to plaque protrusion should never be treated by implantation of additional stents

237. One of the advantages of self-expanding stents is the lack of need to pre-treat the target lesion prior to stent employment:

    a. True
    b. False

238. When using the coronary Wallstent, the selected stent diameter should be equal to the adjacent normal reference diameter, to minimize dissection and restenosis:

    a. True
    b. False

239. Which of the following statements is false concerning the use of balloon angioplasty to predilate a target lesion prior to implantation of a balloon expandable stent:

    a. Predilation with a slightly undersized balloon may reduce the chance of dissection, preserve the shoulders of the lesion, but increase procedural cost
    b. Predilation can confirm that the balloon can be fully inflated, suggesting that stent deployment is feasible
    c. Failure to fully expand a balloon during predilation suggests the presence of a rigid stenosis and is a clear indication for immediate stenting to reduce abrupt closure

240. Acceptable techniques for enhancing stent delivery in the presence of proximal vessel tortuosity include all of the following except:

    a. The use of "power" guiding catheters to enhance coaxial alignment and backup support
    b. The use of heavy duty or extra support guide wires
    c. The use of a "buddy wire" approach to straighten tortuous segments
    d. "Jack-hammering" the stent to facilitate delivery

241. Implantation of the Gianturco-Roubin stent and the Palmaz-Schatz coronary stent share all of the following features except:

    a. Routine predilation of the target lesion
    b. Stent deployment by balloon inflation
    c. Retraction of the delivery sheath before stent deployment
    d. Post-stent adjunctive angioplasty using high pressure balloons

242. Which of the following statements is false concerning the use of adjunctive balloon angioplasty after stent deployment:

    a. Adjunctive angioplasty with high pressure balloons is not necessary if the angiographic appearance suggests "perfect" stent deployment
    b. Adjunctive angioplasty should be routinely performed after stent deployment using high pressure balloons matched to the normal reference diameter and inflated to 14-20 ATM
    c. Intravascular ultrasound is sometimes useful to identify the true reference vessel diameter
    d. Predilation, stent deployment, and adjunctive PTCA can sometimes be achieved using a single balloon

243. All of the following are potential advantages of the radial artery technique for stent implantation except:

    a. Enhanced patient comfort compared to the femoral approach
    b. A lower incidence of bleeding and vascular complications when performed by experienced operators
    c. Reliable delivery of virtually all coronary and biliary stents using 6-French guiding catheters

244. All of the following stents are constructed of stainless steel except:

    a. The coronary Wallstent
    b. The Palmaz-Schatz coronary stent
    c. The Gianturco-Roubin stent
    d. The Multilink stent
    e. The Wiktor stent
    f. The Micro stent

245. Which of the following stents has the greatest metal surface area:

    a. The coronary Wallstent
    b. The Palmaz-Schatz coronary stent
    c. The Multilink stent
    d. The Radius stent
    e. The Micro stent

246. Which of the following statements are false concerning treatment of a rigid stenosis which is targeted for stent implantation:

    a. Rotablator should be avoided because of potential no-reflow and stent thrombosis
    b. Directional atherectomy can be used to unroof the rigid plaque and facilitate stent implantation
    c. Acceptable angioplasty techniques are the use of high pressure balloons or force-focused angioplasty with a parallel guidewire
    d. A rigid lesion should never be treated by stent implantation because of the excessive risk of stent thrombosis

247. Which of the following strategies is least useful when the Palmaz-Schatz stent delivery system will not cross the target lesion:

    a. Retract the stent delivery balloon inside the sheath to facilitate stent delivery
    b. Pre-dilate the target lesion with a larger balloon or at a higher pressure
    c. Change guiding catheters to improve support and coaxial alignment
    d. Exchange the guidewire for a heavy-duty or extra support guidewire
    e. Consider a "buddy" wire approach
    f. Slightly advance the stent delivery balloon to ensure a tapered transition
    g. Consider a bare stent on a lower profile balloon
    h. Use the "stentless" delivery sheath technique

Questions

248. Which of the following statements are true concerning management of sidebranch occlusion after stent deployment:

   a. Predilation of the sidebranch prior to stent deployment may preserve sidebranch patency
   b. Most sidebranches cannot be retrieved after stent implantation and attempting to do so increases the risk of complications
   c. There is a potential risk for balloon entrapment when attempting to retrieve occluded sidebranches
   d. Virtually any balloon can be used to retrieve an occluded branch if necessary
   e. After stent deployment, further dilation with high pressure balloons may then facilitate access to the sidebranch
   f. When sidebranch occlusion occurs after stent deployment, adjunctive angioplasty with high pressure balloons should never be performed inside the stent because of the risk of permanent sidebranch occlusion

249. Which of the following statements are true concerning "suboptimal" stenting:

   a. Intravascular ultrasound may be useful
   b. Repeat balloon inflations with a larger balloon rarely results in incremental benefit
   c. Additional stents should always be avoided because of the potential for stent thrombosis
   d. Most cases of suboptimal stenting are due to mechanical and geometric problems which can be overcome by additional angioplasty or stenting
   e. Intracoronary thrombolytic therapy is recommended to prevent stent thrombosis
   f. Coronary artery bypass surgery is generally necessary to prevent ischemic complications

250. Which of the following statements are true concerning the loss of guidewire position after stent deployment:

   a. If the angiographic result is excellent, no further intervention is necessary even if the stent has not been expanded with a high pressure balloon
   b. If guidewire position is lost prior to high pressure adjunctive angioplasty, the stented segment should routinely be re-crossed with a guidewire and further expanded with a high pressure balloon
   c. An extra support or heavy duty guidewire can be used safely to steer the wire around the stent struts
   d. A flexible guidewire with a J-tip should be used to recross the stented segment

— 61 —

251. Which of the following statements are false concerning the use of articulated stents in angulated lesions:

    a. The stent articulation should be positioned directly on the angle vertex to ensure ideal conformability
    b. Excellent guiding catheter support and heavy-duty guidewires are frequently necessary to facilitate stent deployment
    c. Disarticulated stents should never be used because of the risk of stent embolization
    d. Angulated lesions should never be targeted for treatment with articulated stents

252. Which of the following statements are true concerning the use of stents for aorto-ostial lesions:

    a. The use of an aggressive guiding catheter is more important than coaxial alignment
    b. Predilation of the target lesion should be performed with an undersized balloon to reduce the chance of dissection of the aorta
    c. Heavy duty or extra support guidewires are frequently useful
    d. Calcification of ostial lesions is an absolute contraindication to stent implantation
    e. Embolic stroke and aortic insufficiency are well described complications of stenting ostial lesions
    f. The proximal edge of the stent should reside 1-2 mm in the aorta to ensure complete coverage of the ostium

253. Potentially useful strategies to deal with rupture of the stent deployment balloon include:

    a. Gentle advancement and then slow retraction of the delivery balloon to ease it out of the vessel
    b. Rapid hand inflation with full strength contrast to further expand the stent
    c. Use of a power injector to achieve rapid inflation of the deployment balloon and facilitate further stent expansion
    d. Use incremental increases in balloon size with low profile balloons to further expand the stent after removal of the deployment balloon
    e. Repeat angiography to assess the vessel for perforation
    f. Rupture of the deployment balloon suggests that further balloon inflations are contraindicated because of the risk of complications

254. The following approaches are reasonable to deal with the problem of removing an undeployed Palmaz-Schatz coronary stent when utilizing the stent delivery system:

a. If the stent is inside the delivery sheath, simply remove the entire delivery system over the guidewire

b. If the delivery sheath has been retracted, simply pull the stent back into the delivery sheath and then remove the entire delivery system over the guidewire

c. If the stent delivery sheath has been retracted, simply readvance the delivery sheath over the stent and then remove the entire delivery system over the guidewire

d. If the delivery sheath has been retracted, simply pull the system back into the guiding catheter without manipulating the delivery sheath

e. If the delivery sheath has been retracted, the stent should then be retracted up to but not inside the guiding catheter, followed by removal en-bloc of the guide, stent, and delivery sheath over the guidewire

255. Which of the following observations are consistent with optimal stent deployment using IVUS criteria:

a. Cross sectional area index > 0.8

b. Complete stent apposition defined as a maximum gap < 0.1 mm between the stent strut and vessel wall

c. Symmetry index < 0.7

d. No identifiable plaque within the stented segment

256. Based on the results of randomized clinical trials, the superiority of stenting compared to balloon angioplasty has been demonstrated for the following situations:

a. Abrupt closure

b. Focal de novo lesions in native vessels ≥ 3mm

c. Degenerated vein grafts

d. Restenotic lesions

e. Lesions > 20 mm in length

257. Although stents are superior to conventional balloon angioplasty for reversal of abrupt closure, the randomized trial of angioplasty and stents in Canada (TASC-II) demonstrated that perfusion balloon angioplasty and stenting were equivalent for treatment of abrupt closure:

a. True

b. False

258. Which of the following statements are true concerning the use of stents for abrupt closure:

    a. Patient morbidity and mortality have been essentially eliminated; the risks of bail-out stenting are identical to those of elective stenting
    b. Bail-out stenting is associated with a higher incidence of adverse in-hospital events than elective stenting
    c. Most adverse events are attributed to stent failure or stent-related complications
    d. While focal dissections are ideally suited for single stent implantation, long spiral dissections are poorly treated by stent implantation and should be managed by emergency bypass surgery

259. Vessel occlusion which is definitely due to thrombotic occlusion is best managed by stent implantation:

    a. True
    b. False

260. Which of the following statements are true concerning the use of stents for threatened abrupt closure:

    a. The risk of ischemic complications is lower when stents are used for threatened abrupt closure compared to established abrupt closure
    b. Immediate, pre-emptive stenting for threatened abrupt closure has been shown to be superior to conventional therapy without stenting
    c. The in-hospital cost of bail-out stenting is less than the cost of emergency bypass surgery
    d. Temporary stents using the flow support catheter and heat activated recoverable temporary stent have been shown to be as effective as permanent stent implantation for threatened abrupt closure

261. Randomized studies of the Palmaz-Schatz coronary stent confirm that baseline lesion morphology is an important determinant of immediate and long-term results after stenting:

    a. True
    b. False

262. The following factors readily explain the lower risk of restenosis after stenting compared to conventional balloon angioplasty:

    a. Less elastic recoil
    b. Better immediate lumen enlargement
    c. Less intimal proliferation
    d. Elimination of arterial remodeling

263. The randomized STRESS and BENESTENT trials both confirmed the higher procedural success rates and lower restenosis rates for stenting compared to balloon angioplasty. However, although angiographic restenosis rates were lower for stenting, the need for repeat target vessel revascularization for stents and angioplasty were similar:

    a. True
    b. False

264. The BENESTENT and STRESS trials demonstrated lower rates of restenosis at 6 months for stenting, but at 1 year the need for target lesion revascularization was similar for stent and angioplasty groups:

    a. True
    b. False

265. Numerous studies confirm that between 6 months and 3 years after stent implantation, there is progressive loss of in-stent minimal lumen diameter, which was associated with a marked increase in the need for target lesion revascularization 1-3 years after stenting:

    a. True
    b. False

266. Recurrent ischemia which occurs more than 12 months after successful stent implantation is usually due to progressive disease in a non-stented vessel:

    a. True
    b. False

267. Which of the following statements are true concerning the STRESS and BENESTENT randomized trials:

    a. Procedural success for stenting was significantly higher than angioplasty in the STRESS trial, but not in the BENESTENT trial
    b. Final diameter stenosis was significantly lower for stenting than angioplasty in both trials
    c. The incidence of major ischemic complications in-hospital was significantly less for stent patients than angioplasty patients
    d. Bleeding and vascular complications were more frequent in stent patients
    e. Length of in-hospital stay was significantly longer for stent patients
    f. Angiographic restenosis rates were lower for stents

268. Factors which appear to be correlated with the development of stent restenosis are:

    a. Implantation of multiple stents
    b. Target vessel diameter < 3mm
    c. Target lesion is a restenotic lesion
    d. Lesion length > 10 mm
    e. Residual stenosis > 10% after stent implantation

269. Numerous studies suggest that stent restenosis most commonly involves the proximal and distal margins of the stent and in-stent restenosis is extremely rare:

    a. True
    b. False

270. Which of the following statements are true regarding in-stent restenosis:

    a. Rotablator has been established as the treatment of choice for diffuse in-stent restenosis
    b. PTCA generally results in further stent expansion
    c. Regardless of percutaneous intervention, a repeat course of therapy with Ticlopidine is routinely recommended to prevent stent thrombosis
    d. Cases of burr entrapment after Rotablator have been observed
    e. Directional atherectomy can excise stent struts
    f. After treatment of in-stent restenosis, the recurrent restenosis rate is nearly 50%

Questions

271. Which of the following statements are true regarding Palmaz-Schatz coronary stents and Palmaz biliary stents in vein grafts:

   a. Successful stent delivery can be accomplished in 95-100% of lesions with a low incidence of stent thrombosis, emergency surgery, and ischemic complications when used in non-degenerated vein grafts
   b. When used in focal lesions in nondegenerated grafts, restenosis has been virtually eliminated
   c. Intra-graft urokinase is recommended prior to stent implantation to reduce the chance of distal embolization and no-reflow
   d. After successful stenting, 2 year event-free survival exceeds 90%

272. Reasonable strategies for dealing with revascularization of degenerated vein grafts include:

   a. Multiple overlapping inflations with long balloons
   b. Implantation of overlapping Wallstents without predilation
   c. Initial debulking with devices such as TEC atherectomy followed by deferred stenting 2-6 weeks later
   d. Re-do coronary artery bypass surgery
   e. Medical therapy alone without further revascularization

273. Which of the following statements are true concerning the use of stents in bifurcation lesions:

   a. Experimental and clinical studies suggest a high incidence of sidebranch occlusion after stenting
   b. Stents should never be implanted in lesions which involve the origin of significant sidebranches
   c. Unlike conventional PTCA, the risk of sidebranch occlusion after stenting is extremely high, even if the origin of the sidebranch is not diseased
   d. Stenting across acute marginal branches of the right coronary artery, small diagonal branches of the LAD, and small obtuse marginal branches of the left circumflex do not represent significant contraindications to stent implantation
   e. "Kissing stents" can sometimes be employed for treating selected bifurcation lesions
   f. ReoPro has been shown to be beneficial for reducing complications when stenting bifurcation lesions

274. Which of the following statements are true concerning the use of stents for aorto-ostial lesions:

   a. Several randomized studies confirm the immediate and long-term benefits of stenting compared to other techniques for treatment of aorto-ostial lesions

b. Heavy calcification of aorto-ostial lesions is an absolute contraindication to stenting

c. Stent implantation in aorto-ostial lesions is technically challenging because of difficulties seating the guiding catheter and ensuring proper stent position to adequately cover the lesion

d. Stents should never be implanted in protected ostial left main lesions because of the high-risk of ischemic complications

275. Several studies have confirmed the superiority of stenting lesions at the origin of the LAD compared to directional atherectomy:

a. True

b. False

276. Several randomized studies confirm that for chronic total occlusions, the immediate and long-term results of stenting are superior to those of conventional balloon angioplasty:

a. True

b. False

277. Which of the following statements are true concerning the use of stents in lesions with gross thrombus:

a. Stenting should never be performed in lesions with gross thrombus

b. Clinical studies confirm the superiority of TEC atherectomy to intra-coronary thrombolytic infusion for debulking thrombus prior to stent implantation

c. For patients who are clinically stable, a 3-7 day heparin infusion or a 2-3 week course of warfarin may "clean-up" the vessel and permit stent implantation

d. Stenting is the treatment of choice for thrombotic lesions

278. Which of the following statements are true concerning the use of stents in patients with acute myocardial infarction:

a. Except in extraordinary cases requiring bail-out stenting, stents should never be used in the setting of acute MI because of stent thrombosis

b. When stents are used for bail-out indications in the acute MI setting, the incidence of major in-hospital complications is much higher than those observed after bail-out stenting without MI

c. In contrast to elective stenting, the proper medical regimen after stenting in acute MI includes aspirin, warfarin, Ticlopidine, and subcutaneous heparin

d. Stent implantation in acute MI should only be performed with heparin-bonded stents

e. Observational studies suggest that stents may be implanted in acute MI without excessive risk of stent thrombosis

279. In patients with unstable angina, stent implantation should only be considered if intravenous ReoPro is administered prior to stent implantation:

a. True

b. False

280. When considering implantation of stents in patients with a single patent coronary artery or bypass graft, the following factors are most important:

a. Target vessel caliber

b. Distal run off

c. Target vessel

d. Age of the patient

281. Commercially available covered stents are now widely available and are the treatment of choice for virtually all cases of acute coronary artery perforation:

a. True

b. False

282. Which of the following statements are true concerning the ideal anticoagulation and antiplatelet regimen following stent implantation:

a. After optimal stenting, the incidence of stent thrombosis and subsequent ischemic complications is lower in patients treated with aspirin and Ticlopidine than in patients treated with aspirin alone

b. For optimal stenting, the incidence of stent thrombosis is similar for patients treated with aspirin and Ticlopidine compared to aspirin plus Coumadin

c. The recent ISAR trial confirmed the advantage of aspirin and Ticlopidine over aspirin plus Warfarin after stenting in high-risk patients

d. Soluble aspirin has been shown to be more effective than enteric coated aspirin in preventing stent thrombosis in all patient subgroups

e. The role of low molecular weight heparin injections has not been fully defined after stent implantation

283. Randomized trials have shown clear benefit of intravenous Dextran infusions during stent implantation to prevent stent thrombosis:

a. True
b. False

284. Multiple studies have clearly demonstrated a lower incidence of bleeding, vascular complications, and blood transfusion when aspirin and Ticlopidine are prescribed compared to Warfarin-based regimens after stenting, but these beneficial effects are achieved at the expense of a higher incidence of stent thrombosis:

a. True
b. False

285. After successful stent implantation with optimal results, intravenous administration of Protamine is generally recommended to decrease the risk of bleeding and vascular complications:

a. True
b. False

286. Which of the following statements are true when prolonged intravenous heparin infusions are recommended after stent implantation:

a. Monitoring of PTT is recommended rather than monitoring ACT
b. The ideal PTT should be maintained between 50-80 seconds
c. Patient ambulation is recommended 8 hours after sheath removal to decrease the risk of venous thromboembolism
d. Prolonged groin compression or vascular sealing devices may be useful to prevent vascular complications

287 Which of the following statements are true regarding the use of intravascular ultrasound:

a. IVUS provides accurate measurements of vessel dimensions

b. Assessment of the degree and distribution of calcium is feasible
c. The adequacy of lesion coverage by stents can be easily assessed
d. Parameters for optimal stent implantation can be evaluated
e. IVUS is the best method for assessment of intraluminal thrombus

288. Studies following stent implantation confirm that IVUS is essential before recommending treatment with aspirin and Ticlopidine without prolonged heparin and Warfarin:

a. True
b. False

289. Which of the following statements are true regarding the use of intravascular ultrasound after stenting:

a. IVUS adds procedural cost and time
b. Routine use of high pressure angioplasty does not ensure optimal stent implantation by IVUS criteria
c. Even after high pressure angioplasty, IVUS may reveal inadequate stent expansion and apposition
d. The discrepancy between IVUS and quantitative coronary angiography decreases with higher inflation pressures
e. The prospective AVID trial confirmed that use of IVUS resulted in better angiographic results and improvement in 30 day clinical events compared to patients who did not undergo IVUS

290. Which of the following statements are true concerning the impact of intravascular ultrasound on stent complications:

a. IVUS decreases the risk of in-hospital subacute thrombosis and emergency bypass surgery after stenting
b. Using IVUS criteria, final balloon sizing should be performed with a balloon-to-artery ratio > 12
c. The precise role of IVUS is still uncertain and further study is required

291. Intracoronary urokinase infusion is routinely recommended prior to Wallstent implantation, but is not recommended during implantation of balloon expandable stents:

a. True
b. False

292. Intracoronary urokinase may be useful as an adjunct to recanalize vessels with stent thrombosis, but is not recommended for intraluminal haziness alone:

    a. True
    b. False

293. Randomized trials have confirmed the value of long-acting nitrates and calcium channel blockers for 6 weeks after successful stent implantation to reduce chest pain and recurrent ischemia:

    a. True
    b. False

294. It is reasonable to prescribe prophylactic antibiotics for patients who require dental procedures and endoscopy within 3 months of stent implantation:

    a. True
    b. False

295. Which of the following statements are true regarding stent thrombosis:

    a. Stent thrombosis is associated with a high incidence of ischemic complications including death, myocardial infarction, and emergency bypass surgery
    b. Most episodes of stent thrombosis occur within the first 2 days after stent implantation
    c. The risk of stent thrombosis increases if there is significant unstented disease or dissection distal to the stent
    d. There is an increased risk of stent thrombosis if the stent has not been treated with high pressure inflations, even if the angiographic result is perfect immediately after stent deployment

296. Stent thrombosis is a simple matter of interaction between intravascular metals and blood elements; the degree of anticoagulation is the most important factor in preventing stent thrombosis:

    a. True
    b. False

297. Which of the following factors characterize "optimal stenting" using angiographic criteria without intravascular ultrasound:

a. Complete coverage of the lesion
b. Final diameter stenosis < 50% after stenting
c. Adjunctive angioplasty using high pressure balloons inflated to at least 15 ATM after stent deployment
d. Absence of intraluminal filling defects or haziness inside the stent

298. Which of the following are considered acceptable strategies in the management of stent thrombosis:

a. Intravenous administration of thrombolytic agents without cardiac catheterization
b. Implantation of additional stents
c. Crossing the occluded stent with a guidewire and performing immediate balloon angioplasty
d. Intracoronary administration of urokinase after PTCA
e. Intravenous administration of ReoPro and immediate PTCA

299. Multiple studies have reported less bleeding and vascular complications when aspirin and ticlopidine are used after stent implantation, but the risk of stent thrombosis is increased in such patients compared to those treated with warfarin-based therapies:

a. True
b. False

300. Stent embolization is an infrequent complication, and is usually managed by stent deployment at the site of embolization since stent retrieval is often difficult:

a. True
b. False

301. Which of the following factors may contribute to the observation of coronary artery perforation after stent implantation:

a. Coronary artery perforation does not occur after stent implantation
b. Oversized balloons during stent deployment or subsequent high pressure PTCA
c. Stent deployment in vessels with significant tapering
d. Stenting a contained perforation which resulted from use of another device
e. Subintimal passage of a guidewire followed by stent implantation

302. Which of the following statements are true concerning the cost of stenting:

   a. When used for elective purposes, procedural cost and total hospital cost are increased after stenting compared to PTCA
   b. The STRESS and BENESTENT trials confirmed that at 1 year, stents were more cost-effective than PTCA
   c. The major factor contributing to the high cost of stenting is length of hospital stay, which may decrease with less intensive antiplatelet regimens
   d. Intravascular ultrasound has been shown to be a cost-effective adjunct to stenting

303. You are planning to deploy a Palmaz-Schatz coronary stent in the distal left circumflex coronary artery, which is a moderately tortuous vessel. After engaging the ostium of the left coronary artery with a JL-4 guiding catheter, attempts to slightly advance the guide result in its disengagement from the ostium. Assuming that there is nothing unusual about the patient or the aortic root, appropriate maneuvers at this point include:

   a. Exchange the JL-4 guiding catheter for a geometric catheter to achieve better back-up support
   b. Exchange the JL-4 guide for a JL-3.5 guide
   c. Change to a JL-4 guiding catheter with side holes
   d. Plan to deploy the stent using an extra support or heavy duty guidewire

304. Which of the following statements are true concerning deployment of balloon-expandable and self-expanding stents:

   a. Predilation of the target lesion is recommended before stent deployment
   b. The final stent diameter can be altered by using a different size balloon after stent deployment
   c. After stent deployment, adjunctive angioplasty is recommended using high pressure balloons
   d. When the need for overlapping stents is anticipated, stent deployment should occur from distal to proximal, if possible

305 A severe stenosis in the mid LAD is predilated with a 3.5 mm high-pressure balloon followed by deployment of a 3.5 mm Palmaz-Schatz coronary stent at 7 ATM. After deploying the stent, the same 3.5 mm high pressure balloon will not pass into the stented segment. The reference diameter is 3.5 mm and the angiographic result is perfect. Appropriate strategies at this point include:

   a. Since the angiographic result is perfect, the procedure may be terminated at this point
   b. Attempt to "jack-hammer" the high-pressure balloon into the stented segment, and if this is unsuccessful the procedure may be terminated

c. Attempt to re-wrap the high-pressure balloon and then re-insert it into the stented segment

d. Use an uninflated 3.5 mm high pressure balloon to dilate the stent at a high pressure

e. Exchange the guidewire for a heavy duty guidewire to see if this will facilitate passage of the high pressure balloon

f. Post-dilate the stent with a low profile compliant balloon to "tack up" the edges of the stent followed by further inflation with the high pressure balloon

306. Which of the following statements are true concerning the Palmaz-Schatz coronary stent delivery system:

a. The delivery sheath is designed to protect the stent during insertion and facilitate delivery to the target lesion

b. The stent delivery sheath increases the profile of the delivery system

c. The relative positions of the stent delivery sheath and the stent delivery balloon should never be altered prior to retraction of the delivery sheath at the time of stent deployment

d. Availability of the delivery sheath has decreased the incidence of stent embolization

307. The 3.0 mm, 3.5 mm, and 4.0 mm Palmaz-Schatz coronary stents are virtually identical to each other and represent the same stent mounted on different delivery balloons:

a. True

b. False

308. The 3.0 mm, 3.5 mm, and 4.0 mm Gianturco-Roubin stents are virtually identical to each other and represent the same stent mounted on different delivery balloons:

a. True

b. False

309. Which of the following statements are true concerning stent implantation in a focal lesion in a 4 mm vessel:

a. A 3.0 mm Palmaz-Schatz stent is the only stent available in your inventory; this stent should not be implanted and the patient should be rescheduled at a later date

b. A 3.0 mm Palmaz-Schatz coronary stent is the only stent in your inventory; this stent can be readily deployed and post-dilated with a 4.0 mm high pressure balloon

c. A 3.0 mm Gianturco-Roubin stent is the only stent in your inventory; this stent should not be implanted and the patient should be rescheduled at a later date

d. A 3.0 mm Gianturco-Roubin stent is the only stent in your inventory; this stent should be implanted and post-dilated with a 4.0 mm high pressure balloon

310. Prior to stent implantation in highly eccentric lesions, directional atherectomy or Rotablator is strongly recommended to achieve optimal stent implantation:

a. True
b. False

311. A 4.0 mm Palmaz-Schatz stent is implanted in a focal lesion in a saphenous vein graft. After high pressure balloon inflations, there is no residual stenosis inside the stent, but antegrade flow is severely impaired. The patient is hypotensive and bradycardic. Appropriate measures at this point include:

a. Immediate insertion of a perfusion balloon catheter
b. Refer the patient for immediate coronary artery bypass surgery
c. Insert a pacemaker and intra-aortic balloon pump to stabilize the patient
d. Administer intracoronary nitroglycerin
e. Administer intracoronary verapamil
f. Deploy additional stents until TIMI flow = 3

312. A single Palmaz-Schatz stent is deployed in the mid LAD. After high pressure balloon inflations there is a severe focal dissection at the distal stent margin. Appropriate strategies at this point include:

a. Deployment of another stent distal to the first stent in an attempt to "tack up" the dissection
b. The patient should be referred for emergency bypass surgery since attempts to deploy a stent through a more proximal stent are almost always fruitless
c. Verify that the ACT is greater than 300 seconds to ensure optimal heparin effect
d. As long as the patient does not have clinical evidence for ischemia, the procedure may be terminated and an aggressive anticoagulation regimen with prolonged heparin and warfarin is recommended

313. Which of the following are characteristic of the Gianturco-Roubin stent:

    a. Compatible with a 0.018 inch guidewire
    b. Does not require pre-dilation or post-dilation
    c. The stent can be manually removed from the stent delivery balloon and remounted on any other suitable balloon catheter
    d. Overlapping stents should be avoided because of the risk of damage to the stent coils

314. In contrast to the first generation Gianturco-Roubin stent, the newer second generation stent has the following characteristics:

    a. A flat wire construction to enhance trackability and prevent distortion of the coils
    b. Distinct radiopaque markers at the proximal and distal end of the stent
    c. New heparin bonding to reduce the risk of stent thrombosis
    d. Lower profile delivery balloon to enhance successful stent delivery

315. In contrast to the Palmaz-Schatz coronary stent, intravenous ReoPro has been shown to be important to reduce ischemic complications after deployment of Gianturco-Roubin stents for abrupt closure:

    a. True
    b. False

316. Which of the following statements are true concerning the use of the Gianturco-Roubin stent for bifurcation lesions:

    a. The Gianturco-Roubin stent should never be used in bifurcation lesions
    b. If sidebranch occlusion occurs after implantation of the Gianturco-Roubin stent, conventional balloon angioplasty should not be used to retrieve the sidebranch because of the high likelihood of damage to the coil stent
    c. The risk of sidebranch occlusion is greatest when the branch has disease at its ostium
    d. If sidebranch occlusion occurs after implantation of the Gianturco-Roubin stent, high pressure balloon inflations should not be performed within the stent since it would be impossible to retrieve the sidebranch

317. When implanting the Gianturco-Roubin stent in a native coronary artery because of a severe focal dissection, adjunctive angioplasty should not be performed with high pressure balloons because of the risk of extending the dissection:

a. True
b. False

ROTABLATOR

318. Which of the following statements is true concerning the Rotablator system:

   a. The Rotablator burr is completely covered with diamond chips to ensure plaque ablation during advancement and retraction of the rotating burr
   b. The drive shaft is enclosed in a flexible teflon sheath which protects the arterial wall from the rotating drive shaft and cools and irrigates the system during operation
   c. The speed of burr rotation is controlled by a foot pedal
   d. The Rotablator burr is compatible with virtually all 0.014-inch angioplasty guidewires

319. Differential cutting is an important principle of operation of the Rotablator and is defined as selective ablation of one material while maintaining the integrity of another, based on differences in substrate composition:

   a. True
   b. False

320. Orthogonal displacement of friction is an important principle of operation of the Rotablator, and refers to virtual elimination of the longitudinal friction vector which permits easy passage of the burr during activation:

   a. True
   b. False

321. Several studies confirm that the Rotablator is extremely effective at ablation of calcified plaque, but acceleration of atherosclerosis in adjacent areas is an important limitation of the device:

   a. True
   b. False

322. Which of the following factors influences the size of microparticulate debris generated by the Rotablator:

    a. Burr size
    b. Rotational speed
    c. The pressure and force of burr advancement
    d. Stenosis severity

323. Which of the following statements are true concerning the impact of microparticulate debris generated by the Rotablator:

    a. Most microparticles are smaller than red blood cells and pass harmlessly through the circulation and are cleared by the liver, lungs and spleen
    b. Most imaging studies suggest that Rotablator atherectomy routinely results in hemodynamic dysfunction which often requires pharmacologic or mechanical support
    c. Imaging studies suggest that Rotablator atherectomy results in transient wall motion abnormalities which last 30-40 minutes and may be due to myocardial stunning

324. Which of the following statements are true concerning plaque ablation during rotational atherectomy:

    a. Quantitative angiography suggests that Rotablator atherectomy is extremely efficient, with lumen dimensions equivalent to 90% of the burr diameter
    b. Immediate elastic recoil and vasospasm may improve within 24-hours following atherectomy, resulting in larger lumen dimensions than were observed immediately after the procedure
    c. Intravascular ultrasound confirms that lumen enlargement after Rotablator is due to equal contributions of plaque ablation and vessel expansion
    d. Adjunctive PTCA after Rotablator results in further vessel expansion but no additional plaque removal

325. In several randomized trials, Rotablator is associated with an increase in procedural cost compared to PTCA, but the marked decrease in restenosis after Rotablator results in overall cost effectiveness compared to PTCA:

    a. True
    b. False

326. Which of the following recommendations are reasonable concerning patient preparation prior to Rotablator atherectomy:

 a. Prophylactic administration of intravenous atropine or placement of a temporary transvenous pacemaker are recommended for target lesions in a dominant right coronary artery or dominant circumflex

 b. Because of the potential for transient myocardial dysfunction, continuous monitoring of pulmonary artery pressure and placement of an intra-aortic balloon pump are recommended when Rotablator atherectomy is used in patients with severe baseline left ventricular dysfunction

 c. Bradycardia and heart block are never observed during Rotablator atherectomy of target lesions in the LAD, so temporary pacemakers are not necessary

327. Which of the following statements are true concerning the use of adjunctive medical therapy before and after rotational atherectomy:

 a. Prior to atherectomy, patients should be vigorously treated with diuretics to facilitate "wash out" of particulate debris during atherectomy

 b. Because rotational atherectomy results in a smooth lumen, the target ACT during the procedure is usually 250 seconds

 c. Generous doses of intracoronary nitroglycerin are recommended during the procedure to vasodilate the target vessel and decrease vasospasm

 d. Intracoronary calcium channel blockers may be helpful in reversing no-reflow after Rotablator atherectomy, but should be withheld from patients with baseline left ventricular dysfunction

 e. A "cocktail" of nitroglycerin, verapamil, and heparin in the flush solution may reduce the incidence of no-reflow during Rotablation

328. Which of the following statements is true concerning selection of guiding catheters for Rotablator atherectomy:

 a. The most important principle in selecting a guiding catheter is to achieve coaxial alignment with the target vessel

 b. The most important principle of guiding catheter selection is to achieve a "power position"

 c. With the exception of the 2.5 mm burr, all other burrs can be easily advanced through an 8 French giant lumen guiding catheter (ID $\geq$ 0.086 inches)

329. Which of the following statements are true concerning selection and placement of Rotablator burrs:

    a. An initial burr/artery ratio of 0.8 is often recommended followed by incremental increases in burr size by 0.25 to 0.5 mm
    b. During burr rotation, radiographic contrast should be administered intermittently to monitor the flow of contrast around the burr and to confirm adequate burr position
    c. Failure to neutralize forward tension on the Rotablator before activation can result in vessel dissection
    d. The ideal platform speed is 160,000 RPM for burrs > 2 mm and 180,000 RPM for burrs ≤ 2 mm

330. During rotational atherectomy, you observe that the burr rotational speed decreases from 170,000 RPM to 150,000 RPM. As the burr decelerates, appropriate interventions include:

    a. Instruct the technician to increase the rotational speed up to 170,000 RPM
    b. Instruct the technician to increase the rotational speed to 165,000 RPM, which is within the acceptable limit of 5,000 RPM below the desired speed
    c. Simply place more pressure on the advancing burr to "pop it" through the lesion
    d. Step off the foot pedal so the ablation procedure is immediately terminated
    e. Gently withdraw the burr slightly while allowing it to rotate, which usually results in a slight increase in rotational speed

331. Which of the following statements are true concerning contrast injections during rotational ablation while the burr is spinning:

    a. Contrast injections should never be done while the burr is spinning because of the risk of distal embolization
    b. Contrast injections are useful to provide visual assessment of burr advancement
    c. Contrast injections may be useful to help identify the borders of the original target lesion and the orientation of the rotating burr in tortuous vessel segments
    d. Contrast injections may induce reactive hyperemia
    e. Egress of contrast should never be observed during burr rotation to ensure adequate contact of the burr with the target lesion

332. Which of the following statements are true concerning the optimal duration of Rotablator ablation:

    a. The ideal duration of ablation is based on lesion morphology, distal runoff, hemodynamic performance and clinical factors

b. In general, ideal ablation runs should last 15-30 seconds

c. Since patients with chronic total occlusions usually have adequate collateral circulation, the ideal ablation run is 1-2 minutes

d. The duration between ablation runs should normally be 30-120 seconds to allow particle clearance, administration of vasodilators, and observation of clinical and electrocardiographic changes

333. Which of the following statements are true concerning the use of adjunctive therapies immediately following Rotablator atherectomy:

   a. Because of the high efficiency of lumen enlargement after Rotablator, use of large burrs without adjunctive angioplasty is frequently all that is necessary in most lesions

   b. When adjunctive angioplasty is performed after Rotablator atherectomy, randomized trials have confirmed the restenosis advantage for using slightly oversized balloons at low pressure

   c. Balloon angioplasty, directional atherectomy, and stenting have all been successfully applied as adjunctive treatments immediately following Rotablator

   d. Intravascular ultrasound may be useful to assess the extent and distribution of lesion calcium and guide interventional therapy

334. After uncomplicated Rotablator cases with target lesions in the right coronary artery, the temporary pacemaker should normally be left in place for 12-24 hours, in case the patient develops delayed symptomatic bradycardia or heart block:

   a. True
   b. False

335. Which of the following statements are true concerning the immediate results of Rotablator atherectomy:

   a. Adjunctive devices are required to achieve definitive lumen enlargements in approximately 90% of cases

   b. The degree of lumen enlargement and overall procedural success is not related to baseline lesion morphology

   c. Further lumen enlargement may occur 24 hours after Rotablator suggesting release of elastic recoil and/or resolution of vasospasm

   d. Immediate results of Rotablator are highly dependent on operator technique

336. Which of the following statements are true concerning restenosis after Rotablator atherectomy:

   a. Randomized trials have demonstrated lower rates of restenosis following Rotablator compared to conventional balloon angioplasty
   b. In contrast to restenosis after balloon angioplasty, the restenosis rate after Rotablator of long lesions is similar to that for focal lesions
   c. Restenosis rates are lower for calcified lesions than for non-calcified lesions
   d. Randomized trials have confirmed the restenosis advantage for using slightly oversized balloons at minimal inflation pressure after Rotablator atherectomy
   e. No studies have yet confirmed a restenosis advantage for Rotablator atherectomy compared to balloon angioplasty

337. In considering the application of conventional balloon angioplasty, all available atherectomy devices, and stents, Rotablator is considered the treatment of choice in which of the following lesions:

   a. Complex lesions
   b. Long lesions
   c. Ostial lesions
   d. Chronic total occlusions
   e. Undilatable lesions
   f. Restenotic lesions
   g. Angulated lesions

338. Which of the following statements are true concerning the use of Rotablator atherectomy:

   a. Rotablator is not recommended for lesions containing thrombus
   b. Rotablator atherectomy may be used in selected saphenous vein grafts with rigid nondilatable lesions or severe stenosis involving the ostium
   c. Lesions at the distal anastomosis of vein grafts to native coronary arteries should not be treated with Rotablator atherectomy because of the risk of perforation
   d. In treating highly angulated lesions, lesions located on the outer curve of a vessel may be better suited for Rotablator than lesions on an inner curve
   e. Rotablator atherectomy is considered the treatment of choice for true bifurcation lesions, since there is essentially no risk of side branch occlusion

339. The "dynaglide" function on the foot pedal controls the following functions:

a. Controlled burr rotation at 50-90,000 RPM when "dynaglide" is activated

b. The "dynaglide" function must be deactivated in order to permit full-speed burr rotation for ablation

c. If the "dynaglide" light cannot be extinguished there may be insufficient pressure in the gas tank

d. The "dynaglide" foot pedal is absolutely required in order to safely remove the burr while it is rotating

340. The new Rotablator burrs have been designed so that burrs ≤ 2.38 mm in diameter can be advanced through guiding catheters with internal diameters ≥ 0.086 inches:

a. True

b. False

341. Which of the following statements are true concerning guidewire bias:

a. Guidewire bias is defined as an eccentric orientation of the Rotablator guidewire

b. The presence of guidewire bias often mandates modification in burr sizing strategy and technique

c. Common causes of guidewire bias include non-coaxial alignment of the guiding catheter, presence of a tortuous target vessel, or the presence of an angulated target lesion

d. Failure to recognize the presence of guidewire bias can lead to significant complications

342. Rotablator is not recommended in the setting of acute myocardial infarctions or in clinical situations where thrombus is likely to be present:

a. True

b. False

343. Which of the following statements are true concerning the use of Rotablator atherectomy for angulated lesions:

a. Severely angulated lesions should not be routinely considered for Rotablator

b. For angulated lesions that are highly calcified, initial debulking may be considered using a burr/artery ratio of 0.5

c. Guidewire bias may result in tangential ablation which can increase the risk of perforation

d. Lesions located on the outer curve may be better suited for Rotablator than lesions on the inner curve

e. When a moderate residual stenosis persists after Rotablator of a highly angulated lesion, further lumen enlargement with conventional balloon angioplasty is recommended rather than the use of large burrs

344. Which of the following statements are true concerning the use of Rotablator atherectomy for bifurcation lesions:

a. The sidebranch may be protected by a nitinol guidewire to reduce the chance of sidebranch occlusion

b. The presence of a significant bifurcation lesion is an absolute contraindication to Rotablator atherectomy

c. Gentle predilation of the sidebranch before Rotablator of the parent vessel may decrease the risk of sidebranch occlusion

d. Some bifurcation lesions may be treated in sequence by Rotablator atherectomy of both the parent and branch vessels

345. Which of the following statements are true concerning the Rotablator approach to calcified lesions:

a. Compared to other techniques, Rotablator atherectomy results in the best lumen enlargement in lesions with heavy superficial calcification

b. Rotablator ablation may liberate large amounts of microparticles in heavily calcified lesions

c. To minimize microparticle embolization, initial use of a single large burr is strongly recommended

d. Optimal technique requires that the burr be advanced as rapidly as possible through the calcified lesion to minimize microembolization

e. Extended time intervals between runs may be required until hemodynamics and ECG normalize and symptoms resolve

346. Rotablator of focal lesions < 10 mm in length should be treated with extremely rapid ablation runs to minimize the time of burr activation and decrease the risk of no-reflow:

a. True
b. False

347. Which of the following statements are true concerning the Rotablator approach to lesions > 15 mm in length:

    a. The entire lesion should be traversed by the Rotablator during the first ablation pass
    b. It is not necessary to traverse the entire lesion during the first pass; a segmental ablation technique is recommended
    c. Because of the long lesion length, RPM surveillance is not necessary
    d. Ablation runs should not exceed 15-30 seconds
    e. The time interval between runs should be less than with Rotablator of focal lesions
    f. A stepped burr approach is recommended

348. Under certain circumstances, Rotablator ablation of a heavily calcified but focal lesion may require longer ablation times than a noncalcified long lesion:

    a. True
    b. False

349. Which of the following statements are true concerning the Rotablator approach to eccentric lesions:

    a. Eccentric lesions should not be treated with the Rotablator because of unfavorable guidewire bias
    b. Rotablator atherectomy of eccentric lesions is feasible but may require technical modifications
    c. Careful reposition of the guiding catheter or guidewire may result in favorable guidewire bias
    d. An active guidewire technique may improve the angiographic outcome for eccentric lesions, resulting in "directional rotational atherectomy"

350. Conventional PTCA is attempted on a focal lesion in the mid-LAD but the balloon fails to fully expand despite high inflation pressures. Which of the following statements are true concerning the Rotablator approach at this time:

    a. Rotablator atherectomy should never be performed immediately after unsuccessful angioplasty
    b. The patient should be discharged from the hospital and readmitted for Rotablator atherectomy in 3-4 weeks
    c. The angioplasty balloon should be removed and repeat angiography performed; if there is no angiographic evidence for dissection, Rotablator atherectomy may be performed at this time
    d. If angioplasty results in significant dissection, Rotablator should not be performed

351. Which of the following statements are true concerning the Rotablator approach to ostial lesions:

    a. Since the guiding catheter must reside proximal to the ostium, coaxial guiding catheter alignment is irrelevant
    b. Power guides which result in strong guiding catheter positions are most useful for Rotablator atherectomy of ostial lesions
    c. Allowing the guiding catheter to "kick out" of the ostium is acceptable as long as the guidewire alignment remains coaxial
    d. Initial burr activation must occur while the burr is engaged with the ostial lesion to minimize the chance of injury to the guiding catheter
    e. Since there is no platform segment, it is not necessary to adjust the platform speed to achieve the ideal ablation speed

352. In some restenotic lesions, an acceptable approach is to use a burr size 0.25 mm larger than the burr size that would have been used for a de novo lesion:

    a. True
    b. False

353. Which of the following statements are true concerning Rotablator atherectomy of saphenous vein graft lesions:

    a. Rotablator is absolutely contraindicated in all vein graft lesions
    b. Rotablator may be useful for rigid and fibrotic lesions at the ostium or at the distal anastomosis
    c. Lesions in the body of vein grafts which appear to be associated with soft grumous should not be treated with Rotablator atherectomy
    d. Ostial lesions identified within 6 weeks of surgery are ideal targets for Rotablator atherectomy

354. Which of the following observations are true concerning the behavior of the Rotablator in very tortuous vessels:

    a. Severe proximal tortuosity can significantly impact the results of Rotablator
    b. The Rotablator floppy guidewire may result in less vessel deformity and facilitate advancement of the Rotablator burr through the target vessel
    c. Pseudolesions are commonly observed and may be confused with true lesions, spasm, or dissection
    d. In some cases, activation of the burr at low speeds (100,000 RPM) may facilitate passage of the burr through tortuous segments proximal to the target lesion

355. In chronic total occlusions which cannot be crossed with a guidewire, Rotablator atherectomy is the treatment of choice to debulk rigid plaque:

   a. True
   b. False

356. Which of the following statements are true concerning no-reflow during Rotablator atherectomy:

   a. The development of no-reflow is expected and bears no impact on the need for further Rotablator ablation
   b. Transient "slow flow" (TIMI flow = 2) is an absolute contraindication to further Rotablator atherectomy
   c. Severe chest pain without ECG changes or flow impairment may be due to distal micro-embolization
   d. Intravenous calcium channel blockers are effective for reversing no-reflow after Rotablator

357. Which of the following approaches are reasonable if no reflow occurs during Rotablator atherectomy:

   a. Avoidance of further Rotablator passes
   b. Administration of nitroglycerin 200 mcg IC
   c. Administration of Diltiazem 2 mg IC
   d. Addition of 5 mg of verapamil to the Rotablator flush solution, followed by further Rotablator passes to facilitate delivery of verapamil to the distal microvascular bed
   e. Adenosine 10-15 mg IC

358. Which of the following statements are true concerning the administration of intracoronary calcium channel blockers to reverse no-reflow:

   a. When TIMI flow is ≤ 1, calcium channel blockers should be administered through the guiding catheter and vigorously flushed
   b. When there is no antegrade flow, the calcium channel blockers must be delivered to the distal coronary bed using a suitable transport catheter or deflated balloon catheter
   c. The combination of intracoronary calcium channel blockers and urokinase is superior to calcium channel blockers alone
   d. If no-reflow cannot be immediately reversed, the patient should be referred for emergency bypass surgery

359. Which of the following statements are true concerning dissection or perforation during Rotablator atherectomy:

   a. Frequent small contrast injections should never be used to assess Rotablator action because of the risk of causing contrast-induced dissection
   b. Relative oversizing of the burr compared to the target lesion may be a factor in creating dissection
   c. In highly eccentric and angulated lesions, unfavorable guidewire bias may lead to dissection or perforation
   d. Excessive burr deceleration may lead to no-reflow but is not an important cause of dissection

360. When burr detachment occurs, the burr can usually be retrieved by removing the guidewire:

   a. True
   b. False

361. Which of the following factors may contribute to burr stall:

   a. A kink in the compressed gas line
   b. Over tightening the Y-connector which crimps the drive shaft
   c. An empty gas tank
   d. Aggressive burr advancement into a rigid lesion
   e. A kink in the fiberoptic cable which controls burr speed

362. Which of the following steps are useful to prevent guidewire fracture during Rotablator atherectomy:

   a. Always use the wire clip, especially when depressing the brake-defeat button
   b. It is best to prolapse the Rotablator guidewire into a small branch to avoid injury to a major vessel
   c. Avoid prolonged ablation runs at a single point on the guidewire to avoid excessive guidewire wear
   d. If a loop is identified in the guidewire outside the vessel ostium, do not rotate the burr and simply pull back the guidewire

DIRECTIONAL ATHERECTOMY

363. Contemporary designs of the Simpson AtheroCath now permit routine use of large-lumen 8 French guiding catheters:

a. True
b. False

364. After insertion of the arterial sheath sufficient heparin is recommended prior to directional atherectomy to achieve an ACT > 300 seconds:

a. True
b. False

365. Which of the following statements are true concerning sizing of the AtheroCath:

a. A "stepped" approach is generally recommended, beginning with a 5 or 6 French AtheroCath and then increasing to a 7 French AtheroCath if necessary
b. A 6 French AtheroCath may be slightly undersized for a vessel measuring 3.4 mm in normal diameter
c. "Optimal" directional atherectomy recommendations include the use of larger atherectomy devices than are currently recommended on the product label

366. Which of the following statements are true concerning preparation of the AtheroCath immediately prior to atherectomy:

a. Full strength (100%) contrast is recommended to prep the balloon inflation port
b. A pressure bag with heparinized saline should be hooked up to the flush port
c. Virtually any 0.014 inch guidewire is compatible with the directional atherectomy device
d. If a bare guidewire technique is used to cross the target lesion, an exchange length or extendable guidewire is required
e. The motor drive unit should be attached to the AtheroCath and the cutter locked in closed position prior to advancing the AtheroCath into the guiding catheter

367. For directional atherectomy, match the appropriate guiding catheter based on target vessel and aortic root:

a.	LAD; narrow aortic root	1.	JL 3.5
b.	LCx; wide aortic root	2.	JL 5.0
c.	RCA; normal aortic root	3.	JR 4.0
d.	RCA; Shepherd crook	4.	JRG
e.	SVG to OM; superior origin	5.	JLG
f.	SVG to R-PDA; inferior origin	6.	Multipurpose

368. Once the guiding catheter is engaged in the vessel ostium, over-rotation and deep-seating are recommended to ensure strong guiding catheter support:

    a. True
    b. False

369. Prior to directional atherectomy, routine predilation is generally required for most lesions:

    a. True
    b. False

370. Which of the following statements are true concerning advancement of the AtheroCath into the target lesion:

    a. The AtheroCath should be advanced into the lesion by applying forward pressure on the device; a gentle "screwing motion" should be avoided to reduce the chance of vessel injury
    b. If it is necessary to rotate the AtheroCath to advance it into the lesion, alternating clockwise and counterclockwise rotation is recommended to facilitate delivery of the device to the target lesion
    c. If the AtheroCath does not easily cross the target lesion, "jack hammering" is reasonable to move the housing forward across the stenosis
    d. Co-axial alignment of the guiding catheter is the most important factor when advancing the AtheroCath into the target vessel

371. Which of the following statements are true concerning guidewire manipulation during directional atherectomy:

a. In general the guidewire tip should reside in a straight portion of a major artery and extend 3-5 cm beyond the distal tip of the AtheroCath

b. During atherectomy it is important to confirm that the guidewire does not move freely

c. Guidewire entrapment in a branch vessel may increase the risk of wire fracture after activation of the motor drive unit

d. During each atherectomy cut it is reasonable to hold the guidewire to prevent proximal migration

372. Which of the following statements is true concerning performance of directional atherectomy cuts:

a. Initial cuts should be directed towards angiographically-apparent plaque

b. The balloon on the AtheroCath is designed to further dilate the target lesion and can be inflated to inflation pressures greater than 8 atm

c. The cutter can be briefly activated to facilitate retraction of the cutter in the housing window

d. Cutter activation should proceed until the cutter traverses the entire housing window and reaches the mechanical cutter stop

373. Which of the following statements are true concerning failure to fully advance the cutter during an atherectomy cut:

a. Removal of the AtheroCath when the cutter is not fully advanced increases the risk of tissue embolization

b. If a cut cannot be completed, it is reasonable to partially deflate the balloon and then attempt again to fully advance the cutter

c. If significant residual stenosis persists after initial atherectomy at low pressure, it is reasonable to perform further atherectomy at higher inflation pressures before changing to a larger AtheroCath

d. It is reasonable to empty the collection chamber after a series of 5-7 cuts

e. Immobility of the guidewire may indicate that the collection chamber is full

374. Which of the following statements are true regarding "optimal directional atherectomy:"
a. In general the procedure should be terminated when residual diameter stenosis is < 30%
b. Adjunctive angioplasty is rarely recommended because it increases the risk of dissection
c. When adjunctive angioplasty is recommended after directional atherectomy, undersized balloons are used to prevent complications
d. If a significant residual stenosis persists after initial atherectomy, reasonable strategies include the use of higher inflation pressures, larger AtheroCaths, adjunctive angioplasty, or stenting

375. Which of the following are characteristics of "optimal directional atherectomy" in a target vessel measuring 3.5 mm in diameter:

    a. Final residual stenosis of 25% after a 6 French AtheroCath
    b. Final residual stenosis of 25% after a 7 French AtheroCath
    c. Final residual stenosis < 10% after a 6 French AtheroCath and a 3.5 mm balloon
    d. 0% residual stenosis after a single pass and 3 cuts with a 7 French AtheroCath

376. To achieve optimal directional atherectomy, which of the following steps are reasonable when a residual stenosis of 30% persists in a 3.5 mm vessel after initial atherectomy with a 6 French cutter at 1 atm:

    a. Empty the AtheroCath and reinsert the same device, performing additional cuts at 2 atm
    b. Change to a 7 French AtheroCath and perform additional cuts at 1-2 atm
    c. Abandon atherectomy and dilate the target lesion with a 3.5 mm balloon at 6-8 atm
    d Implant a stent for further definitive lumenal enlargement

377. Although ReoPro has been shown to improve outcome when used at the time of conventional balloon angioplasty, it has not been shown to be beneficial in patients undergoing directional coronary atherectomy:

    a. True
    b. False

378. Which of the following problems are potentially observed when considering directional coronary atherectomy for patients with acute myocardial infarction:

    a. The presence of acute total occlusion may preclude accurate assessment of vessel diameter, making sizing decisions more complex
    b. Directional atherectomy of thrombotic lesions may be associated with no-reflow
    c. Intravenous ReoPro may be useful

379. Which of the following are true concerning the use of directional atherectomy for angulated lesions:

    a. Lesions with moderate or severe angulation are absolute contraindications to directional atherectomy

b. Use of extra support or heavy duty guidewires may facilitate passage of the AtheroCath into angulated lesions

c. Short window atherectomy devices should not be used because of the risk of perforation

d. Operators should have a low threshold for using adjunctive angioplasty to achieve optimal results

380. Which of the following are true concerning the use of directional coronary atherectomy for bifurcation lesions:

a. Compared to conventional balloon angioplasty, directional atherectomy may result in less shifting plaque and "snowplow" injury

b. Use of a nitinol guidewire permits sidebranch protection during directional atherectomy of the parent vessel

c. For sidebranches > 2.5 mm in diameter, conventional angioplasty should be used in preference to directional atherectomy to decrease the risk of dissection

d. As with conventional balloon angioplasty, the risk of sidebranch occlusion after directional atherectomy is greatest when the ostium of the sidebranch has a significant stenosis

381. Which of the following statements are true concerning the use of directional atherectomy for calcified lesions:

a. When calcification is evident by fluoroscopy, intravascular ultrasound may be useful to identify the depth and extent of calcification

b. Extensive superficial calcification is predictive of failure of directional atherectomy

c. Rotablator atherectomy may be useful prior to directional atherectomy when heavy superficial calcification is present

d. All guiding catheters for directional coronary atherectomy can accommodate all Rotablator burr sizes

382. Which of the following characteristics favor successful directional atherectomy for treatment of dissections induced by conventional balloon angioplasty:

a. Focal intimal dissections which protrude into the lumen and obstruct flow

b. Extensive medial dissection with contrast straining

c. Long spiral dissections

d. Target vessel diameter > 3 mm

e. The proximal and distal extent of dissection are readily identified by angiography

383. When directional atherectomy is used for stabilization of dissection, a relatively undersized AtheroCath is recommended to avoid coronary perforation:

    a. True
    b. False

384. Which of the following statements are true concerning the use of directional coronary atherectomy for aorto-ostial lesions:

    a. Predilation with a 2 mm balloon may be necessary to facilitate passage of the AtheroCath
    b. Co-axial alignment of the guiding catheter is preferable to power guide positions
    c. Extra support or heavy duty guidewires may facilitate access to the target lesion
    d. Short cut devices may be useful in difficult anatomic situations
    e. Adjunctive PTCA or stenting may be necessary to achieve definitive lumen enlargement

385. When treating branch ostial lesions with directional atherectomy, short cut devices may be useful to facilitate cornering of the device and limit resection of non-diseased vessel wall components:

    a. True
    b. False

386. Directional atherectomy of degenerated vein grafts is preferred over conventional balloon angioplasty to reduce the risk of no-reflow and myocardial infarction:

    a. True
    b. False

387. Which of the following techniques can be useful when treating tortuous vessels with directional atherectomy:

    a. Guiding catheters with ideal co-axial alignment
    b. Use of extra support or heavy duty 0.014-inch guidewires
    c. Use of short window AtheroCaths
    d. Continuous rotation of the AtheroCath during advancement to reduce longitudinal friction
    e. Predilation of the target lesion

388. Which of the following techniques are useful when the AtheroCath fails to track into the target lesion:

    a. Change to a guiding catheter which provides ideal co-axial alignment
    b. Optimize guidewire support by using an extra support or heavy duty guidewire
    c. Down size to a smaller AtheroCath
    d. Use a short window AtheroCath
    e. Predilate the target lesion with a 2 mm balloon

389. The GTO AtheroCath is a third generation device which has a redesigned shaft to provide better support and torque control than previous AtheroCath generations:

    a. True
    b. False

390. Which of the following adjunctive medical therapies are useful with directional atherectomy:

    a. Aspirin
    b. Prolonged intravenous heparin infusion after successful atherectomy
    c. Intravenous dextran infusion for high risk lesions
    d. Bolus and infusion of ReoPro to decrease complications and possibly restenosis

391. Which of the following statements are true concerning the use of intravascular ultrasound with directional coronary atherectomy:

    a. IVUS may be useful in identifying the extent and distribution of calcium
    b. IVUS is required to achieve "optimal" atherectomy
    c. Randomized trials have confirmed that when intravascular ultrasound is used with directional atherectomy, immediate lumen enlargement is better and restenosis rates are lower than when IVUS is not employed
    d. IVUS may be useful to identify the true reference vessel diameter and help guide selection of proper device size

392. Studies of the mechanisms of lumen enlargement after directional atherectomy suggest that at least half of the lumen enlargement is due to tissue removal, and the rest is due to angioplasty effect:

    a. True
    b. False

393. Which of the following statements are true concerning the three large multicenter randomized trials of directional atherectomy and PTCA (CAVEAT I, CAVEAT II, CCAT):

    a. Directional coronary atherectomy resulted in better immediate lumen enlargement than PTCA
    b. Immediate procedural success rates were similar for directional coronary atherectomy and PTCA
    c. Major complications were more frequent after directional coronary atherectomy
    d. Adjunctive PTCA was discouraged

394. Although dissection is the most common cause of abrupt closure after conventional balloon angioplasty, both dissection and thrombosis occur with nearly equal frequency in cases of abrupt closure after directional atherectomy:

    a. True
    b. False

395. In CAVEAT-I abrupt closure was more common after directional atherectomy than PTCA, but approximately 40% of these abrupt closures after atherectomy occurred at sites other than the target lesion:

    a. True
    b. False

396. Which of the following are true concerning coronary artery perforation after directional atherectomy:

    a. The incidence of perforation after directional atherectomy is higher than after PTCA
    b. Most perforations after directional atherectomy occurred after excision of flow-limiting dissection flaps
    c. Undersized AtheroCaths and low-pressure balloon inflations are recommended to minimize perforation when directional atherectomy is used for resection of dissection flaps
    d. When atherectomy leads to perforation, emergency surgery is always indicated

397. Which of the following statements are true concerning clinical complications after directional atherectomy:

    a. The incidence of death, Q-wave myocardial infarction, and emergency bypass surgery is similar to those after conventional balloon angioplasty

    b. Some studies suggest a higher incidence of asymptomatic elevation of cardiac enzymes after directional atherectomy than after PTCA

    c. The clinical significance of asymptomatic elevation of cardiac enzymes after otherwise uncomplicated procedures is controversial

    d. Intravenous ReoPro may be useful to decrease the incidence of non-Q-wave myocardial infarction after directional atherectomy

398. Which of the following statements are true concerning earlier randomized trials (CAVEAT and CCAT) and more recent trials of optimal atherectomy (OARS and BOAT):

    a. The more contemporary studies includes operators with greater atherectomy experience

    b. Second and third generation atherectomy devices were available in the more contemporary trials, whereas first and second generation devices were available in the earlier randomized trials

    c. Adjunctive balloon angioplasty was encouraged in the more recent contemporary trials, but was specifically discouraged in the earlier trials

    d. More contemporary trials demonstrate a definite restenosis advantage for directional atherectomy compared to balloon angioplasty

    e. Intravascular ultrasound is necessary to achieve optimal directional atherectomy results

399. With directional atherectomy, recovery of deep wall components (media and adventitial) is common and is associated with a higher incidence of restenosis:

    a. True

    b. False

400. In CAVEAT-II, directional atherectomy resulted in better lumen enlargement and higher procedural success than conventional PTCA in vein grafts, but no difference in angiographic restenosis, target lesion revascularization, or event-free survival at 6 months:

    a. True

    b. False

401. Tissue analysis after directional atherectomy indicates that intimal proliferation is highly specific for restenosis and is virtually never observed in other clinical circumstances:

    a. True
    b. False

TRANSLUMINAL EXTRACTION ATHERECTOMY

402. Which of the following correctly identify the equipment necessary for TEC atherectomy:

    a. Specialized TEC cutters ranging from 1.8 to 2.5 mm in diameter (5.5 - 7.5 F)
    b. Special 10F tungsten-braided soft tip guiding catheters in a variety of sizes and configurations
    c. Any conventional 0.014 inch guidewire
    d. Any large bore rotating hemostatic valve

403. TEC cutters ≤ 6.5 F (2.2 mm) may be advanced through any large lumen 9 F guiding catheter:

    a. True
    b. False

404. Specialized TEC guiding catheters should be used to obtain strong power positions in the vessel ostium by over-rotation and deep-seating to facilitate passage of the cutter into the target vessel:

    a. True
    b. False

405. Which of the following statements are true concerning the special TEC guidewire:

    a. The TEC guidewire is made of stainless steel and is 300 cm in length
    b. The TEC guidewire is stiff and should only be used as the platform for the TEC cutter when a conventional 0.014 inch guidewire does not provide sufficient support
    c. Pseudolesions may be observed when the TEC guidewire is in position
    d. When exchanging the specialized 0.014 inch TEC guidewire, a transfer catheter must have an internal diameter ≥ 0.021 inches

406. Which of the following statements are true concerning selection and deployment of TEC cutters:

    a. In general, undersized cutters are recommended to achieve a cutter/artery ratio of 0.5-0.7
    b. To minimize the chance of proximal vessel dissection, the TEC cutter should only be activated when it is within the target lesion
    c. Adequate removal of thrombus and atheroma require rapid advancement and retraction of the cutter through the target lesion, which maximizes tissue removal and minimizes distal embolization
    d. After 2-5 passes through the target lesion, the TEC cutter should be retracted into the guiding catheter and the lesion reassessed for further intervention

407. Which of the following adjunctive medical treatments are routinely recommended prior to or during TEC atherectomy:

    a. Aspirin
    b. Heparin
    c. Intracoronary nitroglycerin
    d. Intracoronary urokinase
    e. Intravenous ReoPro

408. Which of the following statements are true concerning the mechanisms of action of TEC atherectomy:

    a. Angioscopy studies demonstrate partial or complete thrombus removal in > 75% of thrombotic lesions
    b. Non-flow-limiting intimal dissections are rare after TEC
    c. Tissue analysis suggests that the TEC cutter is an extremely efficient device for removal of atherosclerotic tissue
    d. There is virtually no "Dotter" effect after TEC atherectomy

409. Which of the following identifies the role of adjunctive PTCA after TEC atherectomy in native coronary arteries:

    a. Treatment of suboptimal angiographic results
    b. Salvage technical failures
    c. Achieve definitive lumen enlargement
    d. Manage TEC-induced vessel occlusion

Questions

410. The extent of the elastic recoil after TEC is similar to that after conventional PTCA:

    a. True
    b. False

411. TEC atherectomy has been shown to be the treatment of choice in degenerated vein grafts due to elimination of distal embolization and no reflow:

    a. True
    b. False

412. In saphenous vein grafts, TEC atherectomy with PTCA results in substantially lower rates of restenosis compared to PTCA alone:

    a. True
    b. False

413. Compared to PTCA alone in patients with acute ischemic syndromes, the combination of TEC and adjunctive angioplasty may result in less asymptomatic elevation of cardiac enzymes:

    a. True
    b. False

414. Angiographic thrombus increases the risk of adverse outcomes in virtually all studies of percutaneous interventional devices, including TEC atherectomy:

    a. True
    b. False

415. Which of the following conditions are contraindications to TEC atherectomy:

    a. Heavy calcification
    b. Severe lesion angulation
    c. Target vessel diameter < 2 mm
    d. Significant dissection due to another device

e. A true bifurcation lesion

416. The TEC cutter must be advanced over the guidewire after first positioning the guidewire beyond the target lesion, using a bare guidewire technique:

a. True
b. False

DOPPLER FLOW MEASUREMENTS

417. Which of the following statements are true concerning coronary blood flow:

a. Coronary blood flow is primarily regulated by vascular resistance at the level of the coronary arteriole
b. With exercise a decrease in coronary vascular resistance leads to an increase in coronary blood flow
c. In the presence of a severe epicardial coronary artery stenosis, resting basal blood flow may be normal but maximal hyperemic flow is impaired
d. Measurements of coronary flow reserve may identify conditions which impair the normal hyperemic response to exercise and increase myocardial oxygen demand
e. The Doppler flow wire provides online measurements of absolute coronary blood flow

418. Which of the following statements are true concerning evaluation of coronary blood flow using the Doppler flow guidewire:

a. Measurements are of coronary blood flow velocity rather than volumetric flow
b. If the cross sectional area of the artery remains constant, changes in blood flow velocity are parallel to changes in volumetric flow
c. Intracoronary nitroglycerin or other vasodilators are commonly used to minimize differences in vessel diameter between basal and hyperemic conditions
d. Measurement of coronary flow reserve is an important parameter in assessing the functional significance of a lesion

419. Which of the following statements are true concerning coronary flow reserve:

    a. Coronary flow reserve is defined as the ratio of hyperemic to baseline coronary blood flow velocity
    b. Coronary flow reserve < 2 is diagnostic of a significant epicardial stenosis
    c. Impairment in function of the distal microvascular bed can interfere with interpretation of coronary flow reserve
    d. Papaverine or adenosine may be utilized to induce reactive hyperemia

420. Situations in which interpretation of coronary flow reserve may be significantly impaired when evaluating coronary artery disease include:

    a. Longstanding insulin-dependent diabetes
    b. Recent acute myocardial infarction
    c. Severe left ventricular hypertrophy due to aortic stenosis
    d. Severe single vessel coronary artery disease

421. The physiologic assessment of a "borderline lesion" is better evaluated by a Doppler flow wire than intravascular ultrasound:

    a. True
    b. False

422. Which of the following are more commonly associated with the Doppler flow wire than intravascular ultrasound:

    a. Cause ischemia
    b. Provide online information of coronary blood flow
    c. "Trending" to predict ischemic complications after coronary intervention
    d. Assessment of microvascular disease

423. Which of the following statements are true concerning the observation of normal coronary flow reserve in an angiographically borderline lesion:

    a. Normal flow reserve is predictive of a favorable short term prognosis
    b. Normal flow reserve is highly correlated with normal perfusion scans
    c. Normal flow reserve does not exclude the possibility of significant microvascular disease

d. Normal flow reserve suggests that the borderline lesion is not physiologically significant

424. Which of the following parameters are characteristic of "successful" percutaneous intervention:

a. Diastolic predominance of the diastolic/systolic velocity ratio (DSVR)
b. Proximal to distal mean velocity ratio < 1.5
c. Coronary flow reserve > 2.5
d. Hyperemic average peak velocity equal to 20 cm/second

425. A patient with single vessel disease undergoes PTCA of the mid-LAD. Microvascular disease can be excluded as a cause of persistent impairment of coronary flow reserve if the coronary flow reserve in the normal right coronary artery is > 2.5:

a. True
b. False

426. Match the Doppler-flow pattern with the cause:

a. Abrupt flow acceleration
b. Abrupt flow cessation
c. Abrupt flow deceleration
d. Cyclical flow variations

1. Vasovagal reaction
2. Transient spasm
3. Abrupt closure/thrombus
4. Abrupt closure/dissection

EXCIMER LASER CORONARY ANGIOPLASTY

427. Which of the following statements are true concerning excimer laser ablation:

a. The excimer laser emits pulsed ultraviolet light at a wavelength of 308 mm
b. In vivo mechanisms of tissue ablation include photochemical, thermal, and mechanical effects
c. Lasing in blood can induce acoustic effects resulting in tissue injury and dissection
d. Excimer laser ablation in a field of radiographic contrast is preferred to minimize tissue injury

Questions

428. Which of the following statements are true concerning excimer laser catheters:

a. Excimer laser catheters are compatible with conventional angioplasty guidewires
b. Currently available concentric excimer laser catheters consist of more than 200 individual laser fibers, which decreases dead space and increases fiber flexibility
c. An eccentric excimer laser catheter permits directional excimer laser ablation
d. Because of the availability of a wide range of laser catheter dimensions, adjunctive PTCA is rarely necessary

429. In contrast to other percutaneous interventional devices, the currently available excimer laser catheters can be used to revascularize total occlusions which cannot be crossed with a guidewire:

a. True
b. False

430. Which of the following statements are true concerning results of currently available randomized trials of excimer laser and balloon angioplasty:

a. Randomized trials demonstrate a definite restenosis advantage for excimer laser compared to PTCA, but not to Rotablator
b. The saline infusion technique was not routinely employed in earlier randomized trials
c. Long lesions and chronic total occlusions were frequently excluded from earlier trials
d. The incidence of major in-hospital ischemic complications was similar for PTCA and ELCA

431. Which of the following factors may decrease complications due to excimer laser ablation:

a. Use of the saline infusion technique
b. Use of smaller laser fibers
c. Use of the directional laser for highly eccentric lesions
d. Intermittent contrast injections during laser ablation

432. Which of the following represent potential indications for the excimer laser guidewire:

a. Chronic total occlusion which cannot be crossed with a guidewire
b. A rigid nondilatable lesion by PTCA
c. Marked elastic recoil
d. Heavy calcification of an ostial lesion

433. A 1.7 mm excimer laser fiber is used to treat a focal lesion in the mid-LAD at a fluence of 40 mJ/mm and a frequency of 20 Hz. Which of the following techniques are reasonable if the laser catheter will not cross the lesion:

    a. Exchange for a 1.4 mm catheter and attempt again to ablate the lesion
    b. Increase the fluence to 60 mJ/mm
    c. Increase the frequency to 30 Hz
    d. Exchange the laser catheter for a Rotablator burr

434. Which of the following statements are true concerning use of the saline infusion technique:

    a. A special pressurized flush solution is necessary to perform this technique properly
    b. The saline infusion technique has been shown to increase the procedure success rate
    c. The saline infusion technique has been shown to decrease the incidence of dissection
    d. The saline infusion technique has been shown to decrease the incidence of restenosis and target lesion revascularization

435. Which of the following adjunctive medications are recommended prior to and during excimer laser ablation:

    a. Aspirin
    b. Heparin to achieve an ACT > 300 seconds during the procedure
    c. Intravenous ReoPro
    d. Intracoronary verapamil

436. Which of the following guiding catheter characteristics are important for excimer laser ablation:

    a. Co-axial alignment is more important than a "power guide"
    b. Guiding catheters with side holes are recommended to maintain passive perfusion during laser ablation
    c. A 2.0 mm laser catheter requires a guiding catheter with an ID ≥ 0.092 inches
    d. Special Spectranetics guiding catheters are recommended

437. All available excimer laser catheters are compatible with 0.014 inch angioplasty guidewires:

    a. True
    b. False

438. Which of the following statements are true concerning the energy levels for excimer laser ablation:

    a. The excimer laser energy level is dependent on plaque composition

    b. The excimer laser energy level is dependent on whether the target lesion is in a native vessel or saphenous vein graft

    c. In general, if lesion resistance is encountered, fluence should be increased prior to increasing the repetition rate

    d. Ostial and calcified lesions may require higher energy levels than other lesions

    e. Current system software does not permit adjustment of energy parameters without first recalibrating the system

439. In contrast to the Rotablator, excimer laser ablation is initiated when the laser catheter is in full contact with the target lesion at the time of lasing:

    a. True

    b. False

440. Immediately prior to initiation of laser ablation, it is imperative to leave a small amount of radiographic contrast between the laser catheter and the target lesion, to minimize dissection:

    a. True

    b. False

441. Which of the following statements are true concerning the lasing train:

    a. In general the lasing train should last for 2-5 seconds and the laser catheter should be advanced approximately 1 mm per second

    b. For long lesions, the lasing train should be increased to 15-30 seconds and advancement should be at 2 mm per second

    c. The first lasing train should be performed with the saline infusion technique, but subsequent trains do not require repeats saline infusion

    d. Repeated contrast injections should be performed immediately prior to each lasing train

    e. If the operator decides to change the energy level, the laser catheter must first be completely removed from the patient to adjust the energy settings

442. The saline infusion technique should be utilized for all laser procedures to minimize acoustic injury and dissection:

a. True
b. False

443. True bifurcation lesions should be treated with devices other than the excimer laser, since the presence of the bifurcation lesion is an important predictor of complications:

a. True
b. False

444. Which of the following are true concerning the use of excimer laser angioplasty for calcified lesions:

a. Mild lesion calcification is amenable to excimer laser angioplasty using short laser trains and high energy densities
b. Heavily calcified lesions are not readily amenable to excimer laser angioplasty using currently recommended energy densities
c. Excimer laser angioplasty and Rotablator atherectomy are equally effective techniques for heavily calcified lesions

445. Which of the following statements are true concerning the use of excimer laser angioplasty for highly eccentric lesions:

a. The eccentric laser catheter may be better suited for highly eccentric lesions than the concentric laser catheters, to maximize efficiency of laser ablation and minimize vessel injury
b. In general, the maximum laser fiber diameter should be < 70% of the normal reference vessel diameter
c. Laser trains of 3-5 seconds at energy densities of 50 mJ/mm are recommended
d. Most eccentric lesions are readily treated by stand alone excimer laser angioplasty without the need for adjunctive PTCA or other devices

446. Focal lesions < 10 mm in length are readily treated by excimer laser angioplasty, which has been shown to have a safety and restenosis advantage compared to conventional PTCA:

a. True
b. False

447. Which of the following statements are true concerning excimer laser angioplasty of lesions > 10 mm in length:

    a. The maximum recommended laser fiber diameter should not exceed 70% of the normal reference vessel diameter
    b. Laser trains should be continued for 15-30 seconds to permit complete ablation of the entire length of the lesion
    c. The laser trains should be decreased to < 3 seconds when the laser fiber nears the end of the lesion, to minimize injury to the normal vessel segment
    d. Excimer laser angioplasty of long lesions is associated with fewer complications and lower restenosis rates compared to conventional balloon angioplasty

448. Which of the following statements are true concerning excimer laser angioplasty of aorto-ostial lesions:

    a. Power guiding catheters are required to ensure adequate laser ablation
    b. Excimer laser angioplasty is contraindicated in ostial saphenous vein graft lesions
    c. A fluence of 60 mJ/mm may be necessary for calcified ostial lesions
    d. The saline infusion technique cannot be applied to ostial lesions

449. Ostial lesions located in an acute bend at the origin of a sidebranch are particularly well-suited for excimer laser angioplasty compared to other devices:

    a. True
    b. False

450. Excimer laser angioplasty may be used in nondegenerated saphenous vein grafts but is absolutely contraindicated in the presence of degenerated vein grafts:

    a. True
    b. False

451. When subintimal passage of a guidewire occurs during recanalization of a chronic total occlusion, excimer laser angioplasty is recommended to create a small pilot channel prior to more definitive revascularization with other devices:

    a. True
    b. False

CORONARY INTRAVASCULAR ULTRASOUND

452. Which of the following statements are true concerning currently available intravascular ultrasound equipment:

 a. IVUS catheters range in size from 2.9-3.5F and are compatible with 8F guiding catheters
 b. High operating frequency (20-30 MHz) and close proximity of the transducer to the target result in excellent image quality
 c. Ultrasound images are transferred from the catheter tip by fiberoptic cables and are displayed on the video monitor
 d. All intravascular ultrasound systems generate 3 dimensional ultrasound images

453. Which of the following statements are true concerning mechanical types of ultrasound transducers:

 a. An external motor and drive shaft rotate a single transducer at the catheter tip
 b. Most produce images at 30 frames/second
 c. Typical operating frequencies are approximately 30 MHz
 d. Image quality is generally superior to synthetic phased array transducers

454. Advantages of synthetic phased array transducers compared to mechanical transducers include:

 a. Excellent flexibility
 b. Absence of rotational artifacts
 c. An annular array of 32-64 elements near the tip of the catheter
 d. Excellent potential to be readily coupled to a variety of interventional devices for immediate on-line ultrasound imaging.

455. When imaging a normal coronary artery at 20 MHz, the vessel lumen is usually sonolucent, or at frequencies ≥ 30 MHz blood appears as a finely textured specular echo that moves with blood flow:

 a. True
 b. False

456. Which of the following statements are true concerning normal coronary artery morphology by intravascular ultrasound:

    a. A circular lumen is surrounded by distinct layers exhibiting variable echogenicity

    b. Some normal arteries demonstrate three discrete vessel wall layers, whereas other normal coronary arteries have a mono-layered appearance.

    c   When three layers are identified, the middle layer is usually sonolucent and represents the media

    d. Blood echogenicity is often useful in image interpretation by identifying the path of blood flow

457. All of the following characteristics are advantages of intravascular ultrasound except:

    a. Precise quantitative assessment of lumen diameter and cross sectional area

    b. Accurate measurement of "normal" vessel diameter

    c. Precise delineation of the depth and extent of calcification

    d. Precise evaluation of intraluminal thrombus

    e. Greater sensitivity than angiography in evaluating the severity of dissection

458. Intravascular ultrasound is more sensitive than contrast angiography in detecting mild atherosclerotic lesions:

    a. True

    b. False

459. Which of the following characterize calcific plaque by ultrasound criteria:

    a. Greater echogenicity than the surrounding adventia

    b. Accentuation of the ultrasound signal beyond the calcified plaque

    c. Acoustic shadowing

    d. Acoustic oscillations that obscure the near field imaging

460. Non-uniform rotational distortion (NURD) arises when the ultrasound beam is not perpendicular to the vessel wall and makes the circular lumen appear elliptical:

    a. True

    b. False

461. Ring down artifact may decrease the ability to image structures immediately adjacent to the transducer, due to acoustic oscillations that obscure the near field imaging:

    a. True
    b. False

462. The evaluation of ultrasound images is most dependent upon differences in acoustic properties of adjacent structures rather than the true histologic composition of those structures:

    a. True
    b. False

463. Which of the following imaging artifacts is associated with ultrasound interrogation of calcified lesions:

    a. NURD
    b. Ring down artifact
    c. Acoustic shadowing
    d. Geometric distortion

464. All of the following are potential limitations of intravascular ultrasound except:

    a. Added cost
    b. Imaging artifacts
    c. Requires imaging in a blood-free field
    d. Unreliable evaluation of thrombus

465. Which of the following statements are true concerning intravascular ultrasound evaluation of intracoronary thrombus:

    a. A sonolucent lesion is virtually diagnostic of intracoronary thrombus
    b. Identification of thrombus by IVUS is less reliable than angioscopy
    c. Intravascular ultrasound imaging is a reliable technique for dissolution of thrombus
    d. The absence of a sonolucent lesion by IVUS effectively rules out intracoronary thrombus

Questions

466. Which of the following statements are true concerning the safety of intravascular ultrasound:

a. Serious complications are unusual
b. Transient coronary spasm generally responds to intracoronary nitroglycerin
c. The imaging transducer may obstruct coronary blood flow and cause ischemia
d. It is not necessary to administer intravenous heparin when intravascular ultrasound is planned

467. Which of the following statements are true concerning intravascular ultrasound imaging:

a. Arteries which are angiographically normal are virtually always normal by intravascular ultrasound
b. IVUS may be useful for assessment of lesions of borderline severity by angiographic criteria
c. Allograft vasculopathy is readily identified by IVUS
d. IVUS is the imaging method of choice for quantitating the severity of left main stenoses

468. All of the following are important interventional applications of IVUS except:

a. Characterization of plaque composition for device selection
b. Understanding the mechanisms of lumen enlargement of various devices
c. Help guide "optimal" stenting or atherectomy
d. Reliable identification of thrombus, particularly in saphenous vein grafts
e. Precise vessel sizing during stent implantation

469. Which of the following statements are true concerning IVUS guided stenting or atherectomy:

a. IVUS guidance facilitates greater lumen enlargement
b. IVUS has been shown to decrease the incidence of in-hospital major ischemic complications
c. IVUS has been shown to decrease the incidence of restenosis and late target vessel revascularization
d. Although early equipment costs are increased, IVUS has been shown to be cost effective because of its other beneficial effects

470. Which of the following statements are true concerning the mechanisms of lumen enlargement using ultrasound criteria:

a. Lumen enlargement by plaque compression is an important mechanism of PTCA

    b.   About 50% of the lumen enlargement after directional atherectomy is due to tissue removal

    c.   Plaque ablation is an important mechanism of lumen enlargement for Rotablator

    d.   Dissection is an important mechanism of lumen enlargement after PTCA

471. Which of the following statements are true concerning quantitative measurements of vessel dimensions by IVUS:

    a.   Precise quantitation of vascular dimensions is possible with IVUS

    b.   Computerized quantitative angiography and IVUS after PTCA show a strong correlation for measurement of final lumen diameter

    c.   Occult atherosclerosis by angiographic criteria is readily identified by intravascular ultrasound

    d.   Precise quantitative measurements achieved by IVUS have led to improved safety and reduction in complications

472. Optimal atherectomy studies have confirmed that intravascular ultrasound guidance results in better lumen enlargement and fewer complications compared to angiographic guidance alone:

    a.   True

    b.   False

473. Which of the following statements are true concerning optimal stent deployment:

    a.   Stents which appear to be perfectly deployed by angiographic criteria are often suboptimally deployed by IVUS criteria

    b.   When optimal stenting is confirmed by ultrasound criteria, warfarin may be safely omitted from the anticoagulation regimen

    c.   Antiplatelet therapy alone without warfarin should not be prescribed for stent patients unless optimal stenting has been confirmed by IVUS

    d.   Randomized trials have confirmed the benefit of IVUS in reducing late clinical events in stent patients.

474. This IVUS image (next page) after stent deployment shows:

    a.   Optimal stent deployment

    b.   Suboptimal stent deployment due to plaque protrusion

    c.   Suboptimal stent deployment due to poor stent apposition

    d.   Suboptimal stent deployment requiring additional stenting

e. Suboptimal stent deployment requiring high-pressure adjunctive PTCA

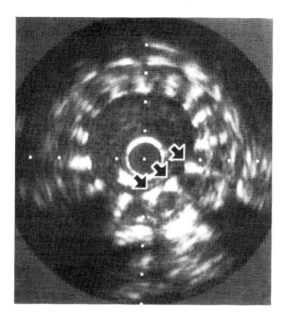

475. Which of the following is least likely to cause ischemia:

a. Angioscopy
b. Intravascular ultrasound
c. Doppler flow wire
d. Ultrasound guided atherectomy

476. Intravascular ultrasound is an excellent device for studying microvascular disease and "Syndrome X:"

a. True
b. False

477. Which of the following are readily studied by intravascular ultrasound:

a. Coronary blood flow
b. Diffuse atherosclerosis
c. Suboptimal angiographic results after intervention
d. Dissection
e. Borderline lesions

478. Match the following IVUS imagess with these IVUS findings:

    a. Non-uniform rotational distortion (NURD)
    b. Calcified atheroma with acoustic shadowing
    c. Soft sonolucent atheroma
    d. Normal coronary artery
    e. Lumen irergularity after PTCA
    f. Underestimation of atherosclerosis by angiography

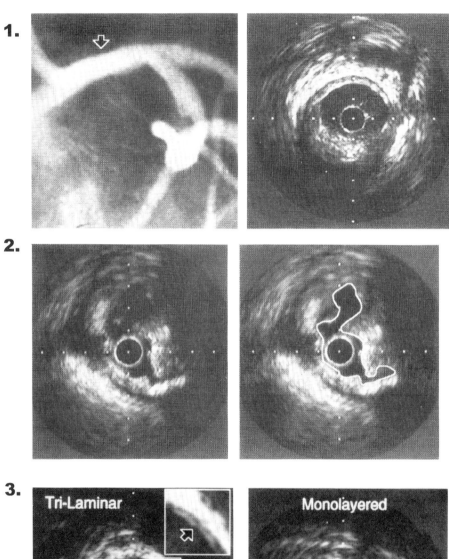

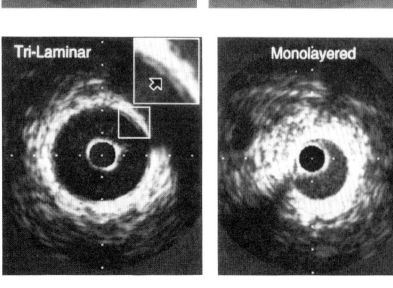

4.

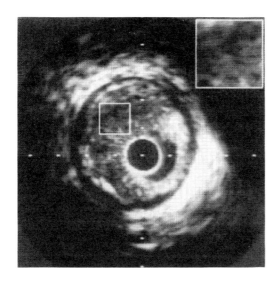

5.

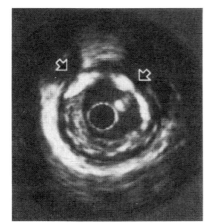 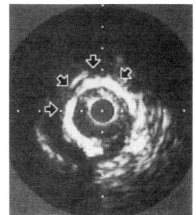

6.

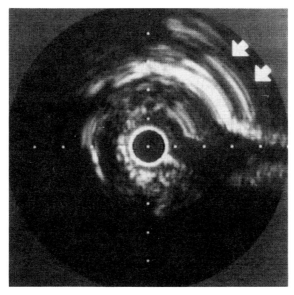

479. Intravascular ultrasound catheters are intended for ultrasound examination of native coronary arteries, but should not be used in saphenous vein bypass grafts because of the risk of no-reflow:

a. True
b. False

480. Which of the following are potential complications of intravascular ultrasound:

a. Dissection
b. Abrupt closure
c. Death
d. Ventricular fibrillation
e. Air embolism

PERIPHERAL VASCULAR DISEASE

481. Peripheral vascular obstruction is commonly described in three discrete anatomic zones, including the inflow tract, the outflow tract, and the runoff bed:

a. True
b. False

482. The abdominal aorta and common and external iliac arteries make up the outflow tract to the lower extremities:

a. True
b. False

483. Which of the following statement are true concerning peripheral vascular atherosclerosis:

a. The most common site of atherosclerosis is above the renal arteries
b. The most severe atherosclerotic lesions are typically located at the aortic bifurcation and involve the origin of the common iliac arteries and the iliac artery bifurcation
c. Aorto-iliac disease never causes calf claudication

d. The presence of good femoral artery pulses excludes the possibility of significant vascular obstruction in the distal aorta and the iliac arteries

484. When considering peripheral vascular obstruction, the outflow tract consists of the anterior tibial artery, posterior tibial artery, and peroneal artery:

a. True
b. False

485. Which of the following statements are true concerning peripheral vascular obstruction between the inguinal ligament and the knee:

a. The common femoral artery is frequently involved with severe atherosclerosis
b. The mid portion of the popliteal artery is often spared significant atherosclerosis
c. The superficial femoral artery is rarely diffusely diseased
d. The most critical lesions in the superficial femoral artery generally occur near the adductor hiatus

486. The runoff bed for the peripheral circulation to the lower extremity consists of the anterior tibial artery, posterior tibial artery, and peroneal artery:

a. True
b. False

487. The proximal segments of the trifurcation vessel system to the lower extremity are frequent sites of atherosclerotic obstruction which limit runoff to the foot:

a. True
b. False

488. Which of the following statements are true concerning peripheral vascular disease in patients with diabetes:

a. Diabetic patients comprise a unique patient population with respect to peripheral vascular disease

b. Approximately ⅓ of diabetics with peripheral vascular disease have severe atherosclerosis limited to the runoff bed

c. Approximately ⅓ of diabetic patients have atherosclerotic disease limited to the inflow and outflow tract vessels

d. Approximately ⅓ of diabetic patients have multiple segmental disease involving the aorta, iliac, and femoral arteries, and trifurcation vessel system

489. Isolated trifurcation vessel disease in diabetic patients is often not amenable to surgical revascularization, but percutaneous intervention using coronary angioplasty balloon catheters may be feasible:

a. True
b. False

490. In evaluating patients with peripheral vascular disease, the clinical history is useful to determine the likelihood of ischemia and the degree of functional impairment, but the quality of pulses is most useful for estimating disease severity:

a. True
b. False

491. Which of the following statements are true concerning the ankle brachial index (ABI):

a. The ankle brachial index is defined as the ratio of systolic pressure in the ankle to the upper arm, and provides objective data about lower extremity circulation

b. The brachial systolic pressure should be measured in both arms, but the lower value should be used to calculate the ABI for both lower extremities

c. When measuring the ankle pressure, the blood pressure cuff should be inflated above systolic pressure to temporarily occlude blood flow, and the pressure at which a Doppler flow signal is heard is then recorded as the ankle systolic pressure

d. Specialized blood pressure cuffs are required to accurately measure the ankle systolic pressure

492. Which of the following statements are true concerning the application of duplex ultrasound to patients with peripheral vascular disease:

a. Direct real-time ultrasound imaging of obstructive lesions is feasible

b. Doppler assessment of the hemodynamics significance of vascular stenoses is an important application of duplex ultrasound

c. Duplex ultrasound can be readily applied to superficial vessels such as the carotid arteries and the iliac and femoral arteries, but is unreliable for evaluation of renal and visceral arterial circulation

d. Doppler flow signals can be subjectively graded but stenosis severity is poorly estimated using Doppler velocity spectra

493. The North American Symptomatic Carotid Endarterectomy Trial (NASCET) and Asymptomatic Carotid Artery Stenosis Trial (ACAS) demonstrated benefit for carotid endarterectomy in all patients with asymptomatic carotid bruits:

a. True
b. False

494. Duplex ultrasound criteria for significant carotid artery stenosis suggest that the most sensitive criterion is the absolute peak velocity at end-diastole at the site of stenosis:

a. True
b. False

495. Match the ankle-brachial index (ABI) and severity of stenosis for peripheral vascular disease:

a. ABI > 1.3, indeterminate symptoms
b. ABI 0.9-1.25, asymptomatic
c. ABI 0.6-0.9, claudication
d. ABI 0.3-0.6, claudication
e. ABI 0.15-0.3, rest pain
f. ABI < 0.15, impending tissue loss

1. Multiple segment total occlusion, poor distal runoff
2. Multiple segment total occlusion, good distal runoff
3. Multiple segment disease
4. Single segment stenosis or well-collateralized occlusion
5. No hemodynamically significant lesion
6. Medial wall calcification, nondiagnostic

496. Which of the following statements are true concerning a normal Doppler flow pattern for circulation to the lower extremity:

    a. A normal flow pattern suggests that no significant obstruction is present
    b. A multiphasic flow signal with a brisk, well-defined high pitched systolic peak characterizes a normal flow pattern
    c. Signals during diastole are lower pitched then signals during systole
    d. There may be transient reversal of flow during early diastole

497. Which of the following statements are true concerning a damped Doppler flow signal in the lower extremity:

    a. A damped signal suggests good proximal circulation with poor distal runoff
    b. A damped signal is characterized by a slow systolic upstroke with a poorly defined systolic peak
    c. A slowly diminishing flow pattern from systole through diastole is consistent with significant proximal obstruction
    d. A damped signal is characterized by antegrade flow during the entire cardiac cycle

498. Assuming that the Doppler flow signal is properly recorded, the absence of a flow signal suggests total vessel occlusion and poor collateral reconstitution:

    a. True
    b. False

499. Doppler velocity spectra are unreliable for grading the severity of carotid artery stenosis:

    a. True
    b. False

500. Even in experienced hands, Doppler analysis of the renal and mesenteric vessels is extremely unreliable:

    a. True
    b. False

501. Which of the following statements are true concerning Doppler flow analysis of the aorta:

    a. The Doppler flow signal from the aorta just above the renal artery is used as a reference signal to estimate the renal/aortic ratio
    b. Although relative velocities are used to estimate the significance of renal artery stenosis, absolute velocities are generally used in the celiac trunk and superior mesenteric artery
    c. The best interpretation of Doppler flow signals from the mesenteric circulation is achieved when the patient has been fasting for at least 8 hours prior to abdominal examination

502. In the normal mesenteric circulation, the end-diastolic velocity in the superior mesenteric artery should dramatically fall within 30 minutes of a caloric challenge:

    a. True
    b. False

503. Which of the following statements are true concerning detection of a subclavian artery stenosis:

    a. A systolic pressure difference > 5 mm Hg between the two arms suggests a significant subclavian artery stenosis
    b. Reversal of blood flow in the ipsilateral vertebral artery is highly suggestive of significant subclavian artery stenosis
    c. Identification of post-stenotic turbulence in the subclavian artery suggests the presence of a total occlusion
    d. A damped waveform by duplex ultrasound suggests a critical subclavian artery stenosis

504. Because of the large caliber of peripheral vessels, the use of aspirin prior to percutaneous intervention is optional:

    a. True
    b. False

505. Sublingual nifedipine and intra-arterial nitroglycerin are often recommended when treating lesions in the renal artery or below the knee, to minimize arterial spasm:

    a. True
    b. False

506. Duplex ultrasound criteria have been established for estimating stenosis severity in the carotid artery, but not in the renal and mesenteric circulation:

    a. True
    b. False

507. Which of the following represent absolute contraindications to percutaneous revascularization of the abdominal aorta:

    a. Total occlusion of the abdominal aorta
    b. Focal stenosis of the abdominal aorta associated with a 4.8 cm abdominal aortic aneurysm
    c. Focal stenosis of the infrarenal aorta without other aortic disease
    d. Purple toe syndrome resulting from spontaneous embolization from a large abdominal aortic aneurysm

508. Which of the following represent reasonable indications for peripheral vascular intervention on the iliac arteries:

    a. Persistent claudication despite smoking sensation and regular exercise
    b. To improve inflow to the lower extremity prior to fempop bypass surgery
    c. The presence of a focal stenosis at the distal anastomosis of a bypass graft
    d. To improve the level of amputation in a diabetic foot

509. A reasonable indication for percutaneous revascularization of renal artery stenosis includes deterioration of renal function, asymmetric decrease in renal size, and documented renal artery stenosis > 50%:

    a. True
    b. False

510. Patients with chronic mesenteric ischemia generally have significant stenoses or occlusion of at least 2 mesenteric vessels:

    a. True
    b. False

511. Which of the following statements are true concerning arterial access prior to percutaneous revascularization:

    a.   Arterial access should always be achieved from the contralateral common femoral artery
    b.   Single wall puncture techniques are generally recommended for antegrade femoral techniques and axillary and brachial techniques, to minimize bleeding from the posterior arterial wall
    c.   A micropuncture set may allow arterial catheterization with less arterial spasm
    d.   Placement of arterial sheaths facilitates exchange of catheters and guidewires and minimizes bleeding

512. Catheterization of the contralateral femoral artery often provides better angle of approach for reaching lesions in the distal external iliac and common femoral artery:

    a.   True
    b.   False

513. The antegrade femoral artery approach is often recommended for lesions in the ipsilateral superficial femoral, deep femoral, or popliteal arteries:

    a.   True
    b.   False

514. Retrograde puncture of the common femoral artery should be accomplished so the needle enters the common femoral artery inferior to the inguinal ligament:

    a.   True
    b.   False

515. Antegrade puncture of the common femoral artery should be performed so that the needle enters the common femoral artery superior to the inguinal ligament:

    a.   True
    b.   False

516. The left axillary artery approach may be useful when there is sharp angulation of a target lesion at the origin of the right renal artery:

    a. True
    b. False

517. Conventional angiography of the peripheral circulation relies on frontal projections; oblique views are rarely indicated and should not be done to avoid extra contrast load:

    a. True
    b. False

518. Which of the following statements are true concerning renal artery angioplasty:

    a. Short-acting antihypertensive medications should be substituted for long-acting drugs
    b. Vascular surgery back-up is usually recommended
    c. Guiding catheters help facilitate angioplasty and stent placement, if necessary
    d. High-pressure balloons are rarely necessary, even when stents are implanted
    e. Blood pressure and renal function should be closely monitored following the procedure

519. Which of the following statements are true concerning renal artery angioplasty:

    a. Inability to cross the target lesion or elastic recoil are common causes of angioplasty failure
    b. The results of renal angioplasty are independent of lesion location and underlying pathology
    c. Angioplasty success for ostial renal artery stenosis exceeds 90%
    d. Long-term patency for ostial renal artery stenosis is better than for non-ostial renal artery stenosis

520. Virtually all patients with renovascular hypertension are cured after successful renal artery angioplasty, regardless of etiology:

    a. True
    b. False

Questions

521. Which of the following statements are true concerning angioplasty of the aorta and iliac arteries:

    a.   Success rates in the aorta are higher than in the common iliac artery
    b.   Long-term patency rates are higher in the common iliac artery than in the aorta

522. Which of the following statements are true concerning angioplasty of the external iliac and common femoral arteries:

    a.   Overall results of angioplasty are best in the external iliac and common femoral arteries
    b.   Procedural success is achieved in over 90% of external iliac and femoral arteries
    c.   Three-year patency exceeds 75%
    d.   Long total occlusions are readily treated by angioplasty and results are similar to angioplasty for nontotal occlusions

523. Which of the following statements are true concerning angioplasty of the superficial femoral and popliteal arteries:

    a.   Early and late results of angioplasty are not as good as those in the aorta and iliac arteries
    b.   Initial success is achieved in 85% of patients and 3-year patency is approximately 60%
    c.   The best results are obtained in focal stenoses or total occlusions < 3 cm in length
    d.   Long-term patency is better when angioplasty is performed for claudication compared to limb salvage

524. Which of the following statements are true concerning the use of angioplasty in the circulation below the knee:

    a.   Angioplasty below the knee is absolutely contraindicated
    b.   The availability of coronary angioplasty balloons and guidewires may improve success rates
    c.   In selected cases, angioplasty may be a useful adjunct for limb salvage

525. Which of the following statements are true concerning the use of stents in the iliac arteries:

    a.   Suboptimal results after angioplasty may be treated by stenting
    b.   The only approved stent in the iliac arteries is the Palmaz stent
    c.   The Schneider Wallstent is available in Europe, but is not available in the United States for iliac artery revascularization

526. Which of the following represent reasonable indications for stenting:

    a. Atherosclerotic ostial renal artery stenosis
    b. Residual pressure gradient or significant stenosis in the iliac artery after angioplasty
    c. Severe dissection after angioplasty in the iliac artery
    d. Suboptimal angioplasty result after revascularization of the common iliac artery

527. Which of the following represent contraindications to stenting:

    a. Arterial rupture with contrast extravation
    b. Diffuse intrarenal vascular disease
    c. Coexisting aneurysms in the target lesion, requiring surgical revascularization
    d. Inability to achieve full balloon expansion prior to stent deployment

528. Which of the following statements are true concerning the use of stents for peripheral vascular disease:

    a. Procedural success rates are highest in the iliac and renal arteries
    b. Subclavian and carotid artery stenoses are absolute contraindications to stenting
    c. In the iliac arteries, 5-year patency after stenting is superior to angioplasty
    d. Potential complications of stenting include renal failure, hematoma, and false aneurysm formation

529. Urokinase is currently the most widely used agent for intra-arterial thrombolysis because of shorter infusion time, fewer complications, and lower cost:

    a. True
    b. False

530. With few exceptions, the application of atherectomy to patients with iliac stenosis is likely to replace the use of conventional angioplasty, due to several randomized trials which demonstrate superior immediate and long-term results after atherectomy:

    a. True
    b. False

531. The immediate and long-term results of laser angioplasty are inferior to those for conventional angioplasty:

    a. True
    b. False

BALLOON VALVULOPLASTY

532. Which of the following statements are true concerning the mechanisms of balloon and surgical mitral commissurotomy:

    a. The mechanisms of closed surgical commissurotomy and percutaneous balloon mitral valvuloplasty are similar
    b. Separation of fused commissures can be achieved with open and closed surgical techniques, but not by balloon valvuloplasty
    c. Balloon valvuloplasty may improve subvalvular thickening and chordal involvement, whereas closed commissurotomy will not
    d. Opened surgical commissurotomy is performed under direct vision, but does not require circulatory arrest or cardiopulmonary bypass

533. In patients with mitral stenosis who are considered for balloon valvuloplasty, identification of left atrial thrombus is not necessarily a contraindication to valvuloplasty if resolution of thrombus can be documented by transesophageal echocardiography:

    a. True
    b. False

534. Which of the following characteristics are used to calculate the mitral valve echo score:

    a. Leaflet mobility
    b. Leaflet thickening
    c. Extent of subvalvular disease
    d. Calcification
    e. Severity of mitral regurgitation

535. The antegrade transvenous approach may be used for balloon mitral valvuloplasty, but the retrograde transarterial approach should never be used:

   a. True
   b. False

536. Which of the following statements are true concerning the technique of transseptal left heart catheterization:

   a. A modified Mullins sheath and dilator are commonly employed to advance the Brockenbrough needle
   b. The correct orientation of the Brockenbrough needle is at 5:00 o'clock; this position should never be altered
   c. AP, shallow RAO, and LAO projections may be useful to confirm proper orientation of the needle prior to transseptal puncture
   d. Perforation leading to cardiac tamponade has been reported in approximately 1% of patients during transseptal catheterization

537. After successful balloon mitral valvuloplasty, a typical hemodynamic response is a 50-70% decrease in transmitral gradient and a 50-100% increase in mitral valve area:

   a. True
   b. False

538. In patients with mitral stenosis, valve areas after valvuloplasty with a single balloon are generally smaller than after a double-balloon:

   a. True
   b. False

539. In patients who have recurrent mitral stenosis after prior surgical commissurotomy, balloon mitral valvuloplasty is not recommended because of excessive valvular scarring:

   a. True
   b. False

Questions

540. Which of the following are recognized complications of balloon mitral valvuloplasty:

    a. Death
    b. Stroke
    c. Mitral regurgitation
    d. Cardiac tamponade
    e. Significant left-to-right shunt

541. After successful balloon mitral valvuloplasty, hemodynamic and clinical improvement persist, and restenosis occurs in < 5% of patients within 5-years:

    a. True
    b. False

542. In virtually all studies of balloon mitral valvuloplasty, the echo score is the most important predictor of immediate and long-term outcome:

    a. True
    b. False

543. Important predictors of successful balloon mitral valvuloplasty include:

    a. Age
    b. Rhythm
    c. Echo score
    d. Mitral valve calcification
    e. Balloon size

544. In randomized trials comparing balloon mitral valvuloplasty and surgical commissurotomy, long-term results were better after surgery:

    a. True
    b. False

545. In adults, the most common cause of aortic stenosis is calcification of a rheumatic valve:

    a. True
    b. False

546. In adults with critical aortic stenosis, balloon aortic valvuloplasty has become a viable alternative to aortic valve replacement:

    a. True
    b. False

547. Which of the following statements are true concerning aortic valve replacement (AVR) for isolated aortic stenosis:

    a. Aortic valve replacement is the standard treatment for most adults
    b. Surgery is generally followed by marked hemodynamic improvement and regression of left ventricular hypertrophy, but no improvement in left ventricular performance or survival
    c. Emergency aortic valve replacement may be associated with peri-operative mortality rates as high as 40%
    d. Age > 75 years is considered a relative contraindication to aortic valve replacement

548. Mechanisms of balloon aortic valvuloplasty include fracture of calcified nodules, separation of fused commissures, and stretching of valve leaflets:

    a. True
    b. False

549. Most adults with symptomatic aortic stenosis should undergo echocardiography, right and left heart catheterization, coronary angiography, and aortography:

    a. True
    b. False

550. The retrograde arterial approach is the standard approach to balloon aortic valvuloplasty; the antegrade transvenous approach should never be utilized:

a. True
b. False

551. The retrograde arterial approach to balloon aortic valvuloplasty may be accomplished via the femoral or brachial route:

a. True
b. False

552. The antegrade approach to balloon aortic valvuloplasty does not require transseptal left heart catheterization:

a. True
b. False

553. Balloon aortic valvuloplasty using a double-balloon technique is preferred over the single balloon technique:

a. True
b. False

554. After successful aortic balloon valvuloplasty, most patients have trivial residual aortic stenosis:

a. True
b. False

555. Which of the following major complications may occur after balloon aortic valvuloplasty:

a. Death
b. Stroke
c. Cardiac perforation
d. Aortic insufficiency

e. Hemorrhage

556. After balloon aortic valvuloplasty, procedure-related mortality is more common in acutely decompensated patients with severe LV dysfunction:

a. True
b. False

557. Sudden hemodynamic collapse after aortic valvuloplasty may be due to cardiac tamponade or disruption of the aortic valve:

a. True
b. False

558. Although successful balloon aortic valvuloplasty is associated with significant residual aortic stenosis, follow-up over 1-3 years is associated with a low incidence of cardiac events:

a. True
b. False

559. Which of the following factors may contribute to an adverse long-term result after balloon aortic valvuloplasty:

a. Persistent severe aortic stenosis
b. Restenosis
c. Severe coronary artery disease
d. Noncardiac comorbid diseases

560. The most important determinant of event-free survival after successful aortic valvuloplasty is improvement in aortic valve area:

a. True
b. False

561. Octogenarians with symptomatic aortic stenosis are equally-well treated by balloon aortic valvuloplasty and aortic valve replacement:

    a. True
    b. False

562. Octogenarians with symptomatic aortic stenosis should not be denied the opportunity for balloon aortic valvuloplasty, since aortic valve replacement in this patient population is associated with prohibitive risk:

    a. True
    b. False

563. Which of the following conditions may represent reasonable indications for balloon aortic valvuloplasty prior to consideration of aortic valve replacement:

    a. Critical aortic stenosis and ejection fraction < 15%
    b. Critical aortic stenosis with a transvalvular gradient of 25 mm Hg and a cardiac output of 2.1 liters per minute
    c. Critical aortic stenosis and cardiogenic shock
    d. Critical aortic stenosis and 3-vessel coronary artery disease

564. Available data suggest that routine balloon aortic valvuloplasty is recommended in all patients with asymptomatic aortic stenosis who require noncardiac surgery:

    a. True
    b. False

565. A 60-year-old cardiologist has unstable angina. Coronary angiography demonstrates a mildly calcified tubular stenosis in the mid-LAD (reference vessel = 3.0 mm). Your partner performs conventional PTCA and states that despite inflation pressures of 10 ATM, there is a persistent waist in the PET balloon ("dog-boning").

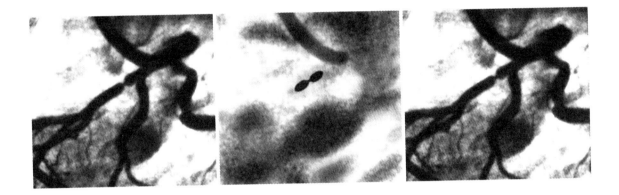

What are reasonable approaches to this lesion at this time:

a. Immediate stent implantation
b. Rotablator atherectomy
c. Cutting balloon angioplasty
d. Force focused angioplasty

566. A saphenous vein graft to the LAD is treated with a 4.5 mm high-pressure balloon (reference vessel = 4.5 mm). Despite inflation pressures up to 16 ATM, the waist in the balloon persists and the lesion is unchanged. All other grafts and left ventricular function are normal.

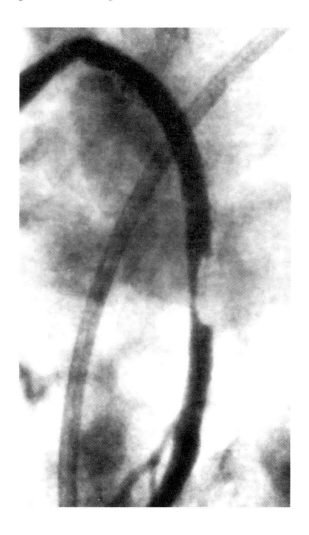

What are reasonable approaches to this lesion now:

a. Immediate stent implantation
b. Redo coronary artery bypass surgery
c. Directional atherectomy
d. Rotablator atherectomy

567. An eccentric lesion in the distal RCA is treated with a 3.5 x 20 mm balloon (reference vessel = 3.5 mm). Despite full balloon expansion at low pressure, the lesion is unchanged. Other vessels and left ventricular function are normal.

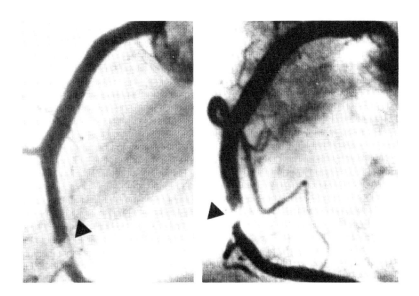

How would you approach this patient at this time:

a. Directional atherectomy
b. Immediate stenting
c. TEC atherectomy
d. Rotablator atherectomy
e. Perfusion balloon angioplasty

568. PTCA of the LAD with a 3.25 x 20 mm balloon is unsuccessful because of "watermelon seeding." There is no apparent lesion calcification by fluoroscopy (reference vessel diameter = 3.2 mm). Other coronary arteries and left ventricular function are normal.

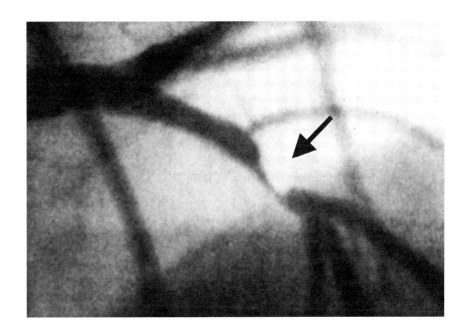

If watermelon seeding persists, how would you approach this lesion now:

a. Prolonged inflation with a 15 mm long balloon
b. Prolonged inflation with a 30-40 mm long balloon
c. Rotablator atherectomy
d. Directional atherectomy
e. Stenting

569. PTCA is performed using a 3.25 mm balloon (reference diameter = 3.1 mm), leaving a residual stenosis of 40% without dissection, thrombus, or impaired flow. Other vessels and left ventricular function are normal. The patient is pain-free.

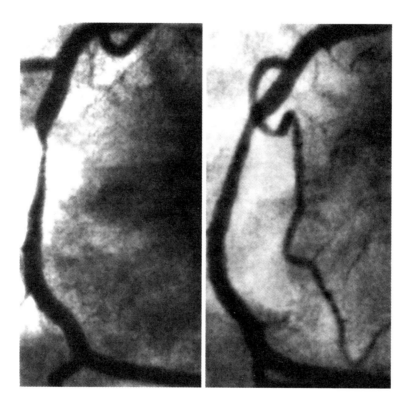

Reasonable approaches to this lesion at this time include:

a. Terminate the procedure and follow the patient clinically
b. Perform a prolonged balloon inflation with a perfusion balloon
c. Use a 3.75 mm balloon at 15 ATM
d. Implant a stent
e. Re-evaluate the lesion with a Doppler wire guidewire

570. Directional atherectomy is performed on this focal vein graft lesion with a 7F AtheroCath (reference diameter = 4.0 mm). After 16 cuts, there is a mild residual stenosis.

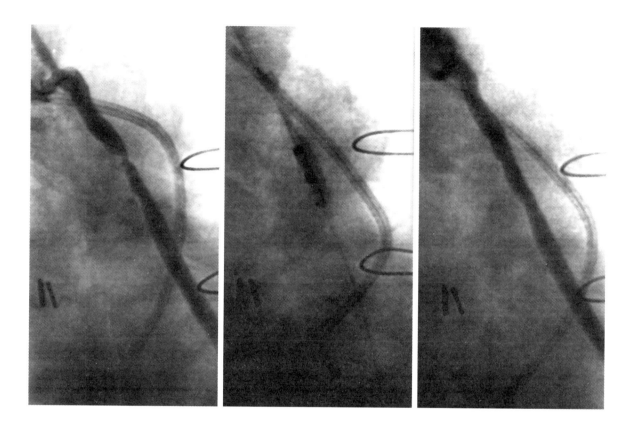

If your goal is to achieve "optimal atherectomy", what would be your next course of action:

a. Perform additional atherectomy at higher pressure
b. Increase the size of the AtheroCath
c. Perform PTCA with a balloon/artery ratio of 1.1
d. Implant a stent
e. Do nothing

571. A 58-year-old man with progressive angina and a severe stenosis in the RCA (left panel, reference diameter = 3.5 mm) is treated by PTCA with a 3.25 mm balloon. Following PTCA, there is a moderate residual stenosis with intraluminal haziness in the orthogonal view (right panel). The patient is pain-free and has no ECG changes. Other vessels and left ventricular function are normal.

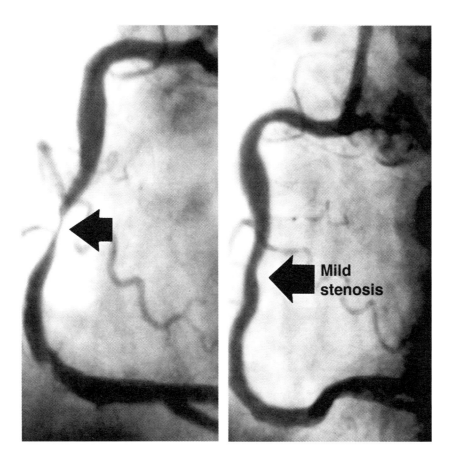

Appropriate recommendations at this point, might include:

a. Confirm that the ACT is ≥ 300 seconds

b. Administer intracoronary lytic therapy

c. Optimize balloon inflations with a balloon/artery ratio ~ 1.0

d. Evaluate the lesion with IVUS or angioscopy

e. Implant a stent

572. A tubular lesion in a vein graft (reference diameter = 4.8 mm) is treated with a 4.5 mm balloon, leaving a moderate residual stenosis with considerable intraluminal filling defects and normal antegrade flow. The patient has mild chest pain and no ECG changes.

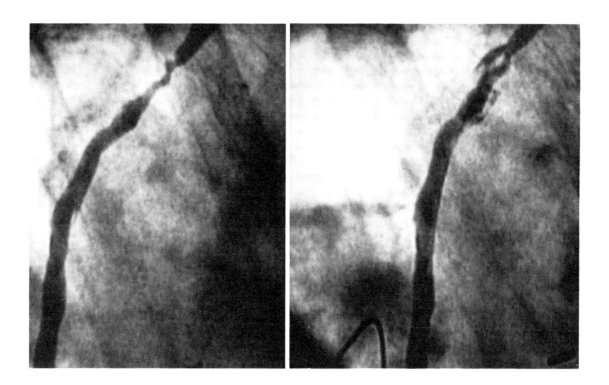

Which of the following statements are true:

a. The angiographic appearance shows definite thrombus
b. ReoPro alone is clearly indicated
c. Implant a stent
d. Intracoronary Urokinase is essential

573. A 58-year-old man undergoes conventional PTCA of a focal stenosis in the proximal LCX, resulting in a non-flow-limitation dissection with an extraluminal "cap".

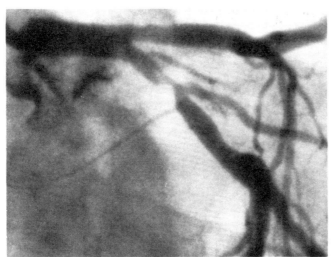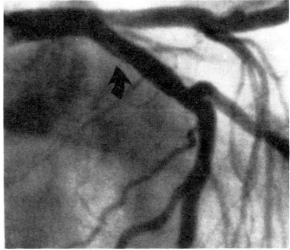

All of the following approaches would be reasonable at this point except:

a. Observe the patient in the Cath Lab for an additional 15 minutes and repeat the angiogram to be certain the result is stable
b. Measure a translesional pressure gradient
c. Perform intravascular ultrasound
d. Measure coronary flow reserve with the Doppler flowire
e. Implant a stent
f. Resect the dissection flap with directional atherectomy

574. A 58-year-old man undergoes conventional PTCA of the proximal LCX (reference vessel = 3.5 mm) for acute myocardial infarction, resulting in restoration of TIMI-3 flow. There is a moderate residual stenosis with a focal "cap" and dye stain (arrow). The patient is asymptomatic and other vessels are normal.

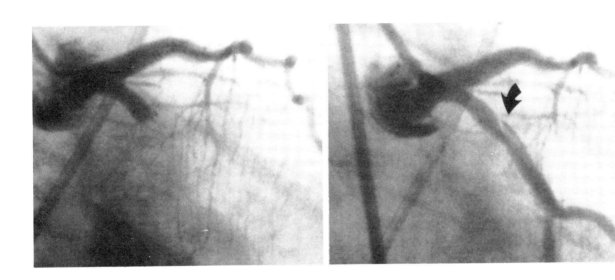

Which of the following statements about this case are true:

a. The risk of recurrent ischemia before discharge is at least 10-15%
b. Assessment of coronary flow reserve with the Doppler flowire is reasonable
c. Stenting is contraindicated because of acute myocardial infarction
d. If stents are implanted, antiplatelet therapy without Coumadin is recommended

575. A 58-year-old man undergoes conventional PTCA of the proximal RCA, which is complicated by a focal dissection and TIMI-2 flow. The patient develops hypotension and bradycardia.

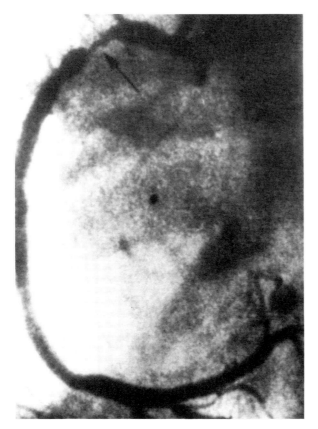 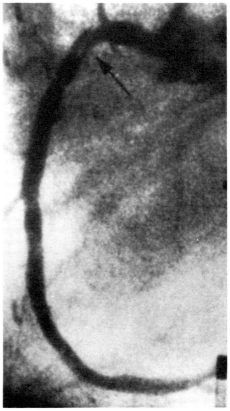

Which of the following statements are true:

a. Directional atherectomy is contraindicated
b. Although stenting is reasonable, a GR-II stent is preferred over a Palmaz-Schatz stent
c. Randomized trials suggest that perfusion balloon angioplasty is equally effective as stenting
d. ReoPro alone is reasonable therapy
e. Intracoronary lytic therapy is of no value in this situation

576. A focal lesion in the mid-RCA (reference = 2.6 mm) is treated by a single 3.0 mm Palmaz-Schatz stent after multiple episodes of restenosis. After stent deployment at 8 ATM there is no residual stenosis. Other vessels and LV function are normal.

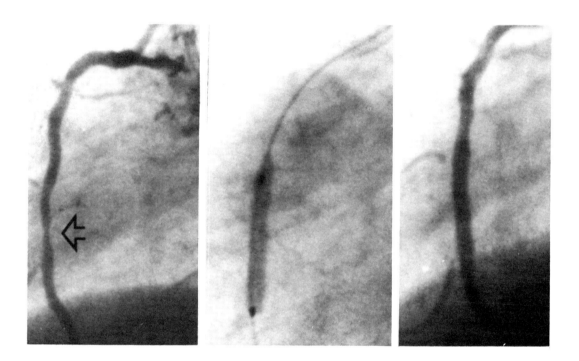

Which of the following is recommended at this time:

a. No further intervention is required and the patient may be discharged within 24 hours
b. Perform IVUS
c. Perform PTCA with a high-pressure balloon at 16 ATM
d. Deploy another stent in the proximal vessel

577. TEC atherectomy is performed on this degenerated saphenous vein graft (reference vessel = 4.2 mm) with a 7.5F cutter, but is complicated by chest pain, ST elevation, and no-reflow (TIMI flow =1).

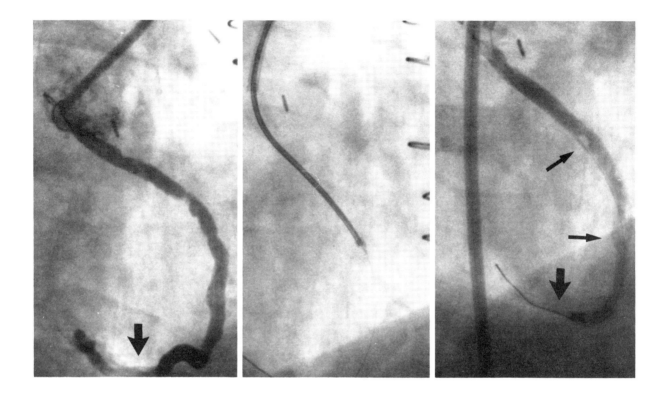

Which of the following statements are true:

a. If normal flow cannot be reestablished, emergency bypass surgery is reasonable
b. Intracoronary calcium antagonists may be useful
c. Intracoronary lytic agents are clearly useful in this situation
d. A long Wallstent is recommended to cover the entire vein graft

578. A 60-year-old woman undergoes atherectomy of the RCA (reference diameter = 2.4 mm), resulting in a jet of free contrast into the pericardium and staining of the right ventricular outflow tract. Other vessels and left ventricular function are normal.

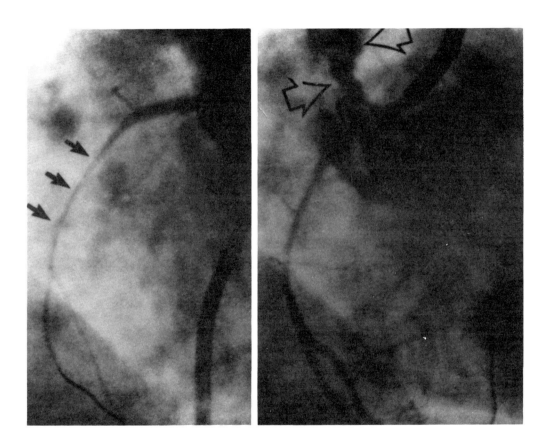

The initial immediate response at this time is:

a. Transfer the patient to the operating room for emergency surgery
b. Perform immediate pericardiocentesis
c. Order an emergency echocardiogram
d. Re-inflate the balloon in the proximal vessel
e. Implant a stent covered with autologous vein

Interventional Cardiology

- Answers -

PTCA EQUIPMENT AND TECHNIQUE

1. Answer: a, d, f, g, h, j, k, l, m

Medical Conditions Requiring Postponement of Elective Intervention

Allergy
- Contrast
- Aspirin

Cardiovascular
- Congestive Heart Failure, decompensated
- Severe Hypertension
- Uncontrolled arrhythmias
- AV block (Type II 2° or 3°)

Pulmonary Disease, decompensated

Diabetes, poorly controlled

Electrolyte abnormalities
- K+ <3.3 or >6.0 mEq/L
- Na+ <125 or > 155 mEq/L

Gastrointestinal
- Acute hepatitis
- Active GI bleeding

Hematologic
- Platelet count <50,000/ul
- Leukocytosis, unexplained
- Hemoglobin <10 gm/dl, acute
- Prothrombin time >16 seconds

Neurologic

- Neurologic deficit, unexplained or progressive
- Cerebral hemorrhage, recent

Renal
- Renal insufficiency, unexplained or progressive

Systemic
- Bacterial infection
- Unexplained Fever

2. Answer: a (true)

References:
1. Schwartz L, Bourassa MG, Lesperance J, et al. Aspirin and Dipyridamole in the prevention of restenosis after percutaneous transluminal coronary angioplasty. N Engl J Med 1988;318:1714-1719.
2. Mufson L, Black A, Roubin G, et al. A randomized trial of aspirin in PTCA: Effect of high vs. low dose aspirin on major complications and restenosis. J Am Coll Cardiol 1988;11:236A.

3. Answer: a, c, e

Over 10% of adults with asthma and 30% of those with asthma and rhinosinusitis develop aspirin sensitivity. Reactions range from exacerbations of nasal congestion, chest tightness, and sneezing to life-threatening bronchospasm and anaphylaxis. Aspirin sensitivity can develop at any time in susceptible individuals; the absence of a prior adverse reaction does not predict continued tolerance. Most aspirin-allergic patients have nasal polyps (>80%), eosinophile and mast cells on nasal smear (>90% and >50%, respectively), and abnormal sinus radiographs (>90%) ranging from mild mucoperiosteal thickening to complete opacification. Scripps Clinic and Research Foundation developed an aspirin desensitization protocol that has proven to be very safe and effective. Desensitization involves the oral administration of progressively larger doses of aspirin at specified time intervals, and results in a refractory period during which aspirin can be safely administered. This desensitization period can be maintained indefinitely as long as aspirin therapy is not interrupted (325 mg every 48 hours or 80 mg QD). If aspirin has not been given for two or more days, repeat desensitization may be necessary. Patients with aspirin allergies who require desensitization should be referred to a center experienced in this technique.

4. Answer: a, c

Despite the success of desensitizing the aspirin-sensitive patient with asthma and rhinosinusitis, desensitization of individuals with aspirin-induced angioedema and/or urticaria remains problematic. These patients should not undergo desensitization. Fortunately, a previous cutaneous reaction to aspirin does not place the individual at increased risk of anaphylaxis upon re-administration of drug. If PTCA is required, aspirin should be prescribed in routine doses. H1 and H2 antagonists can usually control cutaneous symptoms during the periprocedural period.

5. Answer: b (false)

Desensitization has not been reported in individuals who have had an anaphylactic reaction to aspirin; re-administration of aspirin is contraindicated.

6. Answer: b

There is little or no experience with aspirin desensitization in patients with aspirin-induced anaphylaxis. There are isolated case reports of the use of low-molecular weight Dextran, sulfinpyrazone, and dipyridamole in aspirin-allergic patients but there are insufficient data with these drugs to recommend their use in patients with a history of aspirin-induced anaphylaxis. Other more potent platelet inhibitors, such as ticlopidine and clopidogrel, have demonstrated value in unstable angina and unstable cerebral ischemia, and may have value in patients with aspirin-allergy; pretreatment for 2-4 days prior to intervention is recommended to achieve optimal platelet inhibition. ReoPro, a platelet glycoprotein IIb/IIIa receptor antagonist, has recently been shown to reduce ischemic complications following high-risk (EPIC and CAPTURE trials) and elective coronary interventions (EPILOG trial) in patients receiving aspirin; its role in the aspirin-allergic patient has not been defined but is theoretically appealing. Investigational oral platelet receptor antagonists may be useful in the future.

Answers

7. Answer: a, c, d, e, f, I, j, k

Clinical Factors Associated with Increased Risk of Complications and/or Decreased Rate of Success During PTCA

Advanced Age	Severe hypertension
Aortic stenosis	Previous MI
Pulmonary hypertension	Previous CABG
Ejection fraction < 40%	Peripheral vascular disease
Diabetes mellitus	Unstable angina
Female gender	Acute MI
Hypotension	Multiple PVCs

8. Answer: c

Angiographic Factors Associated with Increased Risk of Complications and/or Decreased Rate of Success During PTCA

Multivessel disease	
Left main or equivalent	
Single patent vessel	
Lesion Characteristics:	
Long	Proximal vessel tortuosity
Bend point ($\geq 45°$)	Calcification
Bifurcation	Chronic total occlusion
Thrombus	Ostial location
Eccentric	Diffuse disease
Irregular contour	Degenerated vein graft

9. Answer: d

An activated clotting time (ACT) 300-350 seconds is recommended before advancing PTCA hardware into the coronary artery.

10. Answer: a (true)

Patients who have been receiving continuous heparin prior to the procedure may manifest drug resistance; a higher dose of heparin may be needed in these patients to achieve a therapeutic ACT.

11. Answer: b

The diameter of the final balloon should equal the normal reference segment adjacent to the lesion (balloon/artery ratio ~ 1). The reference diameter is estimated by comparing the target vessel to the guiding catheter (e.g., 7F guide = 2.3mm, 8F = 2.7mm, 9F = 3.0mm, 10F = 3.3mm, 11F = 3.6mm). Although visual estimates of reference diameter are less accurate than digital techniques, they are the simplest and most popular method.

12. Answer: a (true)

Balloon size should be judged carefully; undersizing (balloon/artery ratio <0.9) frequently results in significant residual stenosis and oversizing (balloon/artery ratio ≥ 1.2) increases the risk of emergency bypass surgery and myocardial infarction.[1]

References:
1. Sharma SK, Israel DH, Kamean JL, Bodian CA. Clinical, angiographic, and procedural determinants of major and minor coronary dissection during angioplasty. Am Heart J 1993;126:39-47.

13. Answer: a

14. Answer: b

The guidewire is steered into the distal vessel to provide support for balloon catheter advancement, and should pass smoothly through the stenosis. If buckling occurs, the wire should be retracted and re-advanced rather than forcefully prolapsed beyond the lesion since forceful manipulation increases the risk of dissection.

15. Answer: a (4); b (1); c (3); d (2)

Arterial sheaths commonly used for PTCA are 6-8F in diameter; larger sheaths are required for atherectomy (8-11F), aortic valvuloplasty (12-14F), and percutaneous cardiopulmonary bypass (18-22F).

16. Answer: a, b

The LAD normally arises in an anterior and superior position. A JL4 guide is the catheter of choice in the vast majority of cases. If the ostium of the left main is high or the aortic root is small, a JL 3.5 catheter may be preferred. Once in the left main, gentle counter-clockwise rotation of the guiding catheter will frequently direct it anteriorly. An out-of-plane femoral guiding catheter (30° anterior orientation) is available, though rarely needed. If the left main is short, a short-tip guide may be used to prevent inadvertent obstruction of the circumflex artery. Coaxial alignment between the catheter tip and left main is best confirmed in the LAO (50°)-Caudal (30°) view or in the shallow RAO (5°)-Caudal (20°) view.

17. Answer: a, c

LCX angioplasty is often associated with difficulties in guidewire passage and balloon tracking due to the inherent tortuosity of this vessel. Stable coaxial alignment may be facilitated by gentle clockwise rotation of a JL4 guiding catheter once engaged in the left main. A JL5 may be of benefit in a dilated aortic root or when the tip of a JL4 points anteriorly. An Amplatz left guiding catheter should be considered for a sharply angulated or inferiorly positioned circumflex origin.

18. Answer: b, c

Amplatz catheters can also be extremely useful in providing additional back-up support for balloon advancement when proximal vessel tortuosity, chronic total occlusion, or a distal target lesion is present. If the Amplatz guide becomes deeply engaged, it should be partially withdrawn over an extended balloon to prevent guide-induced injury. Amplatz catheters must be carefully disengaged from the coronary artery; simple withdrawal from the vessel in a manner similar to Judkins guide can cause the tip to advance farther into the vessel. To disengage an Amplatz catheter, it is first advanced slightly to prolapse the tip out of the artery and then rotated away from the ostium prior to withdrawal. Unlike the Amplatz and Judkins curves, which derive their support from the Sinus of Valsalva, the Voda and other geometric guides derive their support from the opposite wall of the aorta.

19. Answer: a

The right coronary artery is more difficult to engage than the left coronary artery, and frequently results in a dampened arterial pressure tracing. For horizontally oriented RCAs and most proximal lesions in gently superior or inferior orientations, a JR4 guiding catheter will usually suffice. However, when additional back-up support is needed a left Amplatz guide or hockey-stick are generally required. For marked superior orientations ("Shepherd's Crook"), a left Amplatz, Hockey-stick, internal mammary, El Gamal, Voda-right, or double-loop Arani catheter (75°) provide better coaxial alignment than a standard Judkin's catheter. Although double-loop Arani catheters provide excellent back-up, they are often very difficult to engage; a Voda-right guide provides similar back-up and is much easier to engage the ostium. Like the left Voda, the right Voda and double-loop Arani derive support from the opposite wall of the aorta rather than the Sinus of Valsalva. For marked inferior orientations, a Multipurpose or Amplatz catheter (left or right) are preferred for better coaxial alignment and backup.

20. Answer: All

Occasionally, guiding catheter engagement obstructs coronary flow, causing an immediate fall in diastolic pressure ("ventricularization") or a fall in both systolic and diastolic pressure ("dampened" pressure). Ventricularization and dampening may be caused by diseased ostium, coronary spasm, non-coaxial alignment of the guide and vessel wall, or mismatch between the vessel diameter and the diameter of the guide; in these instances, forceful contrast injections increase the risk of coronary dissection and must be avoided. When dampening is due to the presence of a small coronary artery or an ostial obstruction, the guiding catheter should be replaced with a sidehole catheter; sideholes allow passive entry of aortic blood into the guiding catheter and coronary artery. If a sidehole catheter is not available, sideholes can be created with a sidehole cutter or the beveled end of the vascular access needle.

21.   Answer: b

Potential problems with sidehole catheters include suboptimal opacification (contrast escapes through the sideholes); decreased back-up support due to weakness of the catheter shaft; and kinking at the sideholes, particularly in giant lumen guides. When sidehole guides are used for ostial lesions, the presence of sideholes will permit passive perfusion, but does not decrease the chance of guiding catheter injury to the vessel ostium.

22.   Answer: a (3); b (1); c (2)

23.   Answer: c

Features to consider when choosing a guidewire include its torque-control, steerability, visibility, flexibility, and support for balloon catheter advancement. Unfortunately, the perfect angioplasty guidewire does not exist: Wires with increased flexibility have decreased steerability; those with increased torque-control have decreased flexibility. Coronary guidewires are available in 0.010, 0.012, 0.014, 0.016, 0.017, and 0.018" diameters. Larger wires (0.016"-0.018") have increased steerability, result in greater straightening of tortuous coronary segments, and provide more support for balloon catheter advancement.

24.   Answer: a, b, e, f

Balloon compliance, defined as the change in balloon diameter per atmosphere of inflation pressure, is an index of the stretchability of a balloon. Balloon materials can be classified as highly-compliant, moderately-compliant, and minimally-compliant; more compliant balloons are generally associated with more "creep", which refers to the tendency of a balloon to enlarge after serial inflations at the same pressure. Balloon compliance ranges from 0.095 mm/ATM (POC balloons) to 0.010 mm/ATM (PET balloons). Although in-vitro testing suggests that PET balloons are less compliant than POC or PE balloons, most studies have found that these differences are not clinically relevant. In fact, high compliance is marketed by some manufactures as an advantage (sizing "flexibility") and by others as a disadvantage ("less predictable" balloon sizing). Concerns about balloon compliance and creep have been heightened by clinical studies suggesting that accurate balloon sizing (ideal balloon/artery ratio = 0.9-1.1) is needed to minimize the risk of dissection, abrupt closure, and major ischemic complications. Despite the recognized importance of proper balloon sizing, there are no data to suggest clear superiority of certain balloon materials: Only two retrospective studies reported different results for compliant and noncompliant balloons; one reported better results for noncompliant balloons, whereas the other reported better results for compliant balloons. In contrast, five nonrandomized studies and two prospective randomized studies (over 4000 lesions in all) failed to show any difference in angiographic results or ischemic complications. Although early studies suggested that angulated lesions may respond better to noncompliant balloons, more recent data from a prospective randomized study suggested no difference in outcome for angulated lesions, lesions > 20 mm, ostial lesions, calcified lesions, or eccentric lesions. Nevertheless, noncompliant balloons are associated with higher burst pressures and are clearly useful in rigid lesions that cannot be dilated at inflation pressures < 10 ATM, and as adjuncts to stenting. Burst pressure (usually reported as rated burst pressure; RBP) is defined as the pressure below which 99.9% of balloons will not rupture. RBP is an important component of product labeling (and as such is monitored by the FDA); it provides the operator with a good idea about the safe range of inflation pressures. RBP commonly ranges from 6-16 ATM. Mean burst pressure (MBP), defined as the pressure at which 50% of balloons will rupture, is higher than RBP and ranges from 10-27 ATM.

25. Answer: b, c, f

Femoral sheaths are removed 4-6 hrs after discontinuing heparin (ACT <150 seconds or PTT < 50 seconds); if thrombolytics have been given, the fibrinogen level should be > 150 mg/dl prior to sheath removal. When uninterrupted anticoagulation is required (e.g., extensive coronary dissection with thrombus), the heparin infusion is decreased by 50% prior to sheath removal. When the ACT is 140-160 seconds, the sheaths are pulled and the site compressed until bleeding stops (usually 30-45 minutes).

BRACHIAL AND RADIAL APPROACH

26. Answer: a, c, e, f

Comparison of Femoral, Brachial, and Radial Catheterization for Coronary Intervention

	Femoral	Brachial	Radial
Physician Factors			
Training	Common	Uncommon	Virtually none
Experience	Extensive	Minimal	Rare
Catheter Manipulation	Easy	More difficult	More difficult
Radiation Exposure	Less	More	More
Superselective intubation	Difficult	Easy	Difficult

	Femoral	Brachial	Radial
Complications			
Bleeding	More common	Less common	Less common
Loss of pulse	Less common	More common	More common
Transfusion	More common	Less common	Less common
Surgical repair	Uncommon	Uncommon	Uncommon
Technical Factors			
Percutaneous	Yes	Yes	Yes
Cut-down/Repair	No	Yes	No
Repeated access	Yes	Limited	Unknown
Bedrest > 8 hours	Common	Not necessary	Not necessary

27. Answer: a, b, c, e

Special indications for brachial and radial techniques include:

Peripheral Vascular Disease. Femoral artery access may be difficult (morbid obesity, extensive post-operative scarring, severe peripheral vascular disease), impossible (aortic occlusion), or relatively contraindicated (coagulopathy). For these patients, the brachial cutdown technique allows an alternative approach for coronary angiography, peripheral aortography, and angioplasty.

Patient Preference. Brachial and radial artery angioplasty allow immediate ambulation; this may be important in selected patients, including those with severe lumbosacral pain aggravated by prolonged bed rest.

Need for Uninterrupted Anticoagulation. Brachial artery repair allows continuous anticoagulation (with heparin or warfarin) and may be useful in decreasing length of stay in stent patients.

Difficult Internal Mammary Artery Cannulation. In some cases, selective angiography of an internal mammary artery conduit cannot be accomplished via the femoral route because of severe tortuosity of the subclavian or brachycephalic arteries. However, selective angiography (and intervention, if necessary) can usually be performed by the ipsilateral (right Judkins or internal mammary artery catheter) or contralateral brachial artery (Simmons catheter).

Severe Coronary Artery Tortuosity. Compared to the femoral approach, the left brachial approach can more readily achieve deep guiding catheter intubation of the target vessel. This may be particularly useful when severe tortuosity of the target vessel precludes advancement of interventional hardware from the femoral approach.

Answers

28. Answer: c

In general, the incidence of peripheral vascular complications associated with brachial cutdown and percutaneous femoral techniques are similar, including significant hematoma (1.3%), retroperitoneal hemorrhage (0.4%), false aneurysm (0.4%), vessel occlusion (0.1%), infection (0.1%), and cholesterol embolization (0.1%).[1] However, femoral vascular complications are usually associated with greater patient morbidity.[2] Compiled data from the TAMI trials show comparable success rates using brachial and femoral access sites, but complication rates were slightly lower from the brachial site.[3-6]

References:
1. Johnson LW, Esenta P, Giambartolomei A, et al. Peripheral vascular complications of coronary angioplasty by the femoral and brachial techniques. Cath Cardiovasc Diagn. 1994;31:165-172.
2. Kiemeneij F, Laarman, GJ. Percutaneous transradial artery approach for coronary stent implantation. Cath Cardiovasc Diagn. 30:173-178, 1993.
3. George BS, Candela RJ, Topol EJ, et al. The brachial approach to emergency cardiac catheterization during thrombolytic therapy for acute myocardial infarction. Cathet Cardiovasc Diagn 1990;20:221-226.
4. Topol EJ, Califf RM, George BS, et al. A randomized trial of immediate vs. delayed elective angioplasty after intravenous tissue plasminogen activator in acute myocardial infarction. N. Engl J Med 317:581-588, 1987.
5. Topol EJ Califf RM, George BS, et al. Coronary arterial thrombolysis with combined infusion of recombinant tissue-type plasminogen activator and urokinase in patients with acute myocardial infarction. Circulation 77:1100-1107, 1988.
6. Topol EJ, George BS, Kereiakes DJ, et al. A randomized controlled trial of intravenous tissue plasminogen activator and early intravenous heparin in acute myocardial infarction. Circulation 79:281-286, 1989.

MULTIVESSEL AND HIGH-RISK INTERVENTION

29. Answer: b, c, d

To determine the optimal revascularization technique for patients with multivessel disease, more than 4000 patients have been randomized in six PTCA vs. CABG trials (Table 1). Specific entry criteria differ between each trial; most excluded patients with previous PTCA or CABG, evolving MI, left main disease, or severe non-cardiac illness. Importantly, less than 10% of patients with symptomatic multivessel disease were actually enrolled into these trials. PTCA was generally confined to diameter stenoses > 50% in vessels > 1.5 mm in diameter supplying viable myocardium and causing ischemia (i.e., complete "functional" revascularization); lesions in small vessels and those supplying nonviable myocardium were generally not dilated. New device intervention was permitted only in CABRI (atherectomy and stents) and BARI (bailout stents). Internal mammary arteries were used in > 75% of CABGs (but only 37% in GABI). Importantly, most patients enrolled into these trials had 2-vessel disease and well-preserved LV function (Table 2).

Table 1. Randomized Trials of PTCA vs. CABG: Inclusion and Exclusion Criteria

Trial	N	Randomized (%)	Criteria
RITA[1]	1011	6	**Inclusion:** 1, 2, or 3-vessel disease (≥ 70% stenosis); lesion supplying ≥ 20% of myocardium; angina or objective evidence of ischemia; equivalent revascularization by PTCA or CABG. **Exclusion:** Previous PTCA or CABG; left main disease, hemodynamically-severe valve disease; noncardiac illness threatening survival.
ERACI[2]	127	9	**Inclusion:** Multivessel disease (≥ 2 vessels with ≥ 70% stenosis) and either significant angina despite medical therapy or a large area of myocardium at risk by exercise testing. **Exclusion:** Dilated ischemic cardiomyopathy; severe 3-vessel disease with EF ≤ 35%; significant left main stenosis; severe valvular or hypertrophic heart disease; evolving acute MI; noncardiac illness threatening survival.
GABI[3]	358	4	**Inclusion:** Age < 75 years; angina ≥ Class 2; multivessel disease (≥ 2 vessels with ≥ 70% stenosis). **Exclusion:** Previous PTCA or CABG; total occlusion; left main stenosis ≥30%; > 50% of LV at risk during abrupt closure; lesion length > 2 cm; diffuse disease; coronary aneurysm, MI within 4 weeks.
CABRI[4]	1054	4.6	**Inclusion:** Age ≤ 76 years with multivessel disease (≥ 2 vessels with ≥ 50% stenosis); clinical ischemia; equivalent degrees of revascularization not required. **Exclusion:** Previous PTCA or CABG; left main stenosis ≥ 50%; last remaining vessel; acute MI within previous 10 days; EF ≤ 35%; overt CHF; recent stroke; severe concomitant illness.
EAST[5]	392	7.6	**Inclusion:** Patients of any age with 2 or 3-vessel disease; angina or objective evidence of ischemia. **Exclusion:** Previous PTCA or CABG; chronic total occlusion > 8 weeks; left main stenosis ≥ 30%; ≥ 2 total occlusions; EF < 25%; MI within 5 days; noncardiac illness threatening survival.
BARI[6]	1829	7	**Inclusion:** Age > 17 and < 80; multivessel disease (≥ vessels with ≥ 50% stenosis); and clinically severe angina (class III-IV or unstable angina; recent non-Q-MI; or class I-II angina either with severe ischemia on exercise testing; recent Q-MI; or EF < 50%), or no angina if severe ischemia on noninvasive testing and either a prior Q-MI or history of angina. **Exclusion:** Emergency revascularization; left main stenosis ≥ 50%; noncardiac illness that was a contraindication to PTCA or CABG or might limit survival; primary coronary spasm; severe ascending aortic calcification; need for other major surgery at same time as revascularization, known or suspected pregnancy.

CONCLUSIONS: Only a small percentage (< 25%) of patients with multivessel disease met inclusion criteria, and even fewer (< 10%) were actually randomized.

Abbreviations: MVD = multivessel disease; LV = left ventricle; EF = ejection fraction; MI = myocardial infarction

Answers

Table 2. Randomized Trials of PTCA vs. CABG: Study Design and Baseline Characteristics

	RITA[1]	ERACI[2]	GABI[3]	CABRI[4]	EAST[5]	BARI[6]
Patients (N)	1011	127	359	1054	392	1829
Study Design						
Planned follow-up (yrs)	10	3	1	5-10	5	10
Complete revascularization required	Yes	No	Yes	No	No	No
Total occlusion eligible	Yes	Yes	No	Yes	No	Yes
New devices	No	No	No	Yes⁺	No	Yes*
IMA (%)	74	77	37	81	90	82
Baseline characteristics						
Age (yrs)	57	57	-	60	61	61
Male (%)	81	54	80	78	73	74
Previous MI (%)	43	31	47	43	41	55
Unstable angina (%)	59	53	14	15	62	65
LVEF (%)	-	61	56	63	62	57
No. diseased vessels (%)						
1	45	0	0	0	0	0
2	43	55	82	58	60	59
3	12	45	18	40	40	41

CONCLUSIONS:
- ▸ Complete revascularization goal varied between trials.
- ▸ Patients with total occlusions were excluded from some trials but not others.
- ▸ Use of new devices and IMA grafting varied between trials.
- ▸ Most patients had 2-vessel disease and normal LV function.

Abbreviations: IMA = internal mammary artery; LVEF = left ventricular ejection fraction; CABG = emergency coronary artery bypass grafting; - = not reported

+   Atherectomy or stenting
*   Bailout stenting
** Complete anatomical revascularization whenever possible

References:
1. Coronary angioplasty versus coronary artery bypass surgery: The randomized intervention treatment of angina (RITA) trial. RITA Trial Participants. Lancet 1993;341:573-80.
2. Rodriguez A, Boullon F, Perez-Balino N. Argentine randomized trial of percutaneous transluminal coronary angioplasty versus coronary artery bypass surgery in multivessel disease (ERACI): In-hospital results and 1-year fellowship. J Am Collage Cardiol 1993;22:1060-1067.
3. Hamm C, Reimers J, Ischinger T, Rupprecht H. A randomized study of coronary angioplasty compared with bypass surgery in patients with symptomatic multivessel coronary disease. N Engl J. Med 1994;331(16):1037-1043.
4. First-year results of CABRI Coronary Angioplasty versus Bypass Revascularization Investigation. CABRI Trial Participants. Lancet 1995;346:1179-84.
5. King S, Lembo N, Weintraub W, Losinski A. A randomized trial comparing coronary angioplasty with coronary bypass surgery. N Engl J. Med 1994;331:1044-1150.
6. The Bypass Angioplasty Revascularization Investigation (BARI): Five-year mortality and morbidity in a randomized study compared CABG and PTCA in patients with multivessel coronary disease. The BARI investigators. N Engl J. Med (submitted).

30.   Answer: a, c, d

Randomized Trials of PTCA vs. CABG: In-Hospital Results

Trial	Group	Complications (%)			Other
		D	**MI**	**CABG**	
RITA[1]	PTCA	0.7	3.5	4.5	Length of stay (4 vs. 12 days)
	CABG	1.2	2.4	-	
ERACI[2]	PTCA	1.5	6.3	1.5	Stroke (1.5% vs. 3.1%)
	CABG	4.6	6.2	-	
GABI[3]	PTCA	1.1	2.3	2.8	Stroke (0% vs. 1.2%); post-op pneumonia (1.1% vs. 10.6%,
	CABG	2.5	8.1*	-	< 0.001); length of stay (5 vs. 19 days); angina (18% vs. 7%, p < 0.005)
CABRI[4]	PTCA	1.3	-	3.3	-
	CABG	1.3	-	-	
EAST[5]	PTCA	1	3	10.1	Stroke (0.5% vs. 1.5%)
	CABG	1	10.3*	-	
BARI[6]	PTCA	1.1	2.1	6.3	Stroke (0.2% vs. 0.8%), respiratory failure (1% vs. 2.2%,
	CABG	1.3	4.6*	-	p < .05)

CONCLUSIONS:
▸   **In-hospital mortality similar between PTCA and CABG groups.**
▸   **In-hospital MI higher in CABG group.**
▸   **Emergency CABG for failed PTCA in 1.5-10%.**
▸   **Length of hospital stay 2-3 fold higher in CABG group.**

Abbreviations: D = death; Q-MI = Q-wave myocardial infarction; CABG = emergency coronary artery bypass grafting; - = Not reported
*   p < 0.01

References:
1.   Coronary angioplasty versus coronary artery bypass surgery: The randomized intervention treatment of angina (RITA) trial. RITA Trial Participants. Lancet 1993;341:573-80.
2.   Rodriguez A, Boullon F, Perez-Balino N. Argentine randomized trial of percutaneous transluminal coronary angioplasty versus coronary artery bypass surgery in multivessel disease (ERACI): In-hospital results and 1-year fellowship. J Am Collage Cardiol 1993;22:1060-1067.
3.   Hamm C, Reimers J, Ischinger T, Rupprecht H. A randomized study of coronary angioplasty compared with bypass surgery in patients with symptomatic multivessel coronary disease. N Engl J. Med 1994;331(16):1037-1043.
4.   First-year results of CABRI Coronary Angioplasty versus Bypass Revascularization Investigation. CABRI Trial Participants. Lancet 1995;346:1179-84.
5.   King S, Lembo N, Weintraub W, Losinski A. A randomized trial comparing coronary angioplasty with coronary bypass surgery. N Engl J. Med 1994;331:1044-1150.
6.   The Bypass Angioplasty Revascularization Investigation (BARI): Five-year mortality and morbidity in a randomized study compared CABG and PTCA in patients with multivessel coronary disease. The BARI investigators. N Engl J. Med (submitted).

Answers

31. Answer: a, b, d

Randomized Trials of PTCA vs. CABG: Late Outcome

Trial	F/U (yrs)	Modality	D / MI / TLR / ASX (%)	Other
RITA[1]	2.5	PTCA CABG	3.1 / 6.1 / 35 / 69 3.6 / 3.9 / 3.8[+] / 79[+]	See 1, below
ERACI[2]	5	PTCA CABG	12.7/ 11.1 / 38 / 54 9.4 / 9.4 / 6.3/ 73	PTCA less expensive the CABG
GABI[3]	3	PTCA CABG	- / - / 37 / 60 - / - / 3.2[+] / 80[+]	
	1	PTCA CABG	2.6 / 4.5 / 44 / 71 6.5 / 9.4 / 6 / 74	See 2, below
CABRI[4]	1	PTCA CABG	3.9 / 4.9 / 35.6/ 67 2.7 / 3.5 / 2.1 / 75[+]	Need for antianginals (84% vs. 65%)
EAST[5]	3	PTCA CABG	7.1 / 14.6/ 54 / 80[†] 6.2 / 19.6 / 13 [+]/ 88[†+]	See 3, below
BARI[6]	5	Overall PTCA CABG	 14/ 8 / 54 / - 11/ 9 / 8[+] / -	See 4, below
		Diabetic[++] PTCA CABG	 35 / - / 62 / - 19 / - / 8[+]/ -	

CONCLUSIONS:
▸ **Infarct-free survival at 1-year similar; diabetics treated with PTCA had higher late mortality.***
▸ **PTCA resulted in more angina, antianginal therapy, and repeat revascularization (3-10 fold) compared to CABG; ~ 20% of PTCA patients required CABG at 1-3 years.**

Abbreviations: ASX = asymptomatic; D = death; Q-MI = Q-wave myocardial infarction; CABG = emergency coronary artery bypass grafting; EF = ejection fraction; - = not reported
* Does not include high mortality among CABG patients during the waiting period (time between randomization and revascularization); +p <0.05, #p < 0.001; ++Patients receiving oral hypoglycemics or insulin at study entry
Other results:
1. PTCA vs. CABG: Death, MI, or reintervention (38% vs. 11%[+]); severe angina 6% in both groups; PTCA less expensive. Pre vs. post-revascularization: 40% of those not working at baseline had returned to work at 6 months; revascularization had no effect on ejection fraction
2. PTCA vs. CABG: Death or MI (5% vs. 11%) [+] [*], antianginals (88% vs 78%)[+]
3. PTCA vs. CABG: Abnormal thallium stress (9.6% vs. 5.7%); use of antianginals (66% vs. 51%) [+] ; costs equal; no difference in LVEF
4. PTCA vs. CABG: Infarct-free survival (79% vs. 80%); 70% of PTCA patients survived 5 years without CABG and at most one repeat PTCA procedure; severe angina present in only 3% of PTCA & CABG groups, but PTCA patients more likely to have angina of all grades

References:
1. Coronary angioplasty versus coronary artery bypass surgery: The randomized intervention treatment of angina (RITA) trial. RITA Trial Participants. Lancet 1993;341:573-80.
2. Mele E, Rodriguez AE, Peyregne E, Boullon F, et al. Final follow-up of argentine randomized trial coronary angioplasty vs. bypass surgery in multivessel disease (ERAC): Clinical outcome and cost analysis. Circulation 1996;84:I-435.
3. Hamm C, Reimers J, Ischinger T, Rupprecht H. A randomized study of coronary angioplasty compared with bypass surgery in patients with symptomatic multivessel coronary disease. N Engl J. Med 1994;331(16):1037-1043.
4. First-year results of CABRI Coronary Angioplasty versus Bypass Revascularization Investigation. CABRI Trial Participants. Lancet 1995;346:1179-84.
5. King S, Lembo N, Weintraub W, Losinski A. A randomized trial comparing coronary angioplasty with coronary bypass surgery. N Engl J. Med 1994;331:1044-1150.
6. The Bypass Angioplasty Revascularization Investigation (BARI): Five-year mortality and morbidity in a randomized study compared CABG and PTCA in patients with multivessel coronary disease. The BARI investigators. N Engl J. Med (submitted).

32. Answer: All

LV dysfunction has also been shown to adversely impact long-term outcome after multivessel PTCA:[1] CABG resulted in more periprocedural stroke and longer hospital study, but improved 5-year event-free survival and less angina compared to PTCA patients. Late outcome, however, was most influenced by *completeness* of revascularization, *not the mode* of revascularization; patients with complete revascularization demonstrated similar event-free survival regardless of treatment mode. These data suggest that CABG may be preferred if PTCA cannot achieve complete revascularization, particularly in patients with diabetes, unstable angina, high-risk lesion morphology, and/or proximal LAD disease.[2,3]

References:
1. O'Keefe JH, Allan JJ, McCallister BD, McConahay DR. Angioplasty versus bypass surgery for multivessel Coronary artery disease with left ventricular ejection fraction <40%. Am J Cardiol 1993;71:897-901.
2. Ellis SG, Vandormael MG, Cowley MJ, et al. Coronary morphologic and clinical determinants of procedural outcome with angioplasty for multivessel coronary disease: Implications for patient selection. Circulation 1990;82:1193-1202.
3. Ellis SG, Cowley MK, DiSciascio G, et al. Determinants of 2-year outcome after coronary angioplasty in patients with multivessel disease on the basis of comprehensive preprocedural evaluation: Implications for patient selection. Circulation 1991;82:1905-1914.

33. Answer: d

Indications for Staging

·   Thrombus prior to or immediately after PTCA
·   Severe dissection or impaired flow after intervention
·   Procedure duration > 3 hrs
·   Contrast volume > 400 cc
·   Borderline lesions (50-70% stenosis) without objective evidence for ischemia

34. Answer: All

Procedures involving high-risk lesions in high-risk patients are best performed at interventional centers experienced in the use of new interventional devices, IABP, and CPS. The need for an experienced operator and support staff cannot be overstated. Intravascular volume depletion exaggerates the hypotensive effects of contrast agents, nitrates and balloon-induced ischemia, and is a risk factor for adverse outcome following acute closure.[1] Aggressive administration of IV fluids (coupled with the negative inotropic effects of contrast agents and balloon-induced ischemia) can readily induce heart failure in patients with marginal LV reserve. Therefore, careful assessment of intravascular volume is mandatory during high-risk intervention; a pulmonary artery catheter is recommended in all patients with labile hemodynamic performance or heart failure. Patients with pre-existing renal insufficiency or a history of renal dysfunction following contrast exposure must be well-hydrated prior to PTCA. In hospitalized patients, aim to maintain urine output > 40 cc/hr with IV crystalloids (100-150 cc/hr starting 8-10 hours prior to the case); supplemental diuretics may be needed to prevent pulmonary congestion when LV dysfunction is present.

Answers

References:
1. Ellis SG, Roubin GS, King SP III et al. In-hospital cardiac mortality after acute closure after coronary angioplasty: Analysis of risk factors from 8,207 procedures. J Am Coll Cardiol 1988;11:211.

35. Answer: a, b

Patients should be transferred to a telemetry unit after high-risk intervention. Overnight observation in a cardiac intensive care unit is preferred if the procedure is complicated by acute closure, a suboptimal angiographic result, or the need for IABP or CPS. Due to a temporal association between heparin withdrawal and acute closure,[1] heparin should be tapered (rather than abruptly discontinued) at a time of day when emergency revascularization is feasible. Recurrent chest pain associated with ECG changes or hemodynamic instability mandates immediate return to the cath lab to exclude abrupt closure.

References:
1. Gabliani G, Deligonul U, Kern MJ, et al. Acute coronary occlusion occurring after successful percutaneous transluminal coronary angioplasty: Temporal relationship to discontinuation of anticoagulation. Am Heart J 1988;16:696.

36. Answer: All

Asymptomatic hypotension may be caused by medications (sedatives, nitrates, calcium channel and β-blockers) and/or mild hypovolemia (NPO status, contrast-induced diuresis); more serious conditions such as tamponade, retroperitoneal bleeding, and sepsis should be considered and promptly excluded.

37. Answer: a, c, d

Left main coronary disease is present in 7% and 15% of patients with stable and unstable angina, respectively. Among 1484 patients enrolled into the CASS Registry with > 50% obstruction of the left main, median survival was 13.3 years for the surgical group, but only 6.6 years for the medical group;[1] the survival benefit was confined mainly to patients with > 60% stenosis, particularly in the presence of LV dysfunction. In another report, 1-year survival was 95% for patients with left main disease and normal LV function, but only 61% when significant LV dysfunction was present.[2] PTCA of unprotected left main disease is technically feasible (success > 90%); however in-hospital and 3-year mortality for elective cases is 9% and 64%, and for acute MI is 50% and 70%.[3] More favorable results with stents have been reported (Table). In a report of 26 patients undergoing unprotected left main DCA, procedural success was 100%, there was no acute closures angiographic restenosis occurred in 33%, and 3-year cardiac survival was 97%.[6] Despite these results, unprotected left main stenosis remains a surgical disease; further studies of percutaneous intervention are required, particularly in patients who refuse surgery or who are poor surgical candidates. In contrast, when the left main is protected, catheter-based interventions can be preformed with acceptable early and late outcomes.[3]

Stenting of Protected and Unprotected Left Main Disease

Series	Protected/Unprotected (n)	In-hospital Results	Follow-up
Silvestria[4] (1997)	0/41	Angiographic success (100%); subacute thrombosis (4.7%); death (4.7%)	10 months: death (2.4%); repeat PTCA (10%)
Laurelle[5] (1997)	0/18	Angiographic success (100%); death (5.5%); emergency CABG (5.5%)	9 months: death (11%); asymptomatic (67%)
Itoh[8] (1996)	33	Success (94%); emergency CABG (3%)	3 months: Death (9%)
Fajadet[7] (1995)	13/21	Success (100%); stent thrombosis (3%)	13 months: Sudden death (3%); repeat PTCA (12%); MI or CABG (0%); asymptomatic (> 90%)

References:
1. Caracciolo EA, Davis KB, Sopko G, et al. Comparison of surgical and medical group survival in patients with left main coronary artery disease. Long-term CASS experience. Circulation 1995;91:2325-2334.
2. Conley MJ, Ely RI, Kisslo J, et al. The prognostic spectrum of left main stenosis. Circulation 178;57:947-952.
3. O'Keefe JH Jr., Hartzler GO, Rutherford BD, et al. Left main coronary angioplasty: early and late results of 127 acute and elective procedures. Am J Cardiol 1989;64:144-7.
4. Silvestri M, Barragan P, Simeoni JB, et al. Stents: Difficult lesion subsets. J Am Coll Cardiol 1997;(Supple A):15A
5. Laruelle CJJ, Brueren GBR, Bal ET, et al. Stenting of "unprotected" left main coronary artery stenosis: Early and late results. J Am Coll Cardiol 1997;(Supple A):15A.
6. Tanaka S, Ueda K, Yung-Sheng H, Kosuga K, Matsui S, et al. Initial and long-term results of directional coronary atherectomy of unprotected left main coronary artery. Circulation 1996;84:I-672.
7. Fajadet J, Brunel P, Jordan C, et al. Is stenting of left main coronary artery a reasonable procedure? Circulation 1995;92:I-355.
8. Itoh A, Colombo A, Hall P, et al. Stenting in protected and unprotected left main coronary artery: Immediate and follow-up results. J Am Coll Cardiol 1996;27:277A.

UNSTABLE ISCHEMIC SYNDROMES

38. Answer: b

39. Answer: c

40. Answer: c

41. Answer: a, c, d, g

Primary PTCA refers to the use of PTCA without prior thrombolytic therapy and is associated with several potential advantages and disadvantages. Primary PTCA results in better acute patency (95-

99% vs. 70-80%), and in high-risk patients, better survival and less recurrent ischemia. In addition, many studies have demonstrated improvement in left ventricular function, and less reperfusion injury, cardiogenic shock and myocardial rupture after primary PTCA compared to thrombolytic therapy. The prognosis of high-risk patients, particularly those with cardiogenic shock, is improved by primary PTCA compared to other treatment modalities. Although older primary PTCA series reported reocclusion rates of 8-15%, contemporary in-hospital and 6-month reocclusion rates are only 4-5% and 9-13% respectively, due to better understanding of the importance of aspirin, heparin, and ionic contrast. [1-9]

Primary (Direct) PTCA

Advantages Compared to Thrombolysis

- Useful in thrombolytic-ineligible patients
- Immediate definition of coronary anatomy
- Early risk stratification
- Superior acute vessel patency and TIMI 3 flow
- Less reocclusion, recurrent ischemia, reinfarction
- Better survival in high-risk patients
- Less reperfusion injury and myocardial rupture
- Lower risk of intracranial hemorrhage
- Shorter length of hospital stay
- Similar cost

Disadvantages Compared to Thrombolysis

- Skilled interventional cardiologist and cath lab must be available
- Logistic delays in mobilizing lab and support staff

References:

1. Zijlstra F, Jan de Boaer M, Hoorntje JCA, Reiffer S, Reiber JHC, Suryapranata H. A comparison of immediate coronary angioplasty with intravenous streptokinase in acute myocardial infarction. N Engl J Med 1993;328:680-684.
2. Griffin J, Grines CL, Marsales D, et al. A prospective, randomized trial evaluating the prophylactic use of balloon pumping in high risk myocardial infarction patients: PAMI-2. J Am Coll Cardiol 1995;25:86A.
3. Brodie BR, Grines CL, Ivanhoe R, Knopf W, Taylor G, O'Keefe J, Weintraub RA, Berdan LG, Tcheng JE, Woodlief LH, Califf RM, O'Neill WW. Six-month clinical and angiographic follow-up after direct angioplasty for acute myocardial infarction. Circulation 1994;90:156-162.
4. O'Neill WW, Weintraub R, Grines CL, Meany TB, Brodie BR, Friedman HZ, Ramos RG, Gangadharan V, Levin RN, Choksi N, Westveer DC, Strzelecki RN, Timmis GC. A prospective placebo-controlled randomized trial of intravenous streptokinase and angioplasty therapy of acute myocardial infarction. Circulation 1992;86:1710-1717.
5. Weaver WD, Parsons L, Every N. Primary coronary angioplasty in hospitals with and without surgery backup. J Invas Cardiol 1995;7:34F-39F
6. Ayres M. Coronary angioplasty for acute myocardial infarction in hospitals without cardiac surgery. J Invas Cardiol 1995;7:40F-46F.
7. Weaver W, Parsons L, Martin JS, Every N. Direct PTCA for treatment of acute myocardial infarction: A community experience in hospitals with and without surgical back-up. Circulation 1995;92:I-138.
8. Wharton TP, Schmitz JM, Fedele FA, McNamara NS, Gladstone AR, Jacobs MI. Primary angioplasty in acute myocardial infarction at community hospitals without cardiac surgery: Experience in 195 cases. Circulation 1995;92:I-138.
9. Grines CL, Browne KF, Marco J, Rothbaum D, Stone GW, O'Keefe J, Overlie P, Donohue B, Chelliah N, Timmis GC, Vlietstra RE, Strelecki M, Puchrowicz-Ochocki S, O'Neill WW. A comparison of immediate angioplasty with thrombolytic therapy for acute myocardial infarction. N Engl J Med 1993;328:673-9.

42. Answer: a (true)

Seventy to seventy-five percent of acute MI patients are ineligible for thrombolytic therapy based on TIMI 2B criteria; these patients are more likely to be older, female, and have prior MI, multivessel coronary disease, lower ejection fraction, and higher in-hospital mortality (18.7% vs 3.9%, $p < 0.001$) compared to lytic-eligible patients.[1] Primary PTCA can be applied to most MI patients irrespective of lytic eligibility;[2,3] however, procedure-related mortality is higher in lytic-ineligible patients due to underlying comorbid disease.[2,3] When lytic eligibility was defined by TIMI-2B criteria, better early and late results were achieved with PTCA than tPA.[4,5]

References:
1. Cragg DR, Friedman HZ, Bonema JD, et al. Outcome of patients with acute myocardial infarction who are ineligible for thrombolytic therapy. Ann Int Med 1991;115:173-177.
2. O'Keefe JO, Bailey WL, Rutherford BD, Hartzler GO. Primary angioplasty for acute myocardial infarction in 1000 consecutive patients. Am J. Cardiol 1993;72:107-G-115G.
3. Brodie BR, Weintraub RA, Stuckey TD, et al. Outcomes of direct coronary angioplasty for acute myocardial infarction in candidates and non-candidates for thrombolytic therapy. Am J Cardiol 1991;67:7-12.
4. Waldecker B, Waas W, Haberbosch W, Voss R, Kistler P, Tillmanns H. Long-term follow-up (2.5 years) of 300 consecutive patients with primary angioplasty for acute myocardial infarction. Circulation 1995;92:I-461.
5. Stone GW, Grines CL, Browne KF, Marco J, Rothbaum D, O'Keefe J, Overlie P, Donohue B, Puchrowicz S, O'Neill WW. Outcome of different reperfusion strategies in thrombolytic "eligible" versus "ineligible" patients with acute myocardial infarction. J Am Coll Cardiol February 1995;401A.

43. Answer: a,b,c,d

Certain patient groups are especially well-suited for primary PTCA including the elderly (less intracranial hemorrhage vs. lytic); patients who present late after symptom onset (higher patency rates with PTCA vs. lytics); patients with vein graft occlusions (low patency rates with IV thrombolytics due to large thrombus burden and stagnant flow);[1,2] and patients without ST-elevation (allows the diagnosis to be confirmed and treatment initiated). The randomized SMART trial (Study of Medicine vs. Angioplasty Reperfusion Trial), which compared PTCA to medicine in thrombolytic-ineligible or undesirable patients, reported less ischemia and reinfarction after PTCA.[3]

Reference:
1. Stone GW, Grines CL, Topol EJ. Update on percutaneous transluminal coronary angioplasty for acute myocardial infarction. Book chapter. Current Review of Interventional Cardiology. Ed. E. Topol, M.D., P. Serruys, M.D., Current Medicine, Philadelphia, PA, 1995. 1-56.
2. Grines CL, Booth D, Nissen S, Gurley J, Bennett K, O'Connor WN, DeMaria A. Mechanism of acute myocardial infarction in patients with prior coronary artery bypass grafting and therapeutic implications. Am J Cardiol 1990;65:1292-96.
3. McKendall GR, Drew TM, Kelsey SF, et al. What is the optimal treatment for thrombolytic ineligible AMI Preliminary results of the Study of Medicine vs. Angioplasty Reperfusion Trial (SMART). J Am Coll Cardiol 1994;1A-484A:225A.

44. Answer: a

Patients in cardiogenic shock are typically taken to the catheterization laboratory for angiography, placement of an intra-aortic balloon pump, and emergency revascularization with PTCA or bypass surgery. Non-randomized studies suggest a survival advantage if PTCA successfully establishes perfusion;[1-18] survival rates in this extremely high-risk patient population are 40-86% after PTCA, 30% after lytic therapy and only 10% after medical therapy. In GUSTO-1, an aggressive revascularization strategy of PTCA or CABG was independently associated with better 30-day survival[15] despite infrequent use of early intervention and balloon pumps.[19] The multicenter randomized trial SHOCK will compare 30-day mortality for patients treated by emergency revascularization (PTCA or CABG) vs. initial medical stabilization and later revascularization if indicated.

References:
1. Kaplan AJ, Bengtson JR, Aronson LG, et al. Reperfusion improves survival in patients with cardiogenic shock after acute myocardial infarction. J Am Coll Cardiol 1990;15:155 (abstr).

2. Lee L, Erbel R, Brown TM, et al. Multicenter registry of angioplasty therapy of cardiogenic shock: initial and long-term survival. J Am Coll Cardiol 1991;17:599-603.

3. Gacioch GM, Ellis SG, Lee L, et al. Cardiogenic shock complicating acute myocardial infarction: the use of coronary angioplasty and the integration of the new support devices into patient management. J Am Coll Cardiol 1992;19:647-653.

4. Bengtson JR, Kaplan AJ, Pieper KS, et al. Prognosis in cardiogenic shock after acute myocardial infarction in the interventional era. J Am Coll Cardiol 1992;20:1482-1489.

5. Hibbard MD, Holmes DR, Gersh BJ, Reeder GS. Coronary angioplasty for acute myocardial infarction complicated by cardiogenic shock. Circulation 1990;82:III-511.

6. Moosvi AR, Villaneuva L, Gheorghiade M, et al. Early revascularization improves survival in cardiogenic shock. Circulation 1990;82:III-308.

7. Eltchaninoff H, Simpendorfer C, Whitlow PL. Coronary angioplasty improves both early and 1 year survival in acute myocardial infarction complicated by cardiogenic shock. J Am Coll Cardiol 1991;17:167.

8. Brown TM, Lannone LA, Gordon DF, et al. Percutaneous myocardial reperfusion reduces mortality in acute myocardial infarction complicated by cardiogenic shock. Circulation 1995;72:III-309.

9. O'Neill WW, Erbel R, Laufer N, et al. Coronary angioplasty therapy of cardiogenic shock complicating acute myocardial infarction. Circulation 1995;72:III-309.

10. Meyer P, Blanc P, Badouy M, Morand P. Treatment de choc cardiogenique primaire par angioplastie transluminale coronarienne a la phase aigue de l'Infarctus. Arch Mal Coeur 1990;83:329-334.

11. Lee L, Bates ER, Pitt B, Walton JA, et al. Percutaneous transluminal coronary angioplasty improves survival in acute myocardial infarction complicated by cardiogenic shock. Circulation 1988;78:145-151.

12. Seydoux C, Goy J-J, Beuret P, et al. Effectiveness of percutaneous transluminal coronary angioplasty in cardiogenic shock during acute myocardial infarction. Am J Cardiol 1992;68:968-969.

13. Heuser RR, Maddoux GL, Goss JE, et al. Coronary angioplasty in the treatment of cardiogenic shock: the therapy of choice. J Am Coll Cardiol 1986;7:219.

14. Shani J, Rivera M, Geengart A, et al. Percutaneous transluminal coronary angioplasty in cardiogenic shock. J Am Coll Cardiol 1986;7:149.

15. Disler L, Haitas B, et al. Cardiogenic shock in evolving myocardial infarction: treatment by angioplasty and streptokinase. Heart Lung 1987;16:649.

16. Verna E, Repetto S, Boscarina M, et al. Emergency coronary angioplasty in patients with severe left ventricular dysfunction of cardiogenic shock after acute myocardial infarction. Eur Heart J 1989;10:958-966.

17. Hochman JS, Boland J, Sleeper LA, Porway M, Brinker J, Col J, Jacobs A, Slater J, Miller D, Wasserman H, Menegus MA, Talley D, McKinlay S, Sanborn T, LeJemtel T, and the SHOCK Registry Investigators. Current spectrum of cardiogenic shock and effect of early revascularization on mortality. Circulation 1995;91:372-881.

18. Holmes DR, Bates ER, Kleiman NS, Sadowski Z, Horgan JHS, Morris DC, Califf RM, Berger PB, Topol EJ. Contemporary reperfusion therapy for cardiogenic shock: The GUSTO-I trial experience. J Am Coll Cardiol 1995;26:668-674.

19. Anderson RD, Stebbins AL, Bates E, Stomel R, Granger CB, Ohman EM. Underutilization of aortic counterpulsation in patients with cardiogenic shock: Observations from the GUSTO-1 study. Circulation 1995;92:I-139.

45. Answer: b (false)

There are few randomized trials of rescue PTCA compared to medical therapy.[1-4] In TAMI-5,[5] rescue PTCA resulted in greater predischarge vessel patency, better wall motion in the infarct zone, and less recurrent ischemia than medical therapy. In the multicenter international RESCUE study (Randomized Evaluation of Salvage angioplasty with Combined Utilization of Endpoints), rescue PTCA patients had better left ventricular function, less congestive heart failure, and lower mortality at 1-month and 1-year than medically-treated patients.[2] Thus, immediate angiography after thrombolytic therapy followed by rescue PTCA of a persistent occlusion is a safe and reasonable strategy.

References:
1. Califf RM, Topol EJ, Stack RS, et al. Evaluation of combination thrombolytic therapy and timing of cardiac catheterization in acute myocardial infarction: results of Thrombolysis and Angioplasty in Myocardial Infarction-Phase 5 randomized trial. Circulation 1991;83:1543-1556.

2. Ellis SG, Ribeiro da Silva E, Heyndrickx G, Talley D, Cernigliaro C, Steg G, Spaulding C, Nobuyoshi M, Erbel R, Vassanelli C, Topol EJ. Randomized comparison of rescue angioplasty with conservative management of patients with early failure of thrombolysis for acute anterior myocardial infarction. Circulation 1994;90:2280-2284.

3. Belenkie I, Traboulsi M, Hall CA, Hansen JL, Roth DL, Manyari D, Filipchuck NG, Schnurr LR, Rosenal TW, Smith ER, Knudtson M. Rescue angioplasty during myocardial infarction has a beneficial effect on mortality: A tenable hypothesis. Can J Cardiol 1992;8:357-362.

4. The CORAMI Study Group. Outcome of attempted rescue coronary angioplasty after failed thrombolysis for acute myocardial infarction. Am J of Cardiol 1994;74:172174.

5. O'Neill W, Timmis GC, Bourdillon PD, Lai P, Ganghadarhan V, Walton J, Ramos R, Laufer N, Gordon S, Schork MA, Pitt B. A prospective randomized clinical trial of intracoronary streptokinase versus coronary angioplasty for acute myocardial infarction. N Engl J Med 1986;314:812-818.

46. Answer: a, b, d

Rescue PTCA improves regional wall motion and LV function, and may reduce the risk of heart failure, shock, and death in patients with a large infarctions. The prognosis of patients after successful rescue PTCA is similar to that after successful thrombolysis. However, patients requiring rescue PTCA are at increased risk for reocclusion compared to patients treated with primary PTCA or successful thrombolytic therapy, and early mortality is high if rescue PTCA is unsuccessful.

47. Answer: b (false)

Even when thrombolysis is successful, a high-grade residual stenosis is present in the majority of patients. The potential value of immediate PTCA is to prevent reocclusion and improve LV function; however, several randomized trials of immediate PTCA after successful thrombolysis have demonstrated that routine PTCA is associated with *more* transfusions and emergency CABG, a trend toward *higher* mortality, and *no* improvement in pre-discharge ejection fraction.[1-6] Therefore, routine PTCA is not recommended after successful thrombolysis when TIMI 3 flow is present. Emergency angiography is often recommended, however, for ongoing ischemia and/or hemodynamic instability; PTCA is then performed when a critical stenosis (> 75%) and impaired (TIMI $\leq$ 2) flow are evident.

References:
1. Califf Rm, Topol EJ, Stack RS, et al. Evaluation of combination thrombolytic therapy and timing of cardiac catheterization in acute myocardial infarction: Results of thrombolysis and angioplasty in myocardial infarction-Phase 5 randomized trial. Circulation 1991;83:1543-1546.
2. Michels KB, Yusif S. Does PTCA in acute myocardial infarction affect mortality and reinfarction rates? A quantitative overview (meta-analysis) of the randomized clinical trials. Circulation 1995;91:476-485.
3. Belenkie I, Traboulsi M, Hall CA, Hansen JL, Roth DL, Manyari D, Filipchuck NG, Schnurr LR, Rosenal TW, Smith ER, Knudtson M. Rescue angioplasty during myocardial infarction has a beneficial effect on mortality: A tenable hypothesis. Can J Cardiol 1992;8:357-362.
4. Rogers WJ, Baim DS, Gore JM, et al for the TIMI-IIA investigators. Comparison of immediate invasive, delayed invasive, and conservative strategies after tissue-type plasminogen activator. Circulation 1990;81:1457-1476.
5. Topol EJ, Califf RM, George BS, et al and the Thrombolysis and Angioplasty in myocardial infarction study group. A randomized trial of immediate versus delayed elective angioplasty after intravenous tissue plasminogen activator in acute myocardial infarction. N Engl J Med 1987;317:581-588.
6. Simoons ML, Arnold AET, Bertiu A, et al. Thrombolysis with tissue plasminogen activator in acute myocardial infarction: No additional benefit from immediate percutaneous coronary angioplasty. Lancet 1988;I:197-202.

48. Answer: b (false)

Several trials[1-5] have compared invasive (routine PTCA before discharge) vs. conservative approaches (PTCA only for spontaneous or inducible ischemia) after successful thrombolysis; pooled data failed to show differences in mortality, reinfarction, or ejection fraction between groups. However, patients treated conservatively had more residual ischemia on predischarge exercise testing, and patients with prior MI treated conservatively had higher in-hospital mortality (12% vs. 4%, p < 0.001).[6] In contrast, in-hospital mortality in diabetic patients without prior MI was lower with the conservative approach (4% vs. 15%, p < 0.001).

References:
1. The TIMI Study Group. Comparison of invasive and conservative strategies after treatment with intravenous tissue plasminogen activator in acute myocardial infarction. Results of the Thrombolysis in Myocardial Infarction (TIMI) Phase II Trial. N Engl J Med 1989;320:
2. SWIFT (Should We Intervene Following Thrombolysis?) Trial Study Group. SWIFT trial of delayed elective intervention vs. conservative treatment after thrombolysis with anistreplase in acute myocardial infarction. Br Med J 1991;302:5550560.
3. Barbash GI, Roth A, Hod H, et al. Randomized controlled trial of late in-hospital angiography and angioplasty versus conservative management after treatment with recombinant tissue-type plasminogen activator in acute myocardial infarction. Am J Cardiol 1990;66:538-545.

4. Van den Brand MJ, Betrui A, Bescos LL, et al. Randomized trial of deferred angioplasty after thrombolysis for acute myocardial infarction. Coronary Artery Disease 1992;3:393-401.

5. Ozbek C, Dyckmans J, Sen S, et al. Comparison of invasive and conservative strategies after treatment with streptokinase in acute myocardial infarction: results of a randomized trial (SIAM). J Am Coll Cardiol 1990;15:63A (abstr).

6. Mueller HS, Cohen LS, Braunwald E, et al, for the TIMI Investigators. Predictors of early morbidity and mortality after thrombolytic therapy of acute myocardial infarction. Analyses of patient subgroups in the Thrombolysis in Myocardial Infarction (TIMI) Trial, Phase II. Circulation 1992;85:1254-1264.

49. Answer: All

Profound hypotension and bradycardia (Bezold-Jarisch reflex from stimulation of vagal afferents) or sudden ventricular fibrillation (VF) may occur after PTCA of an occluded coronary artery, especially the RCA.[1] Bates[2] and Gacioch[3] reported a high incidence of arrhythmia after PTCA-mediated reperfusion, but many of these patients underwent rescue PTCA after failed lytic therapy. One study[4] reported that minor events were more common after primary PTCA for the RCA; major events (death, CPR, defibrillation, cardioversion, IABP, or urgent surgery) were uncommon, except in patients with cardiogenic shock. The PAR registry reported sustained hypotension, bradyarrhythmias, and VT/VF in 16% of RCA infarcts compared to 5% of other infarcts.[5] In PAMI-I,[6] VF occurred in 6.7% of PTCA-treated patients, and was more common in patients with inferior than anterior MI (9.7% vs 1.4%, $p = 0.03$). Slow reperfusion and IV β-blockers were adopted in the PAMI-2 study to reduce severe reperfusion arrhythmias, which resulted in significant reduction in VF (6.7% vs 3.8%, $P = 0.01$).[7]

References:
1. Kaplan B, Safian R, Grines C, et al. Differences in outcome after angioplasty for AMI: The left anterior descending artery vs the right coronary. J Am Coll Cardio 1996;27:166A.

2. Bates ER. Reperfusion therapy in inferior myocardial infarction. J Am Coll Cardiol 1988;12:44A-51A.

3. Gacioch GM, Topol EJ. Sudden paradoxic clinical deterioration during angioplasty of the occluded right coronary artery in acute myocardial infarction. J Am Coll Cardiol 1989;14:1202-9.

4. Kahn JK, Rutherford BD, McConahay DR, et al. Catheterization laboratory events and hospital outcome with direct angioplsty for acute myocardial infarction. Circulation 1990;82:1910-1915.

5. Ohman EM, Califf RM, Topol EJ, et al. Consequences of reocclusion after successful reperfusion therapy in acute myocardial infarction. Circulation 1990;82:781-91.

6. Grines CL, Browne KF, Marco J, Rothbaum D, Stone GW, O'Keefe J, Overlie P, Donohue B, Chelliah N, Timmis GC, Vlietstra RE, Strzelecki M, Puchrowicz-Ochocki S, O'Neill W. A comparison of immediate angioplasty with thrombolytic therapy for acute myocardial infarction. N Engl J Med 1993;328:673-679.

7. Grines CL, Griffin JJ, Brodie BR, Stone GW, Donohue BC, Balestrini CE, Wharton TP, Spain MG, Shimshak T, Jones D, Mason D, Sachs D, O'Neill WW. The second Primary Angioplasty for Myocardial Infarction study (PAMI-II): Preliminary Report. Circulation 1994;90:I-433.

50. Answer: d

Compared to thrombolytic therapy, primary PTCA is associated with less recurrent ischemia (10.6% vs 31.4%) and reinfarction (1.9% vs 8.1%). The low rate of recurrent ischemia after primary PTCA is attributed to the routine use of aspirin prior to PTCA, aggressive heparinization, wide patency of the infarct-related artery, and avoidance of adjunctive thrombolysis.

51. Answer: a

Compared to elective PTCA, PTCA for unstable angina or acute MI is associated with an increase risk of abrupt closure, recurrent MI, and death. Vessel reocclusion after primary PTCA occurs in 5% of patients prior to discharge.[1]

Reference:
1. Griffin J, Grines CL, Marsales D, et al. A prospective, randomized trial evaluating the prophylactic use of balloon pumping in high risk myocardial infarction patients: PAMI-2. J Am Coll Cardiol 1995;25:86A.

52. Answer: d

Reocclusion after successful rescue PTCA is as high as 29%.[1]

Reference:
1. Abbottsmith CW, Topol EJ, George BS, et al. Fate of patients with acute myocardial infarction with patency of the infarct-related vessel achieved with successful thrombolysis versus rescue angioplasty. J Am Coll Cardiol 1990;16:770-778.

53. Answer: c

By 6 months, reocclusion occurs in 10-15% and restenosis in 40%, increasing patient morbidity, mortality, and the need for repeat revascularization.[1-4]

References:
1. Zijlstra F, Jan de Boaer M, Hoorntje JCA, Reiffer S, Reiber JHC, Suryapranata H. A comparison of immediate coronary angioplasty with intravenous streptokinase in acute myocardial infarction. N Engl J Med 1993;328:680-684.
2. Brodie BR, Grines CL, Ivanhoe R, Knopf W, Taylor G, O'Keefe J, Weintraub RA, Berdan LG, Tcheng JE, Woodlief LH, Califf RM, O'Neill WW. Six-month clinical and angiographic follow-up after direct angioplasty for acute myocardial infarction. Circulation 1994;90:156-162.
3. O'Neill WW, Weintraub R, Grines CL, Meany TB, Brodie BR, Friedman HZ, Ramos RG, Gangadharan V, Levin RN, Choksi N, Westveer DC, Strzelecki RN, Timmis GC. A prospective placebo-controlled randomized trial of intravenous streptokinase and angioplasty therapy of acute myocardial infarction. Circulation 1992;86:1710-1717.
4. Nunn C, O'Neill W, Rothbaum D, O'Keefe J, Overlie P, Donohue B, Mason D, Catlin T, Grines C. Primary angioplasty for myocardial infarction improves long-term survival : PAMI-1 follow-up. J Am Coll Cardiol 1996;27:153A.

54. Answer: a

Medical therapy for unstable angina is associated with in-hospital mortality in 1% and myocardial infarction in 7-9%; cardiac events at 1-year include death in 8-18% and myocardial infarction in 14-22%.[1]

Reference:
1. Braunwald E, Mark DB, Jones RH, Cheitlin MD, Fuster V, McCauley K, Edwards C, Green LA, Mushlin AL, Swain JA, Smith EE, Cowan M, Rose GC, Concannon CA, Grines CL, Brown L, Lytle BW, Goldman LA, Topol EJ, Willerson JT, Brown J, Archibald N. Unstable Angina: Diagnosis and Management - Clinical Practice Guidelines. U.S. Department of Health and Human Services. AHCPR Publication No. 94-0682, March 15, 1994.

55. Answer: a (true)

Patients with a history of antecedent angina are more likely to have significant multivessel disease, whereas patients with new onset unstable angina generally have ulceration and thrombus. Early angiography demonstrates a high incidence of complex lesions with ulceration, intraluminal haziness, and thrombus. Many culprit lesions improve with time, due to spontaneous lysis, passivation of platelets (due to aspirin and heparin), and plaque remodeling. Coronary thrombus, plaque rupture, and mural hemorrhage are common findings in patients who die after unstable angina.[1]

Answers

Reference:
1. Roberts W, Kragel A, Gertz S, Roberts S. Coronary arteries in unstable angina, acute myocardial infarction and sudden coronary death. Am J Cardiol 1994;127:1588-1593.

56. Answer: a

Although the technical success rate of PTCA in unstable angina is similar to stable angina, the incidence of periprocedural complications is higher.[1,2] Patients with rest angina and ECG changes have more complications after PTCA[3,4] or new devices.[5-7] The TIMI-3B trial randomized 1473 patients with unstable angina or non-Q MI to PTCA vs. medical therapy.[8] Although there were no differences in death or MI, PTCA allowed earlier discharge, fewer readmissions and less antianginal medication. Medically-treated patients ultimately required angiography in 57% and revascularization in 40% before hospital discharge, which increased to 73% and 58% at 1 year.[9] Thus, most patients ultimately require intervention; early intervention is preferred to reduce cost and improve quality of life.

References:
1. Myler RK, Shaw RE, Stertzer SH, et al. Unstable angina and coronary angioplasty. Circulation 1990;82:II-88-95.
2. Bentivoglio LG, Holubkov R, Kelsey SF et al. Short and long term outcome of percutaneous transluminal coronary angioplasty in unstable versus stable angina pectoris: A report of the 1985-1986 NHLBI PTCA Registry. Cathet Cardiovasc Diagn 1991;23:227.
3. Bittl J, Strong J, Brinker J, et al. Treatment with Bivalirudin (Hirulog) as compared with heparin during coronary angioplasty for unstable or post infarction angina. N Engl J Med 1995;333:764-9.
4. Serruys P, Herrman J, Simon R, et al. A comparison of Hirudin with heparin in the prevention of restenosis after coronary angioplasty. N Engl J Med 1995;333:757-63.
5. Bengtson J, Wilson J. Interventions in unstable angina. In: Interventional Cardiovascular Medicine - Prinicipals and Practice. Eds. Roubin, Califf, O'Neill, Phillips, Stack. Churchill Livingstone, Inc. New York, New York, 1996.
6. Chuang Y, Popma J, Satler et al. Increasing angina predicts an unfavorable outcome after new device angioplasty. J Am Coll Cardiol 1994;289A.
7. Hong M, Popma J, Wong S, et al. Incidence of and factors associated with abrupt closure in patients undergoing elective, new device angioplasty in native coronary arteries. J Am Coll Cardiol 1995;122A.
8. TIMI-3B Investigators. Effects of tissue plasminogen activator and a comparison of early invasive and conservative strategies in unstable angina and non Q-wave myocardial infarction. Circulation 1994;89:1545-1556.
9. Anderson H, Cannon C, Stone P, et al. One year results of the thrombolysis in myocardial infarction (TIMI)3B clinical trial. J Am Coll Cardiol 1995;26:1643-1650.

57. Answer: a, b, c

The role of IABP in the setting of PTCA for unstable ischemic syndromes is somewhat controversial: In some studies, balloon pumps improved LV function and reduced reocclusion from 18-27% to 2-8%;[1,2] in other studies of high risk patients (age > 70 years, 3 vessel disease, EF < 45%, suboptimal PTCA, vein graft, serious arrhythmias), IABP resulted in less ischemia and repeat PTCA, but failed to reduce death, recurrent MI, heart failure, stroke, reocclusion, or LV function at 1 and 6 weeks after acute MI.[3,4] In the PAMI-2 trial,[5] if 2 or more high-risk factors were present, IABP reduced in-hospital heart failure. In CAVEAT, 65% of the patients randomized to DCA had unstable angina. Compared to PTCA, DCA was associated with more non Q-wave MI in-hospital (5.9% vs. 2.5%, p = 0.006) and at 6-months (8.2% vs. 3.8%, p = 0.0031).[6] Unless the lesion is undilatable, Rotablator is not recommended due to the risk of distal embolization of thrombus and no-reflow. Preliminary experience supports the feasibility and safety of stenting in the setting of recent or acute MI; procedural success is > 90%, and the incidence of stent thrombosis is 0-9.6%.[7-15]

References:
1. Ohman GM, George B, White C, et al. Use of aortic counterpulsation to improve sustained coronary patency during acute MI. Results of a randomized trial. Circulation 1994;90:792-799.
2. Ishihara M, Sato H, Tateishi H, et al. Intraaortic balloon pumping as the postangioplasty strategy in acute myocardial infarction. Am Heart J 1991;122:385-389.
3. Griffin J, Grines CL, Marsales D, et al. A prospective, randomized trial evaluating the prophylactic use of balloon pumping in high risk myocardial infarction patients: PAMI-2. J Am Coll Cardiol 1995;25:86A.
4. Grines CL, Brodie BR, Griffin JJ, Donohue BC, Costantini C, Balestrini C, Stone G, Jones DE, Sachs D, O'Neill WW. Prophylactic intraaortic balloon pumping for acute myocardial infarction does not improve left ventricular function. J Am Coll Cardiol 1996;27:167A.
5. Stone GW, Marsalese D, Brodie B, Griffin J, Donohue B, Costantini C, Balestrini C, Wharton, Jones D, Sachs D, Grines CL. The routine use of intra-aortic balloon pumping after primary PTCA improves clinical outcomes in very high risk patients with acute myocardial infarction - Results of the PAMI-2 trial. Circulation 1995;92:I-139.
6. Topol EJ, Leya F, Pinkerton CA, et al. A comparison of directional atherectomy with coronary angioplasty in patients with coronary artery disease. N Engl J Med 1993;329:221-7.
7. Verna E, Castiglioni B, Onofri M, et al. Intracoronary stenting of the infarct-related artery without anticoagulation in acute myocardial infarction. Euro Heart J 1995;16:12.
8. Levy G, deBoisgelin, Volpiliere R, Bouvagnet P. Intracoronary stenting in direction infarct angioplasty: Is it dangerous? Circulation 1995;92:I-139.
9. Romero M, Medina A, Suarez J, et al. Elective Palmaz-Schatz stent implantation in acute coronary syndromes induced by thrombus-containing lesions. Euro Heart J 1995;16:179.
10. Repetto S, Onofri M, Castiglioni B, et al. Stenting of the infarct related artery during complicated angioplasty in acute myocardial infarction. J Invas Cardiol 1996;8:177-183.
11. Rodriguez A, Fernandex M, Santaera O, et al. Coronary stenting in patients undergoing PTCA during acute myocardial infarction. Am J Cardiol 1996;77:685-689.
12. Steinhubl S, Moliterno O, Teirstein P, et al. Stenting for acute myocardial infarction: The early United States multicenter experience. J Am Coll Cardiol 1996;22:279A.
13. Benzuly K, Allen D, Mason D, et al. A prospective pilot study of primary stenting for acute myocardial infarction (STAMI). J Invas Cardiol 1996;8:38.
14. Stone G, Marice M, Brodie B, et al. Primary stenting in acute MI: Interim report from the PAMI-3 stent pilot study. European Congress of Cardiology. August, 1996.
15. Lefkovits J, Anderson K, Weisman H, Topol E. Increased risk of non-Q-MI following DCA: Evidence for a platelet dependant mechanism from the EPIC Trial. Circulation 1994;90:I-214.

58. Answer: a, c, d, f

Aspirin reduces the incidence of acute closure by 30-50% and is considered routine pharmacotherapy prior to and after all percutaneous coronary interventions. However, despite its ability to inhibit cyclooxygenase and the arachidonic acid pathway, platelet aggregation still occurs.[1] In randomized trials, Ticlopidine has been shown to reduce stroke in patients with transient ischemic attacks and to reduce MI in patients with unstable angina.[2] Aspirin and Ticlopidine have shown a synergistic effect in reducing platelet deposition[3] and thrombin generation after PTCA.[4] The EPIC (Evaluation of 7E3 in the Prevention of Ischemic Complications) trial randomized 2099 high-risk PTCA or DCA patients (unstable angina, MI or high risk lesion morphology) to ReoPro bolus, bolus and infusion, or placebo.[5,6] Among the 64 patients enrolled for primary PTCA (n=42) or rescue PTCA (n=22), the acute and 6 month ischemic endpoints were reduced in the ReoPro group.[7] Among the 489 patients with unstable or post-MI angina, the rate of CK elevation was higher in the placebo group (9% vs 1.8%).[8] Although the rate of early death or revascularization was similar, less mortality was observed at 6 months after ReoPro (1.8% vs 6.6%, p = 0.038). In addition, preliminary data from the European CAPTURE trial demonstrated a reduction in the 30-day combined endpoint of death, MI, or urgent reintervention for unstable angina patients treated with ReoPro for 18-24 hrs prior to PTCA; this effect was mainly due to a reduction in CK elevation (placebo 9.4%; ReoPro 4.4%).[9] Intraprocedural heparin dosed to maintain an ACT of 300 seconds during elective PTCA appears adequate to reduce the risk of abrupt closure.[10] However, the "ideal ACT" is not known. Since unstable angina and acute MI patients are hypercoagulable, higher ACT levels may confer additional benefit. An ACT of 300 did not completely suppress thrombin activity in humans, and resistance was predictive of acute ischemic events following PTCA and directional atherectomy.[11-13] Hirudin, a peptide derived from the medicinal leech, has been shown to effectively reduce platelet deposition and restenosis in animal models. In a randomized trial comparing hirudin vs. heparin in 1141 unstable angina patients undergoing PTCA, hirudin was associated with fewer ischemic events within the first 96 hours, but there was no difference in angina, major cardiac events, or restenosis at 7-months.[14] The GUSTO 2-B substudy randomized acute MI patients undergoing primary PTCA to heparin or hirudin; preliminary reports suggest no significant difference in clinical outcomes. Although some studies of unstable angina show immediate angiographic improvement after thrombolytic therapy, multiple recent randomized trials have consistently demonstrated a *worse* clinical outcome for PTCA patients treated with thrombolytic therapy,[15-21] even when angiographic features most likely to benefit from lytics (complex lesions, filling defects) are present! Potential mechanisms by which thrombolytic agents potentiate vessel occlusion include enhanced platelet aggregation[22-24] and intramural hemorrhage.[25-28] Furthermore, coronary dissections that occur during PTCA may be more difficult to "tack-up" when thrombolytics have been given. Based on a large body of data, routine thrombolytic therapy should be avoided in patients undergoing PTCA for unstable angina.

References:
1. Coller BS. Platelets and thrombolytic therapy. N Engl J Med 1990;322:33-42.
2. Sadowski Z, Kuczak D, Dyduszynski. Comparison of ticlopidine and aspirin in unstable angina, presented at European Congress of Cardiology, 1995.
3. Jeong M, Owen W, Staabon, et al. Does ticlopidine effect platelet deposition and acute stent thrombosis? Circulation 1995;92:I-489.
4. Gregorini L, Marco J, Fajadet J, et al. Ticlopidine alternates post-angioplasty thrombin generation . Circulation 1995;92:I-608.
5. EPIC Investigators. Use of a monoclonal antibody directed against the platelet glycoprotein IIb/IIIa receptor in high-risk coronary angioplasty. N Engl J Med 1994;330:956-961.
6. Topol EJ, Califf RM, Weisman HF, Ellis SG, Tcheng JE, Worley S, Ivanhoe R, George BS, Fintel D, Weston M, Sigmon K, Anderson KM, Lee KL, Willerson JT; on behalf of the EPIC investigators. Randomised trial of coronary intervention with antibody against platelet IIb/IIIa integrin for reduction of clinical restenosis: Results at six months. Lancet 1994;343:881-886.
7. Simoons M. The CAPTURE study, as presented at the 45th Annual Session of the American College of Cardiology in Orlando, Florida, USA, March 1996.
8. Linoff AM, Califf R, Anderson , et al. Striking clinical benefit with platelet IIb/IIIa inhibition by C7E3 among patients with unstable angina: Outcome in the EPIC trial. Circulation 1994;90:I-21.
9. Simoons M. The CAPTURE study, as presented at the 45th Annual Session of the American College of Cardiology in Orlando, Florida, USA, March 1996.
10. Ferguson J, Dougherty K, Gaos C, et al. Relation between procedural activated coagulation time and outcome after percutaneous transluminal coronary angioplasty. J Am Coll Caridol 1994;23:1061-1065.
11. Snitzer R, Hiremath Y, Lee J, et al. Suppression of intracoronary thrombin activity by weight-adjusted heparin administration during coronary interventions. Circulation 1995;92:I-609.
12. Winters K, Oltrona L, Hiremath Y, et al. Heparin-resistant thrombin activity is associated with acute ischemic events during high risk coronary interventions. Circulation 1995;92:I-608.
13. Harrington Ra, Leimberer JD, Berdan L, Topol EJ, Califf RM for the CAVEAT Investigators. The ACT index: A method for stratifying likelihood of success and risk of acute complications in coronary intervention. Circulation 1993;88:I-208.
14. Serruys P, Herrman J, Simon R, et al. A comparison of Hirudin with heparin in the prevention of restenosis after coronary angioplasty. N Engl J Med 1995;333:757-63.
15. O'Neill WW, Weintraub R, Grines CL, Meany TB, Brodie BR, Friedman HZ, Ramos RG, Gangadharan V, Levin RN, Choksi N, Westveer DC, Strzelecki RN, Timmis GC. A prospective placebo-controlled randomized trial of intravenous streptokinase and angioplasty therapy of acute myocardial infarction. Circulation 1992;86:1710-1717.
16. Grines C, Brodie B, Griffin J, Donohue B, Sampaoiesi A, Costantini C, Sachs D, Wharton T, Esente P, Spain M, Stone G. Which primary PTCA patients may benefit from new technologies? Circulation, 1995;92:I-146.
17. Spielberg C, Schnitzer L, Linderer T, et al. Influence of catheter technology and adjuvant medication on acute complications in percutaneous coronary angioplasty. Cathet Cardiovasc Diagn, 1990;21:72.
18. Ambrose JA, Torre SR, Sharma SK, et al. Adjuvant urokinase for PTCA in unstable angina: final angiographic results of TAUSA pilot study. Circulation, 1991;84:II-590.
19. Buller CE, Fung AY, Thompson CR, Ricci DR, Thompson B, Schrachtman M, Williams DO. Does pre-treatment with tPA improve safety of coronary angioplasty in acute coronary syndrome? Results from TIMI II-B. Circulation 1994;90:I-22.
20. Ambrose JA, Almeida OD, Sharma SK, Torre SR, Marmur JD, Israel DH, Ratner DE, Weiss MB, Hjemdahl-Monsen CE, Myler TK, Moses J, Unterecker WJ, Grunwald AM, Garrett JS, Cowley MJ, Anwar A, Sobolski J for the TAUSA Investigators. Adjunctive thrombolytic therapy during angioplasty for ischemic rest angina. Results of the TAUSA Trial. Circulation 1994;90:69-77.
21. Mehran R, Ambrose JA, Bongu RM, Almeida OD, Israel DH, Torre S, Sharma SK, Ratner ED for the TAUSA study group. Angioplasty of complex lesions in ischemic rest angina: Results of the Thrombolysis and Angioplasty in UnStable Angina (TAUSA) trial. J Am Coll Cardiol 1995;26:961-966.
22. Kerins DM, Roy L, FitzGerald GA, Pitzgerald DJ. Platelet and vascular function during coronary thrombolysis with tissue-type plasminogen activator. Circulation, 1989;80:1718.
23. Bennett WR, Yawn DH, Migliore PJ, et al. Activation of the complement system by recombinant tissue plasminogen activator. J Am Coll cardiol, 1987;10:627.
24. Fitzgerald DJ, Roy L, Wright F, Fitzgerald GA. Functional significance of platelet activation following coronary thrombolysis. Circulation, 1987;76:IV-153.
25. Castaneda-Zuniga WR, Sibley R, Amplatz K. The pathologic basis of angioplasty. Angiology, 1984;35:195.
26. Kohchi K, Taebayashi S, Block PC. Arterial changes after percutaneous transluminal coronary angioplasty: results at autopsy. J Am Coll Cardiol, 1987;10:592.
27. Waller BF, Rothbaum DA, Pinkerton CA, et al. Status of the myocardium and infarct-related coronary artery in 19 necropsy patients with acute recanalization

using pharmacologic (streptokinase, r-tissue plasminogen activator), mechanical (percutaneous transluminal coronary angioplasty) or combined types of reperfusion therapy. J Am Coll Cardiol, 1987;9:785.

28. Colavita PG, Ideker RE, Reimer KA, et al. The spectrum of pathology associated with percutaneous transluminal coronary angioplasty during acute myocardial infarction. J Am Coll Cardiol, 1986;8:855.

LV DYSFUNCTION

59. Answer: a, b, d, e

Potential Candidates for Supported Angioplasty

- Target vessel supplies the majority of viable myocardium.

- Ejection fraction < 20%.

- Jeopardy score > 3.

- Cardiogenic shock and multivessel disease.

60. Answer: a, c, d

IABPs decrease myocardial oxygen demand, increase coronary perfusion pressure (by augmenting diastolic blood pressure and decreasing left ventricular filling pressure), and increase cardiac output by 20-39%.[1] IABPs were previously associated with a high incidence of vascular complications (9-43%), including AV fistulae, pseudoaneurysms, iliofemoral thrombosis and local bleeding. In contrast, the PAMI-2 study found no increase in vascular complications in patients randomized to IABP after PTCA for acute MI. Complications are more common in patients with pre-existing vascular disease, diabetics, and females (4 times more common than men); however, complication rates are not affected by age, adequacy of anticoagulation, or body surface area.[2] Effective diastolic augmentation requires a stable cardiac rhythm.[3] Moderate hemolysis and thrombocytopenia are common, although platelet counts below 50,000 are quite unusual.

References:

1. Kaltenbach M, Gruentzig A, Rentrop P, et al. In: Transluminal Coronary Angioplasty and Intracoronary Thrombolysis, 1982;145-150.
2. Alderman JD, Gabliani GI, McCabe CH, et al. Incidence and management of limb ischemia with percutaneous wire-guided intraaortic balloon catheters. J Am Coll Cardiol 1987;9:524-530.
3. Fuchs RM, Brin KP, Brinker JA, et al. Augmentation of regional coronary blood flow by intra-aortic balloon counterpulsation in patients with unstable angina. Circulation 1983;68:117-123.

61. Answer: e

For CPS, intravenous heparin, 300 U/kg (average 20,000-25,000 units) is given as a bolus. ACT should be >400 seconds while on CPS. Prophylactic blood transfusions should be considered in patients undergoing CPS if baseline hemoglobin <10gm/dl.

Answers

62. Answer: a (true)

Hypotension is very common within the first few minutes of CPS and usually responds to a bolus of normal saline (100-300 cc) rather than increasing the flow rate. Hypotension occurs secondary to a decrease in systemic vascular resistance from CPS-induced volume shifts or vasodilation. On occasion, decreasing CPS flow may improve systemic vascular resistance and restore blood pressure. When vasopressors are required, Neosynephrine (1 mg) can be given directly thorough the CPS unit.

63. Answer: a, b

CPS provides excellent systemic perfusion independent of ventricular function or intrinsic cardiac rhythm. Patient perception of chest pain is less common in CPS-supported patients, allowing for prolonged balloon inflations.[1] The most significant deficiency of CPS-supported angioplasty is that myocardial ischemia still occurs distal to the inflated balloon; regional wall motion abnormalities and anaerobic metabolism occur during balloon inflation despite CPS.[2] CPS cannot be continued > 6 hrs because of disseminated intravascular coagulation, hemolysis, third-spacing of fluids, hypokalemia, and hypomagnesemia.

References:
1. Vogel RA, Shawl F, Tommaso C, et al. Initial report of the national registry of elective cardiopulmonary bypass supported coronary angioplasty. J Am Coll Cardiol 1990;15:23-29.
2. Stack RK, Pavlides GS, Miller R, et al. Hemodynamic and metabolic effects of venoarterial cardiopulmonary support in coronary artery disease. Am J Cardiol 1991;67:1344-1348.

64. Answer: a (true)

Because of the many drawbacks associated with prophylactic CPS, standby CPS has emerged as an accepted support strategy. When this approach is employed, 5-6F sheaths are usually placed in the left femoral artery and vein after angiographic views demonstrate their suitability for CPS cannulae. Experienced operators can usually prime the support system and insert cannulas in less than 5 minutes.[1] Data from the CPS registry indicate that only 5-10% of patients with standby CPS will actually require initiation of circulatory support. Mortality rates in patients who undergo standby CPS (6%) are similar to those in whom prophylactic placement was performed. Several reports suggest that patient outcome improves when CPS is initiated within 10 minutes of cardiac arrest unresponsive to conventional ACLS measures.

Reference:
1. Overlie PA. Emergency use of portable cardiopulmonary bypass. Cathet Cardiovasc Diagn 1990;20:27-31.

65. Answer: d

Autoperfusion catheters are inserted over 0.014-0.018-inch guidewires; because of differences in profile and trackability, they may be more difficult to place in tortuous vessels or distal coronary segments than nonperfusion balloons. Once properly positioned, inflation pressures > 6 ATM may impair blood flow. The central lumen should be intermittently flushed with heparinized saline to prevent thrombosis. Distal flow is directly related to the perfusion pressure; rates as high as 40-60 ml/min have been reported.[1] However, hypotension must be corrected since flow rates are dependent on arterial pressure; fluids, IABP or vasopressors may be necessary. Subjective and objective evidence of ischemia, ST segment shifts, and segmental wall motion abnormalities improve with autoperfusion catheters.[2] In a nonrandomized series of 31 patients in whom abrupt closure developed after coronary angioplasty, a bail-out catheter was successfully placed before surgery in 61%. Among those in whom a bailout catheter could be properly positioned, there was a lower incidence of Q-wave infarction (9% vs. 75%), less ST segment elevation, and greater subsequent use of internal mammary grafts.[3]

References:
1. Stack RS, Quigley PJ, Collins G, et al. Perfusion balloon catheter. Am J Cardiol 1988;61:77G-80G.
2. Turi ZG, Campbell CA, Gottimukkala MV, et al. Preservation of distal coronary perfusion during prolonged balloon inflation with an autoperfusion angioplasty catheter. Circulation 1987;75:1273-1280.
3. Banka VS, Trivedi A, Patel R, et al. Prevention of myocardial ischemia during coronary angioplasty: a simple new method for distal antegrade arterial blood perfusion. Am Heart J 1989;118:830-836.

PATIENT CHARACTERISTICS

66. Answer: a, b, c, d

Although coronary artery disease typically occurs with advancing age, 3-6% of patients are less than 40 years old. Compared to older patients, young patients typically have more cardiac risk factors and less extensive disease. Compared to younger patients, elderly patients (age 65-75 years) undergoing coronary revascularization are more often female, and are more likely to have diffuse disease, calcified lesions, unstable angina, prior MI, comorbid conditions, and low ejection fractions. Nevertheless, elective use of CABG, PTCA and new devices can be performed with success rates > 90% and major complication rates of 3-13%.[1-10] However, the elderly are at increased risk of death after acute closure; there is also a 2-3 fold risk of peripheral vascular complications (pseudoaneurysm, AV fistula, large hematoma) and blood transfusions. Patients between the ages of 65-75 with symptomatic coronary artery disease should be offered percutaneous or surgical revascularization; CABG and PTCA achieve similar long-term survival rates. However, PTCA is associated with less in-hospital morbidity and mortality, but more repeat procedures are needed to treat recurrent angina. Procedural success can be achieved in 85% of patients > 80 years old. Compared to younger patients, octogenarians have more acute complications and late cardiac death.

References:
1. Hannan E, and Burke J. Effect of age on mortality in coronary artery bypass surgery in New York, 1991-1992. Am Heart J 1994;128:1184-91.
2. O'Keefe J, Sutton M, et al. Coronary angioplasty versus bypass surgery in patients >70 years old matched for ventricular function. J Am Coll Cardiol 1994;24:425-430.
3. Peterson ED, Gollis JG, Bebchuk JD, DeLong ER, et al. Chances in mortality after myocardial revascularization in the elderly. The National Medicare experience. Ann Intern Med. 1994;121:919-927.
4. Lindsay J, Reddy V, et al. Morbidity and mortality rates in elderly patients undergoing percutaneous coronary transluminal angioplasty. Am Heart J 1994;128:697-702.
5. Burnstein S, Sun GW, Hammer JS, Mann JD, et al. Adjusted influence of age and gender on PTCA outcomes and hospital resource consumption. J Am Coll Cardiol 1994;March Special Issue:223A.
6. Jollis JG, Peterson ED, Bebchuk JD, DeLong ER, et al. Coronary angioplasty in 20,006 patients over age 80 in the United States. J Am Coll Cardiol 1995;

Answers

February Special Issue:47A.

7. Elliot JM, MacIsaac AI, Lefkovits J, Horrigan MCG, Franco I, Whitlow PL. New coronary devices in the elderly: Comparison with angioplasty. Circulation 1994;90:4:I-333.

8. Weyrens EJ, Goldenberg I, Fishman MJ, et al. Percutaneous transluminal coronary angioplasty in patients aged > 90 years. Am J Cardiol 1994;74:397-398.

9. Mullany CJ, Brooks M, Kelsey S, et al. Outcome of patients ≥ 65 years undergoing coronary revascularization: A report from bypass angioplasty revascularization investigation (BARI). J Am Coll Cardiol 1997;29 (Suppl A.);73A.

10. Nasser TK, Fry ETA, Peters TF, et al. In-hospital and interim clinical outcome of coronary stents in the elderly. J Am Coll Cardiol 1997;29 (Suppl A):71A.

67. Answer: b (false)

Several studies suggest that females have a higher in-hospital mortality than males.[1-4] However, females are older, and have a higher prevalence of diabetes mellitus, hypertension, unstable angina, and prior MI. After accounting for these differences, gender has little or no independent effect on outcome; a report from BARI suggested improved outcome for females.[5]

References:

1. Peterson ED, Gollis JG, Bebchuk JD, DeLong ER, et al. Chances in mortality after myocardial revascularization in the elderly. The National Medicare experience. Ann Intern Med. 1994;121:919-927.

2. Malenka DJ, O'Connor GAT, Robb J, Kellett M Jr., et al. Is female gender a risk factor for adverse outcomes following PTCA? Circulation 1995;92:I-437.

3. Weintraub WS, Wenger NK, Kosinski AS, et al. Percutaneous transluminal coronary angioplasty in women compared with men. J Am Coll Cardiol 1994;24:81-90.

4. Arnold A, Mick M, et al. Gender differences for coronary angioplasty. Am J Cardiol 1994;74:18-21.

5. Jacobs A, Kelsey SF, Brooks MM, et al. Improved outcome for women undergoing coronary revascularization: A report from the Bypass Angioplasty Revascularization Investigation (BARI). Circulation 1996;94:I-205.

68. Answer: a (true)

Despite greater comorbidity and coronary risk factors among African-Americans, results from the 1985-1986 NHLBI PTCA Registry indicate that PTCA outcome is independent of race.[1] In a report using new devices, procedure-related death was higher among blacks, which may have been due to a higher prevalence of comorbid conditions.[2]

References:

1. Scott, N, Kelsey S, et al. Percutaneous transluminal coronary angioplasty in African-American patients (The National Heart, Lung, and Blood Institute 1985-1986 percutaneous transluminal coronary angioplasty registry). Am J Cardiol 1994;73:1141-1146.

2. Chuang YC, Merritt AJ, Popma JJ, Bucher TA, et al. Do racial differences affect outcome after new device angioplasty? J Am Coll Cardiol 1994;February Special Issue:301A.

69. Answer: a, c

Compared to nondiabetics, patients with diabetes mellitus have a 2-3 fold higher rate of coronary disease, and are at increased risk of myocardial infarction, congestive heart failure and cardiac mortality. Compared to nondiabetics, patients with diabetes have more in-hospital deaths and strokes, lower long-term survival, and more late MI, CABG, and PTCA.[1,2] Approximately 20-25% of diabetics die within 5 years of CABG. Even after correction for differences in baseline characteristics (unstable angina, lower EF, multivessel disease, other comorbidity), diabetes mellitus is still an independent predictor of adverse outcome. Approximately 10-20% patients submitted for percutaneous intervention have diabetes mellitus. Most PTCA series indicate similar success rates (~ 90%) among diabetics and nondiabetics,[3-5] despite more unstable angina, prior MI, prior CABG, peripheral vascular disease, coronary calcification, and lower ejection fractions in diabetics.[6] In the Bypass Angioplasty Revascularization Investigation (BARI) trial, PTCA patients with diabetes had higher 5-year mortality compared to CABG patients with diabetes (35% vs. 19%, p = 0.0024).[1] In CAVEAT-I, compared to non-diabetics undergoing directional atherectomy, diabetics had more angiographic restenosis (60% vs 47%) and more frequent bypass surgery (12.8% vs 8.5%).[7] Results from STRESS I-II trials suggest that stenting maybe preferred to PTCA in diabetics,[8] but restenosis rates after stenting remain higher in diabetics vs. non-diabetics.[8,9]

References:
1. The BARI Investigators. Comparison of coronary bypass surgery with angioplasty in patients with multivessel disease. N Engl J Med 1996;335:217.
2. Uthoff K, Schuerholz T, Mügge A, Schaefers JH, et al. Coronary revascularization in renal risk patients —coronary angioplasty (PTCA) or coronary artery bypass grafting (CABG)? Circulation 1995;92:I-643.
3. Stein B, Weintraub W, et al. Influence of diabetes mellitus on early and late outcome after percutaneous transluminal coronary angioplasty. Circulation 1995;91:979-989.
4. Faxon DP, Kip KE, Currier JW, Yeh W, et al. Diabetics have a significantly poorer eight year outcome after angioplasty. Circulation 1995;92:I-76.
5. Tan K, Sulke N, et al. Clinical and lesion morphologic determinants of coronary angioplasty success and complications: Current experience. J Am Coll Cardiol 1995;25:855-65.
6. Bailey WL, Westerhausen DR, Rutherford BD, McConahay DR, et al. Characteristics and long term outcomes of diabetic patients presenting for coronary angioplasty. J Am Coll Cardiol 1993;21:2:273A.
7. Levin GN, Jacobs Ak, et al. Impact of diabetes mellitus on percutaneous revascularization (CAVEAT-I). Am J Cardiol 1997;79:748-755.
8. Abizaid A, Mehran R, et al. Does diabetes influence clinical recurrence after coronary stent implantation? J Am Coll Cardiol 1997;29 (Suppl A):188A.
9. Elezi S, Schuhlen H, et al. Stent placement in diabetic versus non-diabetic patients. Six-month angigraphic follow. J Am Coll Cardiol 1997;29 (Suppl A):188A.

70. Answer: a (true)

PTCA of chronic dialysis patients is associated with high rates of ischemic and vascular complications, and frequent clinical recurrence.[1,2] In the largest report to date, patients on hemodialysis undergoing PTCA or CABG had 2-3 fold higher mortality at 1 and 12 months compared to the general PTCA population.[3]

Reference:
1. Chang GL, Ghazzail ZMB, Weintraub WS, et al. Coronary revascularization in patients on chronic dialysis. J Am Coll Cardiol 1997;(Suppl A);180A.
2. Gradaus F, Schoebel FC, Ivens K, et al. High rate of restenosis following coronary angioplasty in patients with chronic renal failure. J Am Coll Cardiol 1997;(Suppl A);418A.
3. Ahmed WH, Pashos CL, Ayanian JZ, Bittle JA. 30-day and one-year mortality in hemodialysis patients undergoing coronary revascularization: Results from a national cohort. Circulation 1995;92:I-75.

71. Answer: b

Coronary artery disease is the leading cause of death among patients who survive more than one year after cardiac transplantation, and affects 20-40% of allografts 1-5 years after transplantation. Angiographic abnormalities range from focal stenoses to diffuse involvement of the entire epicardial coronary circulation. Because allograft hearts are denervated, angina pectoris is distinctly uncommon — clinical presentations typically include silent myocardial infarction, heart failure, or sudden death. Unfortunately, medical therapy and surgical revascularization are relatively ineffective: Medical therapy is empiric and consists of risk factor modification, immunosuppressive and antiplatelet agents, diet, and exercise. Diltiazem (30-90 mg orally 3 times/day) [1] and lipid lowering agents may retard the progression of coronary disease and are uniformly recommended. PTCA, atherectomy, and stents have been applied to small numbers of patients. Combined data show success rates of 91% and in-hospital mortality in 5%.[2-6]

Answers

References:
1. Schroeder J, Gao SZ, et al. A preliminary study of diltiazem in the prevention of coronary artery disease in heart-transplant recipients. N Engl J Med 1993;328:164-170.
2. Halle A, DiSciascio G, et al. Coronary angioplasty, atherectomy and bypass surgery in cardiac transplant recipients. J Am Coll Cardiol 1995;26:120-8.
3. Swan JW, Norell M, Yacoub M, et al. Coronary angioplasty in cardiac transplant recipients. Eur Heart J 1993;14:65-70.
4. Sandhu JS, Uretsky BF, Reddy S, et al. Potential limitations of percutaneous transluminal coronary angioplasty in heart transplant recipients. Am J Cardiol 1992;69:1234-1237.
5. Mullins PA, Shapiro LM, Aravot DA, et al. Experience of percutaneous transluminal coronary angioplasty in orthotopic transplant recipients. Eur Heart J 1991;12:1205-1207.
6. Jain SP, Zhang S, Khosia S, et al. Is coronary stenting a better option in palliative treatment of cardiac allograft vasculopathy? J Am Coll Cardiol 1997;(Suppl A):28A.

72. Answer: a (true)

The presence of silent ischemia increases the risk of adverse cardiac events.[1] Findings from the Asymptomatic Cardiac Ischemia Pilot (ACIP) trial suggest that compared to medical therapy alone, revascularization may improve the extent and frequency of exercise-induced ischemia,[2] anginal status, and 1-year survival.[3,4] Elective PTCA on patients with silent ischemia is safe and effective. The ACIP and other ongoing randomized trials will determine whether suppression of silent ischemia by PTCA or bypass surgery improves long-term outcome.

References:
1. Erne P, Evequoz D, Zuber M, Yoon S, Burckhardt D. Swiss interventional study on silent ischemia II (SWISSI II): Study design and preliminary results. Circulation 1995;92:I-80.
2. Chaitman B, Stone P, Knatterud G, et al. Asymptomatic cardiac ischemia pilot (ACIP) study: Impact of anti-ischemia therapy on 12-week rest electrocardiogram and exercise test outcomes. J Am Coll Cardiol 1995;26:585-593.
3. Rogers W, Bourassa M, Andrews T, et al. Asymptomatic cardiac ischemia pilot (ACIP) study: Outcome at 1-year for patients with asymptomatic cardiac ischemia randomized to medical therapy or revascularization. J Am Coll Cardiol 1995;26:594-605.
4. Bourassa M, Pepine C, Forman S, et al. Asymptomatic cardiac ischemia pilot (ACIP) study: Effects of coronary angioplasty and coronary artery bypass graft surgery on recurrent angina and ischemia. J Am Coll Cardiol 1995;26:606-614.

INTRACORONARY THROMBUS

73. Answer: d

Among patients undergoing PTCA for medically-refractory unstable ischemic syndromes, the incidence of thrombus is ~ 40% by angiography and ~ 90% by angioscopy.[1-4]

References:
1. Ambrose JA, Winters SL, Stern A, et Al. Angiographic morphology and the pathogenesis of unstable angina pectoris. J Am Coll Cardiol 1985;5:609-616.
2. Fuster V, Badimon L, Badimon J, et al. The pathogenesis of coronary artery disease and the acute coronary syndromes. N Eng J Med 1992;326:242-250.
3. Cowley MJ, DiSciascio G, Vetrovec GW. Coronary thrombus in unstable angina: Angiographic observations and clinical relevance. In Hugenholtz PG and Goldman BG (eds): Unstable Angina: Current Concepatients and Management. Schattauer Press, Stuttgart, 1985;95-102.
4. Gotoh K, Minamino T, Katoh O, et al. The role of intracoronary thrombus in unstable angina: angiographic assessment and thrombolytic therapy during ongoing anginal attacks. Circulation 1988;77:526-534.

74. Answer: c

The strictest angiographic criteria for thrombus require definite intraluminal globular filling defects in multiple angiographic views, or if the vessel is totally occluded, a convex margin that stains with contrast and persists for several cardiac cycles.[1-3] Numerous studies have demonstrated the poor sensitivity of angiography for detecting intracoronary thrombus (as low as 19%), although specificity approaches 100% when strict definitions are used.[4-11]

References:
1. Ambrose JA, Winters SL, Stern A, et Al. Angiographic morphology and the pathogenesis of unstable angina pectoris. J Am Coll Cardiol 1985;5:609-616.
2. Fuster V, Badimon L, Badimon J, et al. The pathogenesis of coronary artery disease and the acute coronary syndromes. N Eng J Med 1992;326:242-250.
3. Cowley MJ, DiSciascio G, Vetrovec GW. Coronary thrombus in unstable angina: Angiographic observations and clinical relevance. In Hugenholtz PG and Goldman BG (eds): Unstable Angina: Current Concepatients and Management. Schattauer Press, Stuttgart, 1985;95-102.
4. Mizuno K, Satumora K, Miyamoto A, et al. Angioscopic evaluation of coronary-artery thrombi in acute coronary syndromes. New Engl J Med 1992;326:287-291.
5. Mizuno K, Miyamoto A, Satomura K, et al. Angioscopic coronary macromorphology in patients with acute coronary disorders. Lancet 1991;337:809-812.
6. Mizuno K, Hikita H, Miyamoto A, Satomura K, et al. The pathogenesis of an impending infarction and its treatment - an angioscopic analysis. Jpn Circ J 1992, 56:1160-5.
7. Hombach V, Hoher M, Kochs M, Eggeling T, et al. Pathophysiology of unstable angina pectoris-correlations with coronary angioscopic imaging. Eur Heart J 1988,;9:40-5.
8. Waxsman S, Sassower M, Zarich S, et al. Angioscopy can identify lesion specific predictors of early adverse outcome following PTCA in patients with unstable angina. Circulation 1994;90:I-490.
9. Manzo K, Netso R, Sassower M, Leeman D, et al. Coronary lesion morphology by angioscopy vs angiography: the ability to detect thrombi. J Am Coll Cardiol 1994: 955-4023.
10. Annex BH, Ajluni SC, Larkin TJ, O'Neill WW, Safian RD. Angioscopic guided interventions in a saphenous vein bypass graft. Cathet Cardiovasc Diagn 1994;31:330-3.
11. den Heijer P, Foley D, Escaned J, Hillege HL, Serruys PW, Lie KI. Angioscopic versus angiographic detection of intimal dissection and intracoronary thrombus. J Am Coll Cardiol 1994;955-100.

75. Answer: c

Direct visualization by coronary angioscopy provides the best method for detecting intraluminal thrombus, while intravascular ultrasound and angiography are less accurate.[1]

Reference:
1. Siegel RJ, Fischbein MC, Chae JS, Helfant RH, Hickey A, Forrester JS. Comparative studies of angioscopy and ultrasound for the evaluation of arterial disease. Echocardiography 1990;7:495-502.

76. Answer: b (false)

PTCA of thrombotic lesions is associated with an increased incidence acute occlusion, distal embolization and no-reflow.[1-8] Distal embolization and no-reflow are more common in vein graft disease compared to native vessel disease.

References:
1. Shah PB, Ahmed WJ, Ganz P, Bittl JA. Hirulog compared with heparin during coronary angioplasty of thrombus-containing lesions. Circulation 1996;94:I-197.
2. White CJ, Ramee SR, Collins TJ, et al. Coronary thrombi increase PTCA risk: Angioscopy as a clinical tool. Circulation 1996:93:253-258.
3. Hillegass WB, Ohman EM, O'Hanesian MA, et al. The effect of preprocedural intracoronary thrombus on patient outcome after percutaneous coronary intervention. J Am Coll Cardiol 1995;21:94A
4. Tan K, Sulke N, Taub N, Sowton E. Clinical and lesion morphologic determinants of coronary angioplasty success and complications: Current experience. J Am Coll Cardiol 1995;25:855-65.
5. Violaris AG, Herrman JP, Melkert R, et al. Does local thrombus formation increase long term luminal renarrowing following PTCA? A quantitative angiographic analysis. J Am Coll Cardiol 1994;February Special Issue:139A.
6. Tenaglia A, Fortin D, Califf R, Frid D, et al. Predicting the risk of abrupt vessel closure after angioplasty in an individual patient. J Am Coll Cardiol 1994;24:1004-11.
7. Myler R, Shaw R, Stertzer S, Hecht H, et al. Lesion morphology and coronary angioplasty: Current experience and analysis. J Am Coll Cardiol 1992;19:1641-52.
8. Mehran R, Ambrose JA, Bongu M, et al. Angioplasty of complex lesions in ischemic rest angina: Results of the thrombolysis and angioplasty in unstable angina (TAUSA) trial. J Am Coll Cardiol 1995;26:961-966.

Answers

77. Answer: a (true)

78. Answer: a, b

PTCA of thrombus-containing lesions has been associated with acute closure in up to 20% of patients;[1-3] pretreatment with a 2-14 day course of heparin and aspirin has been shown to reduce the risk of PTCA in some studies, but not in others.[4-9] Recent data suggest that high dose intravenous heparin (ACT > 350-400 seconds) is associated with lower rates of abrupt closure. The efficacy of thrombolysis as adjunctive therapy for thrombotic lesions is controversial. Nonrandomized data suggest a role for intracoronary thrombolytic therapy when thrombus is present prior to or after PTCA.[10-13] However, systemic thrombolytic therapy has consistently failed to confer clinical benefit for unstable angina and non-Q-wave myocardial infarction, despite modest angiographic improvement.[14] Thrombolytic therapy in unstable angina has produced a similar degree of angiographic resolution of thrombus as aspirin and heparin therapy.[15]

References:
1.	Mabin TA, Holmes DR, Smith HC. Intracoronary thrombus role in coronary occlusion complicating PTCA. J Am Coll Cardiol 1985;5:198-202.
2.	Sugrue DR, Holmes DR, Smith HC. Coronary artery thrombus as a risk factor for acute vessel occlusion during PTCA: Improved Results. Br Heart J 1986;53:62-66.
3.	Deligonul V, Gabliani GI, Caroles DG, et al. PTCA in patients with intracoronary thrombus. Am J Cardiol 1988;62:474-476.
4.	Jang Y, Lincoff AM, Plow EF, Topol EJ. Cellular adhesion molecules in coronary artery disease. J Am Coll Cardiol 1994;24:1591-601.
5.	Laskey MAL, Deutsch E, Barnathan E, et al. Influence of heparin therapy on percutaneous transluminal coronary angioplasty outcome in unstable angina pectoris. Am J Cardiol 1990;65:1425-1429.
6.	Myler RK, Shaw NE, Stertzer SH, et al. Unstable angina and coronary angioplasty. Circulation 1990;82:88-95.
7.	Hettleman BD, Aplin RA, Sullivan PR, et al. Three days of heparin pretreatment reduces major complications of coronary angioplasty in patients with unstable angina. J Am Coll Cardiol 1990;15:154A.
8.	Pow TK, Varricchione TR, Jacobs AK, et al. Does pretreatment with heparin prevent abrupt closure following PTCA? J Am Coll Cardiol 1988;11:238A.
9.	Lukas MA, Deutsch E, Hirshfeld JW Jr, et al. Influence of heparin therapy on percutaneous transluminal coronary angioplasty outcome in patients with coronary arterial thrombus. Am J Cardiol 1990;65:179-182.
10.	Schieman G, Cohen BM, Kozina J, et al. Intracoronary urokinase for intracoronary thrombus accumulation complicating percutaneous transluminal coronary angioplasty in acute ischemic syndromes. Circulation 1990;82:2052-2060.
11.	Pavlides GS, Schreiber TL, Gangadharan V, et al. Safety and efficacy of urokinase during elective coronary angioplasty. Am Heart J 1991;121:731-736.
12.	Chapekis AT, George BS, Candela RJ. Rapid thrombus dissolution by continuous infusion of urokinase through an intracoronary perfusion wire prior to and following PTCA: Results in native coronaries and patent saphenous vein grafts. Cathet Cardiovasc Diagn 1991;23:89-92.
13.	Kiesz R, Hennecken J, Bailey S. Bolus administration of intracoronary urokinase during PTCA in the presence of intracoronary thrombus. Circulation 1991;84:II-346.
14.	The TIMI IIIB Investigators. Effects of tissue plasminogen activator and a comparison of early invasive and conservative strategies in unstable angina and non Q wave myocardial infarction: Results of the TIMI IIIB trial. Circulation 1994;89:1545-1556.
15.	The TIMI IIIA Investigators. Early effects of tissue-type plasminogen activator added to conventional therapy on the culprit coronary lesion in patients presenting with ischemic cardiac pain at rest. Results of the Thrombolysis in Myocardial Ischemia (TIMI IIIA) Trial. Circulation 1993;87:38-52.

79. Answer: a (true)

In the TAUSA study, the urokinase-treated group had a higher incidence of acute vessel occlusion, even in lesions that were complex or contained filling defects suggestive of thrombus.[1] Similar findings were observed in the PAMI-2 study and other clinical trials of acute MI and unstable angina. Possible explanations for the disappointing results of thrombolysis include thrombolytic-induced platelet aggregation, and medial hemorrhage resulting in a more severe stenosis or bleeding complications. Based on the available data, routine thrombolytics should be avoided before, during, and after interventional procedures in patients with acute ischemic syndromes.

Reference:
1.   Mehran R, Ambrose JA, Bongu M, et al. Angioplasty of complex lesions in ischemic rest angina: Results of the thrombolysis and angioplasty in unstable angina (TAUSA) trial. J Am Coll Cardiol 1995;26:961-966.

BIFURCATION LESIONS

80. Answer: c

The likelihood of significant sidebranch narrowing or closure depends on whether the branch originates from the primary lesion and the degree to which its ostium is narrowed. Branch vessels that do not originate from the parent vessel (but may be transiently covered by balloon inflation) are at low risk (< 1%) for sidebranch occlusion.[1] However, if the sidebranch originates from the parent lesion, the risk of occlusion increases progressively as the sidebranch ostial stenosis increases. In one study, branch-ostial stenoses ≤ 50% had a 12% risk of occlusion compared to 41% with ostial stenoses > 50%.[4] When the primary atheroma obstructs both parent vessel and sidebranch ostium by > 50%, there is a high incidence of branch occlusion (14-34%) [1-3] or stenosis (27-41%)[3-5] unless protected by a guidewire. Predictors of sidebranch occlusion include significant branch-ostial stenosis, parent vessel dissection, and unstable angina; factors not predictive of sidebranch occlusion include branch vessel caliber, success of parent vessel PTCA, and anatomic location of the branch.[2,5-7]

Parent Vessel-Side Branch Relationships[1-3,5,8]

Anatomy	Risk of side branch occlusion	Technical difficulty in passing a wire into branch	Protection required
Branch uninvolved by parent vessel lesion but in jeopardy due to transient occlusion during balloon inflation (Type 2B, 3B)	Low (< 1%)	Low	No
Branch originates from diseased parent vessel segment; branch is normal (Type 1B)	Moderate (1-10%)	Low-Moderate	Probably yes; depends on vessel size, distribution
Ostium of branch vessel > 50% stenosis (Type 1A, 2A, 3A)	High (14-35%)	High	Yes

References:
1.   Meier B, Gruentzig AR, King SB III, et al. Risk of side branch occlusion during coronary angioplasty. Am J Cardiol 1984;53:10-14.
2.   Ciampricutti R, El-Gamol M, Van Golder B, et al. Coronary angioplasty of bifurcation lesions without protection of large sidebranches. Cathet Cardiovasc Diagn 1992;27:191-196.
3.   Weinstein JS, Baim DS, Sipperly ME, et al. Salvage of branch vessels during bifurcation lesion angioplasty. Cathet Cardiovasc Diagn 1991;22:1-6.
4.   Boxt LM, Meyeruvitz MF, Taus RH, et al. Sidebranch occlusion complicating percutanous transluminal coronary angioplasty. Radiology 1986;161:681-683.
5.   Vetrovec GW, Cowley MJ, Wolfgang TC, et al. Effects of percutaneous transluminal coronary angioplasty in lesion associated branches. Am Heart J 1985;109:921-925.
6.   George BS, Myler RK, Stertzer SH, et al. Balloon angioplasty of coronary bifurcation lesions. Cathet Cardiovasc Diagn 1986;12:124-138.
7.   Arora RR, Raymond RE, Dimas AP, et al. Side branch occlusion during coronary angioplasty: incidence, angiographic characteristics, and outcome. Cathet Cardiovasc Diagn 1989;18:210-212.
8.   Renkin J, Wijns W, Hanet C, et al. Angioplasty of coronary bifurcation stenoses. Cathet Cardiovasc Diagn 1991;22:167-173.

81. Answer: a, b, c, e

Need for Sidebranch Protection

Sidebranch Protection Recommended	1.	Any sidebranch > 2.0 mm in diameter that has an ostial stenosis ≥ 50% and originates from the parent vessel lesion (Types 1A, 2A, 3A). "True" bifurcation lesions (Type 1A) are associated with a high incidence of sidebranch occlusion and a low salvage rate when left unprotected.
	2.	Any sidebranch > 2 mm in diameter (without ostial stenosis) originates from the parent vessel lesion (Type 1B). Although it is usually possible to retrieve these occluded sidebranches, their large caliber justifies protection. In such lesions, a double guidewire approach is reasonable; if sidebranch occlusion occurs, sequential PTCA or a kissing balloon technique may be employed.
Protection Probably Not Necessary*	1.	The sidebranch is normal and does not originate from the parent vessel lesion (Type 2B, 3B). Even though the sidebranch may be transiently covered by the inflated balloon in the parent vessel, the risk of occlusion is low.
	2.	The sidebranch is < 1.5 mm in diameter and would not receive a bypass graft during CABG.
	3.	The sidebranch supplies a small amount of viable myocardium.
	4.	Isolated stenoses of the origin of the sidebranch usually do not require protection of the parent vessel (Type 4).

* In these lesions, it may be reasonable to leave the sidebranch unprotected; if sidebranch occlusion does occur, it can be retrieved by conventional PTCA, depending on the clinical situation, or not retrieved at all.

82. Answer: a, b, d

In addition to the usual risks of PTCA, bifurcation angioplasty is associated with sidebranch occlusion, incomplete dilation due to the "snow-plow" effect, and retrograde propagation of dissection from sidebranch to parent vessel. There are no data to suggest a higher risk of aneurysm formation after bifurcation PTCA.

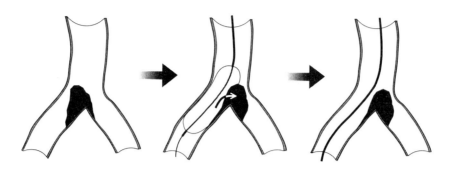

"Snow-Plow" Effect

During PTCA of the parent vessel, shifting plaque causes sidebranch narrowing. Simultaneous dilatation of both limbs of the bifurcation ("kissing-balloon" technique) is often required when the snow-plow effect complicates PTCA.

83. Answer: c

84. Answer: b (false)

In CAVEAT-I, compared to bifurcation lesions treated by PTCA, DCA led to higher success (88% vs. 74%, p < 0.001) and less restenosis (50% vs. 61%, p < 0.001), but more ischemic complications (9.5% vs. 3.7%, p < 0.001).[1]

References:
1. Lewis B, Leya F, Johnson S, et al. Outcoe of angioplasty (PTCA) and atherectomy (DCA) for bifurcation and non-bifurcation lesios in CAVEAT. Circulation 1993;88:I-601.

85. Answer: b (false)

Although stents should be used cautiously in lesions with large sidebranches, high success and acceptable complication rates have been reported. In one study, Gianturco-Roubin stenting resulted in reappearance of sidebranches which were initially occluded after PTCA — the incidence of sidebranch occlusion was 6-18% after initial PTCA but rare after stenting.[1] Another study of the Palmaz-Schatz stent revealed sidebranch occlusion in 10%; two-thirds were associated with initial PTCA and one-third was associated with subsequent stenting.[2] The management of sidebranch occlusion is less complicated after the Gianturco-Roubin stent, since wires and balloons may be passed through the stent coils and into the affected branch. PTCA salvage through slotted stents is feasible, but low-profile balloons are necessary to reduce the risk of balloon entrapment.[3] In a report of 43 cases of sidebranch narrowing treated by PTCA through Palmaz-Schatz and Gianturco-Roubin stent struts or articulation sites, success was achieved in 84% and there were no cases of balloon entrapment.[4] Late (8-month) follow-up after stenting across sidebranches revealed progression and regression of sidebranch narrowing in 19% and 26%, respectively.[5] In another study, all occluded sidebranches after stenting were patent at 6 months.[2] Limited data are available concerning the use of kissing stents; Colombo et al.[6] treated 18 major bifurcation lesions with kissing stents; procedural success was 89%, but ischemic complications and stent thrombosis occurred in 11% and 6%, respectively.[6] In another report, "T" stenting (stent in the ostium of the sidebranch followed by a second stent in the main vessel spanning the sidebranch) was attempted with the Wiktor stent. Success was obtained in 21/21 main branches and 20/21 sidebranches, with angiographic restenosis present in 10% and 15% of main and sidebranches, respectively.[7]

References:
1. Mazur W, Grinstead C, Hakim A, et al. Fate of side branches after intracoronary implantation of the Gianturco-Roubin flex-stent for acute or threatened closure after percutaneous transluminal coronary angioplasty. Am J Cardiol 1994;74:1207-1210.
2. Fischman DL, Savage MP, Leon MB, et al. Fate of lesion-related sidebranches after coronary artery stenting. J Am Coll Cardiol 1993;22:1641-6.
3. Guarneri E, Sklar M, Russo R, Claire D, Schatz R, Teirstein P. Escape from Stent Jail: An in vitro model. Circulation 1995;92:I-688.
4. Caputo RP, Chafizedeh ER, Stoler RC, et al. "Stent Jail" — A minimum security prison. J Invas Cardiol 1996;8.
5. Pan M, Medina A, de Lezo JS, et al. Follow-up patency of sidebranches covered by intracoronary Palmaz-Schatz stent. Am Heart J 1995;129:436-440.
6. Colombo A, Maiello L, Itoh A, et al. Coronary stenting of bifurcation lesions: Immediate and follow-up results. J Am Coll Cardiol 1996; 27:277A.
7. Carrie D, Elbaz M, Mebarkia M, et al. "T" shaped stent placement: A technique for the treatment of coronary bifurcation lesions. J Am Coll Cardiol 1997;(Suppl A):16A.

86. Answer: a, c

Salvage rates depend on whether the affected sidebranch contains a high-grade ostial stenosis, and whether the branch was initially protected by a second wire. Acutely occluded sidebranches without ostial stenoses can be reopened in 75-100% of cases, although salvage rates < 50% have been reported when the ostium of the sidebranch contains a significant stenosis.[1-3] In another report, sidebranch retrieval was successful in 10/11 (91%) protected sidebranch occlusions compared to 11/34 (32%) unprotected branches.[2] When attempting to salvage an occluded sidebranch, excessive or forceful sidebranch probing increases the risk of traumatizing the parent vessel lesion and should be avoided. In addition, it is best to protect the parent vessel with a guidewire in the event of parent vessel closure.

References:
1. Ciampricutti R, El-Gamol M, Van Golder B, et al. Coronary angioplasty of bifurcation lesions without protection of large sidebranches. Cathet Cardiovasc Diagn 1992;27:191-196.
2. Weinstein JS, Baim DS, Sipperly ME, et al. Salvage of branch vessels during bifurcation lesion angioplasty. Cathet Cardiovasc Diagn 1991;22:1-6.
3. Thomas TS, Williams DO, Most AS. Efficacy of coronary angioplasty of bifurcation lesions: immediate and late outcome. Circulation60.

87. Answer: a, c

Sustained patency of the parent vessel is rarely affected by occlusion of its sidebranch; retrograde propagation of dissection from sidebranch to parent vessel is rare.[1] Myocardial infarction is also uncommon after sidebranch occlusion.[1-4] Of 167 patients with sidebranch occlusion after PTCA, chest pain occurred in 13% and Q-wave MI in 8%; septal perforator occlusion, which comprised 27% of all branch closures, was not associated with MI. Among patients with branch occlusion in the 1985-1986 NHLBI PTCA Registry, emergency CABG was required in 11% and death occurred in 3%.[5] When data from several large retrospective series are complied, the overall incidence of death is < 1%.

References:
1. Vetrovec GW, Cowley MJ, Wolfgang TC, et al. Effects of percutaneous transluminal coronary angioplasty in lesion associated branches. Am Heart J 1985;109:921-925.
2. Ciampricutti R, El-Gamol M, Van Golder B, et al. Coronary angioplasty of bifurcation lesions without protection of large sidebranches. Cathet Cardiovasc Diagn 1992;27:191-196.
3. Myler RK, Shaw RE, Stertzer SH, et al. Lesion morphology and coronary angioplasty: current experience and analysis. J Am Coll Cardiol 1992. In press.
4. Meier B, Gruentzig AR, King SB III, et al. Risk of side branch occlusion during coronary angioplasty. Am J Cardiol 1984;53:10-14.
5. Holmes DR JR, Holubkov R, Vlietstra RE, et al. Comparison of complications during percutaneous transluminal coronary angioplasty from 1977 to 1981 and from 1985 to 1986. The National Heart, Lung, and Blood Institute Percutaneous Transluminal Coronary Angioplasty Registry. J Am Coll Cardiol 1988;12:1149-1155.

TORTUOSITY AND ANGULATED LESIONS

88. Answer: All

When balloon angioplasty is performed in vessels with proximal tortuosity, there appears to be an increased incidence of procedural failure (inability to cross the lesion with a guidewire, inadequate guiding catheter support) and more acute complications.[1-4] However, different results in different studies may be due to varying definitions of tortuosity.

Effect of Proximal Tortuosity on Acute PTCA Outcome

Series	N	Anatomic Subgroup	Success (%)	Other (%)	
Tan[1]	965	No tortuosity	93	Acute closure:	3
(1995)	142	Moderate	93		4.2
	50	Severe	84		6
Ellis[2]	189	Type A	92	Acute complications:	2
(1990)	65	Proximal tortuosity	72		15

References:
1. Tan K, Sulke N, Taub N, Sowton E. Clinical and lesion morphologic determinants of coronary angioplasty success and complications: Current experience. J Am Coll Cardiol 1995;25:855-65.
2. Ellis SG, Vandormael MG, Cowley MJ, et al. Coronary morphologic and clinical determinants of procedural outcome with angioplasty for multivessel coronary disease. Implications for patient selection. Circulation 1990;82:1193-1202.
3. Flood RD, Popma JJ, Chuang YC, Salter LF, et al. Incidence, angiographic predictors, and clinical significance of coronary perforation occurring after new device angioplasty. J Am Coll Cardiol 1994;23:301A.
4. Holmes DR, Berdan L, et al. Abrupt closure: The coronary angioplasty versus excisional atherectomy trial (CAVEAT) experience. J Am Coll Cardiol 1994;23:I-585A.

89. Answer: a

Severe proximal vessel tortuosity is problematic for successful use of all atherectomy devices, stents, and lasers, which are more bulky, less flexible, and less trackable than conventional balloon catheters. The Rotablator is the most flexible of the atherectomy devices; activation of the burr may reduce friction and enhance burr movement through moderate-to-severe bends. In one report, Rotablator success was independent of proximal vessel tortuosity,[1] although only 28 such lesions were present. TEC and ELCA are somewhat flexible and may track around moderate bends, but attempts to negotiate extreme tortuosity is potentially dangerous. DCA has long been contraindicated in the setting of extreme tortuosity due to the risk of failure and complications;[2-4] however, the recent availability of small housing devices (5 mm) and AtheroCaths with enhanced torque (GTO device) may facilitate passage into tortuous vessels.

References:
1. Ellis SG, Popma JJ, Buchbinder M, Franco I, et al. Relation of clinical presentation, stenosis morphology, and operator technique to the procedural results of rotational atherectomy and rotational atherectomy-facilitated angioplasty. Circulation 1994;89:882-892.
2. Holmes DR, Berdan L, et al. Abrupt closure: The coronary angioplasty versus excisional atherectomy trial (CAVEAT) experience. J Am Coll Cardiol 1994;23:I-585A.
3. Hinohara T, Rowe MH, Robertson, GC, Selmon MR, et al. Effect of lesion characteristics on outcome of directional coronary atherectomy. J Am Coll Cardiol 1991;17:1112-20.
4. Ellis SG, De Cesare NB, Pinkerton CA, Whitlow P, et al. Relation of stenosis morphology and clinical presentation to the procedural results of directional coronary atherectomy. Circulation 1991;84:644-653.

90. Answer: a, b

PTCA of angulated (> 45-60°) stenoses is associated with increased incidence of procedural failure,[1] major ischemic complications,[1-5] and restenosis. Nevertheless, high procedural success (85-95%) and low complication rates (< 3%) are often reported. Complications are usually due to dissection and abrupt closure, possibly from straightening the vessel during balloon inflation.

References:
1. Ellis SG, Vandormael MG, Cowley MJ, et al. Coronary morphologic and clinical determinants of procedural outcome with angioplasty for multivessel coronary disease. Implications for patient selection. Circulation 1990;82:1193-1202.
2. Hermans WRM, Foley DP, Rensing BJ, Rutsch W, et al. Usefulness of quantitative and qualitative angiographic lesion morphology, and clinical characteristics in predicting major adverse cardiac events during and after native coronary balloon angioplasty. Am J Cardiol 1993;72:14-20.
3. Tenaglia AN, Zidar JP, Jackman JD, Fortin DF, et al. Treatment of long coronary artery narrowings with long angioplasty balloon catheters. Am J Cardiol 1993;71:1274-1277.
4. Van Belle E, Bauters C, Lablanche JM, et al. Angiographic determinants of acute closure after coronary angioplasty: A prospective quantitative coronary angiographic study of 3679 procedures. J Am Coll Cardiol 1994;23:222A.
5. Meckel CR, Ahmed W, Ferguson JJ, Strony J, et al. Angiographic predictors of severe dissection during balloon angioplasty: A report from the Hirulog Angioplasty Study. Circulation 1994;90:I-64.

91. Answer: a (true)

Virtually all atherectomy and laser devices should be avoided in severely angulated lesions because of the risk of dissection or perforation. One study using the Rotablator reported procedural success in 35/41 (85%) moderately angulated lesions (45-60°), but angle > 60° was a powerful predictor of procedural failure, major ischemic complications, and perforation.[1] In a larger report, compared to non-angulated lesions, Rotablator treatment of 123 angulated lesions > 45° resulted in lower success (86% vs 94%), more dissections (36% vs 16%), and a higher mortality rate (2.7% vs 0.3%).[2] DCA has been used with high success (91%) and low complications (3.6%) in lesions with mild angulation (~ 30°),[3] but angulation ≥ 45° was an independent predictor of procedural failure (relative risk 4.8) and major ischemic complications (relative risk 2.7).[4] Likewise, TEC and ELCA should not be used on severely angulated lesions due to the high risk of complications.[1,5,6] Stents can be used to treat mild-moderately angulated lesions, but the value of stenting highly angulated lesions is uncertain and stenting of hinge points has been associated with higher restenosis rates than lesions without hinge points.[7] With coiled wire stents, atheroma may prolapse through the coils leading to suboptimal results and the occasional need for multiple stents. Slotted tubular stents may provide better lumen enlargement but may be difficult to negotiate acute bends. All considered, new device angioplasty of severely angulated lesions has been associated with an increased incidence of acute closure[8] and perforation.[9]

References:

1. Ellis SG, Popma JJ, Buchbinder M, Franco I, et al. Relation of clinical presentation, stenosis morphology, and operator technique to the procedural results of rotational atherectomy and rotational atherectomy-facilitated angioplasty. Circulation 1994;89:882-892.
2. Chevalier B, Commeau P, Favereau X, Gueri Y, et al. Limitations of rotational atherectomy in angulated coronary lesions. J Am Coll Cardiol 1994;23:285A.
3. Hinohara T, Rowe MH, Robertson, GC, Selmon MR, et al. Effect of lesion characteristics on outcome of directional coronary atherectomy. J Am Coll Cardiol 1991;17:1112-20.
4. Ellis SG, De Cesare NB, Pinkerton CA, Whitlow P, et al. Relation of stenosis morphology and clinical presentation to the procedural results of directional coronary atherectomy. Circulation 1991;84:644-653.
5. Ghazzal ZMB, Hearn JA, Litvack F, Goldenberg T, et al. Morphological predictors of acute complications after percutaneous excimer laser coronary angioplasty. Results of a comprehensive angiographic analysis: Importance of the eccentricity index. Circulation 1992;86:820-827.
6. Bittl JA, Sanborn TA, Tcheng JE, Siegel RM, et al. Clinical success, complications, and restenosis rates with excimer laser coronary angioplasty. Am J Cardiol 1992;70:1533-1539.
7. Phillips PS, Alfonso F, Segovia J, Goicolea J, Hernandez R, et al. Effects of Palmaz-Schatz stents on angled coronary arteries. Am J Cardiol 1997;79:1191-193.
8. Hong MK, Popma JJ, Wong SC, Kent KM, et al. Incidence of and factors associated with abrupt closure in patients undergoing elective, new device angioplasty in native coronary arteries. J Am Coll Cardiol 1995;25:122A.
9. Freed M, May M, Lichtenberg A, Strzelecki M, et al. Predictors of angiographic and clinical complications after new device coronary interventions. Circulation 1994;90:I-549.

92. Answer: b (false)

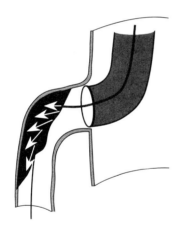 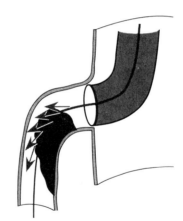

Lesion on Outer Curve:
Device directed into lesion

Lesion on Inner Curve:
Device deflected into disease-free wall

CALCIFIED LESIONS

93. Answer: b (false)

Angiography has poor sensitivity for detecting mild-to-moderate lesion calcium, and only moderate sensitivity for extensive lesion calcium.[1]

Reference:
1. Tan, K., N. Sulke, et al. Clinical and lesion morphologic determinants of coronary angioplasty success and complications: Current experience. J Am Coll Cardiol 1995;25:855-65.

94. Answer: a (true)

In one report, 11% of lesions with angiographic calcium failed to show calcium by IVUS (i.e., false positives).[1]

Reference:
1. Tan, K., N. Sulke, et al. Clinical and lesion morphologic determinants of coronary angioplasty success and complications: Current experience. J Am Coll Cardiol 1995;25:855-65.

95. Answer: a (true)

IVUS has shown that lesion calcium plays a direct role in promoting dissection following PTCA. In a report involving 41 patients undergoing coronary and peripheral angioplasty, both the incidence (88% vs. 53% for non-calcified lesions) and extent of dissection were significantly higher among calcified lesions.[1] When present, the dissection usually originated at the transition between calcified and noncalcified plaque, presumably due to nonuniform shear forces generated by balloon expansion.

Reference:
1. Fitzgerald P, Ports T, Yock P. Contribution of localized calcium deposits to dissection after angioplasty: An observational study using IVUS. Circulation 1992;86:64-70.

96. Answer: b (false)

Most reports have failed to show any association between lesion calcium and restenosis after PTCA.

97. Answer: a, c, d

Rotablator is the treatment of choice for undilatable lesions; other potentially useful techniques include force-focused angioplasty and ELCA.

98. Answer: c

High procedural success (> 90%) and low complication rates (< 5%) can be achieved after Rotablator atherectomy of calcified stenoses.[1-5] In fact, Ellis et al[6] found that lesions *without* calcium were at greater risk for procedural complications compared to lesions with calcium. Rotablator atherectomy preferentially ablates calcified atheroma;[7,8] results in a larger and more concentric lumen with fewer dissections in calcified vs. noncalcified lesions;[9] and produces microfractures in calcified deposits, increasing lesion compliance and rendering them more susceptible to PTCA.[8] Among 67 undilatable lesions treated with the Rotablator (73% of which were calcified), overall procedural success was 96%.[10] After atherectomy, 78% of previously undilatable lesions responded to inflation pressures < 6 atm. In an IVUS study of Rotablator followed by PTCA, DCA, or stents, Rotablator + stent achieved the largest lumen and smallest residual stenosis (Rota + PTCA = 24%; Rota + DCA = 16%; Rota + stent = 12%, p < 0.0001). At the present time, Rotablator atherectomy is the preferred method of revascularizing moderate-to-heavily calcified stenoses.

References:
1. Hoffman R, Mintz GS, Kent KM, et al. Is there an optimal therapy for calcified lesions in large vessels? Comparative acute and follow-up results of rotational atherectomy, stents, or the combination. J Am Coll Cardiol 1997;(Suppl A):68A.
2. Dussaillant GR, Mintz GS, Pichard AD, et al. The optimal strategy for treating calcified lesions in large vessels: Comparison of intravascular ultrasound results of rotational atherectomy + adjunctive PTCA, DCA, or stents. J Am Coll Cardiol 1996;27:153A.
3. Warth D, Leon M, et al. Rotational atherectomy multicenter registry: Acute results, complications and 6-month angiographic follow-up in 709 patients. J Am Coll Cardiol 1994;24:641-648.
4. MacIssac AI, Whitlow PL, Cowley MJ, Buchbinder M. Angiographic predictors of outcome of coronary rotational atherectomy from the completed multicenter registry. J Am Coll Cardiol 1994;March Special Issue:353A.
5. Leon MB, Kent KM, Pichard AD, et al. Percutaneous transluminal coronary rotational angioplasty of calcified lesions. Circulation 1991;84(4):II-521.
6. Ellis S, Popma J, et al. Relation of clinical presentation, stenosis morphology, and operator technique to the procedural results of rotational atherectomy-facilitated angioplasty. Circulation 1994;89:882-892.
7. Mintz G, Potkin B, et al. Intravascular ultrasound evaluation of the effect of rotational atherectomy in obstructive atherosclerotic coronary artery disease. Circulation 1992;86:1383-1393.
8. Kovach J, Mintz G, et al. Sequential intravascular ultrasound characterization of the mechanisms of rotational atherectomy and adjunct balloon angioplasty. J Am Coll Cardiol 1993;22 (4):1024-32.
9. Fitzgerald PJ, Stertzer SH, Hidalgo BO, Myler RK, et al. Plaque characteristics affect lesion and vessel response to coronary rotational atherectomy: An intravascular ultrasound Study. J Am Coll Cardiol 1994;March Special Issue:353A.
10. Reisman M, Devlin PG, Melikian J, Fenner J, Buchbinder M. Undilatable noncompliant lesions treated with the Rotablator: Outcome and angiographic follow-up. Circulation 1993;Speical Issue:2949.

99. Answer: b (false)

Directional Coronary Atherectomy (DCA) has a very limited ability to excise calcified plaque and should be avoided when moderate-to-heavy lesion calcium is present. IVUS studies clearly show that the presence and extent of lesion calcium correlates with ineffective plaque removal after primary DCA.[1-5] Future development of calcium-cutters may improve DCA success. TEC has an extremely limited ability to cut calcium and should not be used on heavily calcified lesions. Because of the excellent flexibility of TEC cutters, vessel calcification proximal to the target lesion is not a contraindication to TEC atherectomy.

References:
1. Popma JJ, Mintz GS, Satler LF, et al. Clinical and angiographic outcome after directional coronary atherectomy. A qualitative and quantitative analysis using coronary arteriography and intravascular ultrasound. Am J Cardiol 1993;72:55E-64E.
2. De Franco AC, Tuzcu EM, Moliterno DJ, et al. "Directional" coronary atherectomy removes atheroma more effectively from concentric than eccentric lesions: Intravascular ultrasound predictors of lesional success. J Am Coll Cardiol 1995;February Special Issue:137A.
3. Matar FA, Mintz GS, Kent KM, et al. Predictors of intravascular ultrasound endpoints after directional coronary atherectomy in 170 patients. J Am Coll Cardiol 1994;February Special Issue:302A.
4. DeLezo JS, Romero M, Medina A, et al. Intraocoronary ultrasound assessment of directional coronary atherectomy: Immediate and follow-up findings. J Am Coll

Answers

Cardiol 1993;21:298-307.

5. Hong MK, Chuang YC, Prunka N, Satler LF. Predictors of early and late cardiac events in patients undergoing saphenous vein graft angioplasty with PTCA and new device modalities. Circulation 1993;88:I-601.

100. Answer: b (false)

Heavy lesion calcium increases the risk of incomplete stent expansion[1] and restenosis; a stent should not be deployed in a calcified lesion if full balloon expansion cannot be achieved, since incomplete stent expansion greatly increases the risk of stent thrombosis.[2] Even when heavily calcified plaque is first modified by the Rotablator, final lumen cross-sectional area after stenting may be smaller than in lesions without calcification,[3] but is still larger than the combination of Rotablator plus by PTCA[4,5] or DCA.[5] Final diameter stenosis and target lesion revascularization appear to be lowest after Rotablator plus stenting compared to stenting alone or Rotablator plus DCA or PTCA.[6,7]

References:
1. Hong MK, Chuang YC, Prunka N, Satler LF. Predictors of early and late cardiac events in patients undergoing saphenous vein graft angioplasty with PTCA and new device modalities. Circulation 1993;88:I-601.
2. Tamura T, Kimura T, Nosaka H, Nobuyoshi M. Predictors of restenosis after Palmaz-Schatz stent implantation. Circulation 1994;90:I-324.
3. Goldberg SL, Hall P, Almagor Y, Maiello L, et al. Intravascular ultrasound guided rotational atherectomy of fibro-calcific plaque prior to intracoronary deployment of Palmaz-Schatz stents. J Am Coll Cardiol 1994;February Special Issue:290A.
4. Mintz GS, Dusaillant GR, Wong SC, Pichard AD, et al. Rotational atherectomy followed by adjunct stents: The preferred therapy for calcified lesions in large vessels? Circulation 1995;92:I-329.
5. Ellis S, Popma J, et al. Relation of clinical presentation, stenosis morphology, and operator technique to the procedural results of rotational atherectomy-facilitated angioplasty. Circulation 1994;89:882-892.
6. Hoffman R, Mintz GS, Kent KM, et al. Is there an optimal therapy for calcified lesions in large vessels? Comparative acute and follow-up results of rotational atherectomy, stents, or the combination. J Am Coll Cardiol 1997;(Suppl A):68A.
7. Dussaillant GR, Mintz GS, Pichard AD, et al. The optimal strategy for treating calcified lesions in large vessels: Comparison of intravascular ultrasound results of rotational atherectomy + adjunctive PTCA, DCA, or stents. J Am Coll Cardiol 1996;27:153A.

101. Answer: b

ELCA is an alternative to Rotablator for superficial lesion calcification; small initial fibers (1.3 mm), high fluence (50-60 mJ/mm^2), and the saline-infusion technique are recommended.

102. Answer: a, d, e

The mechanism of Rotablator atherectomy is tissue displacement by pulvuarization and microembolization. No-reflow is uncommon, and can be virtually eliminated by using a small initial burr, stepwire increments in burr size, ablation runs < 30 sec, careful attention to burr speed with RPM surveillance, and a Rotaflush cocktail of nitrates, calcium blockers, and heparin.

103. Answer: c

Unlike calcium located at the intimal-lumen interface, deep tissue calcium (at or near the medial-adventitial border) does not usually interfere with PTCA, DCA, or stenting. Initial use of Rotablator or ELCA is not generally required, and device selection can be based on associated lesion morphologies. Deep calcium has little or no impact on procedural outcome.

ECCENTRIC LESIONS

104. Answer: b (false)

Contrast angiography has poor predictive value for the detection of eccentric plaque. In one report of angiographically-apparent eccentric lesions, only 30/48 (63%) had eccentric plaque morphology by intravascular ultrasound (IVUS), and 21/30 (70%) of angiographically "concentric" lesions were eccentric by IVUS.[1] In a second report, concordance between IVUS and angiography for assessment of lesion eccentricity was only 53%.[2]

References:
1. Braden GA, Herrington DM, Kerensky RA, et al. Angiography poorly predicts actual lesion eccentricity in severe coronary stenoses: Confirmation by intracoronary ultrasound imaging. J Am Coll Cardiol 1994;Special Issue:413A.
2. Mintz GS, Popma JJ, Pichard AD, Kent KM, et al. Comparison of intravascular ultrasound and coronary angiography in the assessment of target lesion plaque distribution in coronary artery disease. TCT Meeting (Washington DC), February, 1995; Abstract.

105. Answer: a, b, d, e

High success (> 90%) and low complication rates (< 3-4 %) have been consistently reported for PTCA of most eccentric lesions.[1,2] While originally classified as a "Type B" characteristic (procedural success 60-85%, increased risk of acute closure), most data indicate that lesion eccentricity does not adversely affect procedural success or restenosis.[1-3] Observational reports suggest that compared to concentric lesions, PTCA of eccentric lesions may be associated with more elastic recoil, less effective plaque compression, more vasospasm, and suboptimal lumen enlargement;[4-6] the risk of abrupt closure is similar for concentric and eccentric lesions.

References:
1. Tan K, Sulke N, et al. Clinical and lesion morphologic determinants of coronary angioplasty success and complications: Current experience. J Am Coll Cardiol 1995;25:855-65.
2. Myler RK, Shaw RE, Stertzer SH, et al. Lesion morphology and coronary angioplasty: current experience and analysis. J Am Coll Cardiol 1992;19:1641-52.
3. Ellis SG, Vandormael MG, Cowley MJ, et al. Coronary morphologic and clinical determinants of procedural outcome with angioplasty for multivessel coronary disease. Implications for patient selection. Circulation 1990;82:1193-1202.
4. Kimball BP, Eric SB, Cohen EA, et al. Comparison of acute elastic recoil after directional coronary atherectomy versus standard balloon angioplasty. Am Heart J 1992;124:1459.
5. Baptista J, diMario C, Ozaki Y, de Feyter P, deJaegere P , Roelandt J, Serruys PW. Deterinants of lumen and plaque changes after balloon angioplasty: A quantitative ultrasound study. J Am Coll Cardiol 1994;March Special Issue:414A.
6. Fiscell TA, Bausback KN. Effects of luminal eccentricity on spontaneous coronary vasoconstriction after successful percutaneous transluminal coronary angioplasty. Am J Cardiol 1991;68:530.

106. Answer: a (DCA); b (Rotablator); c (TEC atherectomy)

107. Answer: a (true)

Virtually all stent designs are capable of treating lesions with all types of abnormal contour, including eccentric lesions. Stents are unmatched in their ability to enlarge lumen dimensions, resist elastic recoil, and decrease dissection, all of which are important considerations when treating eccentric lesions. The favorable results of simplified anticoagulation regimens (i.e., without warfarin) may make stents the treatment of choice for a wide range of lesions, including those with eccentric morphology.

OSTIAL LESIONS

108. Answer: a (true)

The presence of an ostial stenosis poses a special management problem for the interventional cardiologist. Of all lesions considered for PTCA, ostial lesions are the most likely to be associated with suboptimal angiographic results due to lesion rigidity and elastic recoil. Aggressive efforts to improve lumen dimensions with balloons frequently result in further elastic recoil, dissection, and a high incidence of restenosis. In contrast to non-ostial lesions, the successful treatment of ostial lesions is most dependent on the use of new interventional devices.

109. Answer: a, c, d, e

If pressure damping occurs during intervention on an ostial lesion, a side-hole catheter or larger diameter guide should be used. Smaller diameter guides may have a tendency to engage aorto-ostial lesions more deeply and exacerbate pressure damping, whereas larger diameter guides will tend to sit outside the ostium and result in less pressure damping. In general, coaxial alignment — not aggressive vessel intubation — will minimize ostial injury, permit proper positioning of interventional devices, and facilitate angiographic assessment of the ostium. As long as coaxial alignment is maintained, it is usually possible to advance and center the balloon with the guiding catheter positioned just outside the ostium. Once the balloon is properly positioned, the guiding catheter can be gently retracted 1-2 cm into the aorta; gentle forward pressure on the balloon catheter or low-pressure balloon inflation (1-2 atm) may help maintain proper balloon position while the guide is retracted. The balloon should not be fully inflated if partially inside the guiding catheter due to the risk of balloon rupture, dissection, or air embolism. When the guiding catheter is retracted, short (10-20 mm) balloons may "watermelon-seed" out of the lesion; this can be prevented by using long (30-40 mm) balloons.

110. Answer: a, b, d

To ensure that the stenosis is not due to transient spasm prior to intervention, it is helpful to administer intracoronary nitroglycerin or perform a subselective injection in the Sinus of Valsalva. IVUS can be useful if an adequate angiogram cannot be obtained.

111. Answer: b, d, e, f

Because of the suboptimal results of PTCA alone for ostial lesions, multi-device therapy is recommended, and associated lesion morphology weighs heavily in selecting the optimal method of revascularization. DCA is well-suited for noncalcified ostial stenoses in vessels ≥ 3 mm. Eccentric or ulcerated lesions are also suitable for DCA. However, other devices should be considered in the presence of moderate-to-heavy calcification, large amounts of clot, diffuse disease, vessel diameter < 3.0 mm, or severe angulation. TEC may be useful for ostial vein graft lesions with thrombus, but is contraindicated in the presence of significant calcification, marked eccentricity, extreme angulation, or dissection. The Rotablator may be of particular benefit for ostial lesions with or without calcification, but should be avoided when either dissection, thrombus, or severe angulation is present. ELCA may be useful for noncalcified ostial lesions, particularly those with long (>30 mm) segments of disease, and directional ELCA may be useful for eccentric ostial lesions. However, all lasers should be avoided in severely angulated lesions or in the presence of dissection. Rotablator is preferred for heavily calcified lesions since the results of ELCA are unpredictable in such lesions. Stents can be used for ostial lesions which can be fully expanded by a balloon. Adjunctive balloon angioplasty is frequently required after DCA, and virtually always after TEC, Rotablator, and ELCA of ostial lesions. Some studies demonstrate that compared to PTCA alone, a further 22% gain in lumen diameter is possible when PTCA is preceded by TEC or ELCA, and a 44% incremental gain when PTCA is preceded by Rotablator ("facilitated angioplasty"). There is also growing optimism for using combinations of new devices for ostial lesions ("device synergy"), including Rotablator + stents, Rotablator + DCA, and DCA + stents.

LONG LESIONS

112. Answer: a, b, c

Although angioplasty success declines as lesion length increases,[1-3] procedural success can still be achieved in 74-97% of lesions > 20 mm in length. However, observational data may overestimate success rates since long lesions with other complex features (e.g, calcium, angulation) are often treated with laser, atherectomy devices, or stents. In the randomized Amsterdam Rotterdam (AMRO) trial of ELCA vs. PTCA for long lesions, PTCA success was only 79%.[4] Furthermore, intravascular ultrasound has shown that the residual stenosis is frequently underestimated by contrast angioplasty since the "normal" reference segment used to measure stenosis severity is often diseased itself. The impact of lesion length on major complications is controversial. Several reports indicate that PTCA of long lesions is associated with an increased risk of dissection[3,5,6] and abrupt closure.[1,3,7-9] In these studies, the incidence of abrupt closure was 1-6% for lesions <10 mm and 9-14% for lesions > 10 mm. In contrast, other studies reported no relationship between lesion length and acute closure[10] or major complications.[2,11-13] These divergent results may be due to differences in patient characteristics, the presence of multivessel disease, associated lesion morphologies, and the use of long (30 - 40 mm) balloons and new devices. The influence of lesion length on restenosis risk is controversial. The Multi-Hospital Eastern Atlantic Restenosis Trial (M-HEART) demonstrated a direct relationship between lesion length and restenosis (lesion lengths of 0.3-2.9 mm, 3.0-4.6 mm, 4.7-7.0 mm, and 7.1-28.0 mm showed restenosis rates of 32%, 33%, 42%, and 49%, respectively).[14] Other reports failed to demonstrate an association.[15,16] Although long lesions may result in a greater loss in lumen diameter at 6-months, these observations do not necessarily correlate with clinical restenosis.[17] Considerable clinical experience suggests that long (30-40 mm) balloons might improve acute results by distributing inflation pressure more evenly across the diseased vessel segment and atheroma/vessel junction, which is frequently the site of dissection.

References:

1. Tan K, Sulke N, Taub N, Sowton E. Clinical and lesion morphologic determinants of coronary angioplasty success and complications: Current experience. J Am Coll Cardiol 1995;25: 855-65.
2. Myler R, Shaw R, et al. Lesion morphology and coronary angioplasty: Current experience and analysis. J Am Coll Cardiol 1992;19:1641-1652.
3. Zidar JP, Tenaglia AN, Jackman JD, et al. Improved acute results for PTCA of long coronary lesions using long angioplasty balloon catheters. J Am Coll Cardiol 1992;19:34A.
4. Appleman YEA, Piek JJ, Strikwerda S, et al. Randomized trial of excimer laser angioplasty vs. balloon angioplasty for treatment of obstructive coronary artery disease. Lancet 1996;347:79-84.
5. Raymenants E, Bhandari S, Stammen F, De Scheerder ID, Desmet W, Piessens J. Effects of angioplasty balloon material and lesion characteristics on the incidence of coronary dissection in 2150 dilated lesions. J Am Coll Cardiol 1993;21:291A.
6. Raymenants E, Bhandari S, Stammen F, De Scheerder I, et al. Effects of angioplasty balloon material and lesion characteristics on the incidence of coronary dissection in 2150 dilated lesions. J Am Coll Cardiol 1993;21:291A.
7. Ellis SG, Roubin GS, King SB III, et al. Angiographic and clinical predictors of acute closure after native vessel coronary angioplasty. Circulation 1988;77:372-379.
8. Detre KM, Holmes DR Jr, Holubkov R, et al. Incidence and consequences of periprocedural occlusion. The 1985-1986 National Heart, Lung and Blood Institute Percutaneous Transluminal Coronary Angioplasty Registry. Circulation 1990;82:739-750.
9. Tenaglia AN, Fortin DF, Califf RM, et al. Predicting the risk of abrupt vessel closure after angioplasty in an individual patient. J Am Coll Cardiol 1994;23:1004-1011.
10. de Feyter PJ, van den Brand M, Jaarman G, et al. Acute coronary artery occlusion during and after percutaneous transluminal coronary angioplasty. Frequency, prediction, clinical course, management, and follow-up. Circulation 1991;83:927-936.
11. Hermans WR, Foley D, et al. Usefulness of quantitative and qualitative angiographic lesion morphology, and clinical characteristics in predicting major adverse cardiac events during and after native coronary balloon angioplasty. Am J Cardiol 1993;72:14-20.
12. Savage MP, Goldberg S, Hirshfeld JW, et al, for the M-Heart Investigators. Clinical and angiographic determinants of primary coronary angioplasty success. J Am Coll Cardiol 1991;17:22-8.
13. Commeau P, Zimarino M, Lancelin B, et al. Rotational coronary atherectomy for the treatment of aorto-ostial and branch-ostial lesions. Circulation 1994;90:I-213.
14. Hirshfeld JW Jr, Schwartz JS, Jugo R, et al. Restenosis after coronary angioplasty: A multivariate statistical model to relate lesion and procedure variables to restenosis. J Am Coll Cardiol 1991;18:647-656.
15. Ellis SG, Roubin GS, King SB III, et al. Importance of stenosis morphology in the estimation of restenosis risk after elective percutaneous transluminal coronary angioplasty. Am J Cardiol 1989;63:30-34.
16. Leimgruber PP, Roubin GS, Hollman J, et al. Restenosis after successful coronary angioplasty in patients with single-vessel disease. Circulation 1986;73:710-717.
17. Foley DP, Meilkert R, Umans VA, et al. Is the relationship between luminal increase and subsequent renarrowing linear or non-linear in patients undergoing coronary interventions? J Am Coll Cardiol 1994;Special Issue:302A.

113. Answer: c

Although early Rotablator success was possible in only 70% of long lesions,[1] more recent studies have reported success in more than 90% of lesions 16-25 mm in length.[2-5] However, increasing lesion length has been associated with an increased risk of MI,[1,2,4] coronary artery perforation,[6] and restenosis.[7] Despite these complications, many interventionalists believe that Rotablator atherectomy (with adjunctive PTCA as needed) is the preferred method of revascularizing long lesions, especially those with superficial calcium. In such lesions, it is important to use slow passes with a small burr to minimize microcavitation and the generation of large particulate debris, which can result in slow-flow and ischemic complications.

References:
1. Reisman M, Harms V, Whitlow P, Feldman T, Fortuna R, Buchbinder M. Comparison of early and recent results with rotational atherectomy. J Am Coll Cardiol 1997;29:353-7.
2. Teirstein PS, Warth DC, Haq N, et al. High speed rotational coronary atherectomy for patients with diffuse coronary artery disease. J Am Coll Cardiol 1991;18:1694-1701.
3. Warth D, Leon MB, O'Neill W, Zacca N, Polissar NL, Buchbinder M. Rotational atherectomy multicenter registry: Acute results, complications and 6-month angiographic follow-up in 709 patients. J Am Coll Cardiol 1994;24: 641-648.
4. Ellis, S., J. Popma, et al. Relation of clinical presentation, stenosis morphology, and operator technique to the procedural results of rotational atherectomy-facilitated angioplasty. Circulation 1994;89:882-892.
5. Reisman M, Cohen B, Warth D, Fenner J, Gocka IT, Buchbinder M. Outcome of long lesions treated with high speed rotational ablation. J Am Coll Cardiol 1993;21:443A.
6. Cohen BM, Weber VJ, Bass TA, et al. Coronary perforation during rotational ablation: Angiographic determinants and clinical outcome. J Am Coll Cardiol 1994;February Special Issue:354A.
7. Leguizamón JH, Chambre DF, Torresani EM, et al. High-speed coronary rotational atherectomy. Are angiographic factors predictive of failure, major complications or restenosis? A multivariate analysis. J Am Coll Cardiol 1995;February Special Issue:95A.

114. Answer: a (true)

In an early report by Robertson et al,[1] DCA of long lesions resulted in lower success, more emergency CABG, and higher restenosis rates compared to DCA of focal stenoses. In another early report, lesion length independently predicted abrupt closure, which occurred in 3%, 4%, and 7% of lesions < 10 mm, 10-20 mm, and ≥ 20 mm in length, respectively.[2] In the CAVEAT trial, lesion length and calcification predicted DCA failure.[3] More recently, Mooney et al. demonstrated procedural success in 97% of long lesions by making a series of longitudinal cuts through the entire length of the lesion; this allowed better DCA positioning (and less ischemia) during remaining circumferential cuts. Lesions were highly selected for favorable morphology; highly calcified or angulated lesions, and vessels < 3 mm in diameter were excluded.

References:
1. Robertson GC, Selmon MR, Hinohara T, et al. The effect of lesion length on outcome of directional coronary atherectomy. Circulation 1990;82:III-623.
2. Popma J, Topol E, et al. Abrupt vessel closure after directional coronary atherectomy. J Am Coll Cardiol 1992;19:1372-1379.
3. Lincoff AM, Ellis SG, Leya F, Masden RR, et al. Are clinical and angiographic correlates of success the same during directional coronary atherectomy and balloon angioplasty? The CAVEAT Experience. Circulation 1993;88:I-601.
4. Mooney, M., J. Mooney-Fishman, et al. Directional atherectomy for long lesions: Improved results. Cathet Cardiovasc Diagn. 1993;1:26-30.

115. Answer: a, b, d

In the first 3000 patients enrolled into the ELCA Registry, procedural success was 90% for short and long lesions.[1] Importantly, procedural success was independent of lesion length and was achieved in 89% and 87% of lesions > 20 mm and > 30 mm in length, respectively. Although dissections were more common in long lesions,[2] major ischemic complications occurred with equal frequency among short and long lesions.[1-3] Randomized trials comparing ELCA vs. PTCA (AMRO trial), and ELCA vs. PTCA vs. Rotablator (ERBAC trial) for long lesions are now complete. In the **AM**sterdam **RO**tterdam (AMRO) trial, 308 patients with 325 lesions ≥ 10 mm were randomized to ELCA (without saline infusion) or balloon angioplasty. No differences in procedural success, late clinical events, or functional status were observed.[4,5] However, ELCA was associated with more acute closure (8% vs. 0.8%, p = 0.005), a trend towards more restenosis (52% vs 41%, p = 0.13),[4] and incremental costs of $4476 per treated segment.[6] In the Excimer-Laser **R**otablator **B**alloon **A**ngioplasty for **C**-Lesions (ERBAC) trial, both ELCA and Rotablator resulted in better immediate lumen enlargement than PTCA, but no difference in restenosis at 6 months.[7]

Answers

The efficacy of ELCA for long lesions with heavy calcification, marked angulation, or thrombus awaits further study.

References:
1. Litvack F, Eigler N, Margolis J, et al. Percutaneous excimer laser coronary angioplasty: Results in the first consecutive 3,000 patients. J Am Coll Cardiol 1994;23:323-9.
2. Baumbach A, Bittl J, Fleck E, et al. Acute complications of excimer laser coronary angioplasty: A detailed analysis of multicenter results. J Am Coll Cardiol 1994;23:1305-1313.
3. Ghazzal, Z., J. Hearn, et al. Morphological predictors of acute complications after percutaneous excimer laser coronary angioplasty. Results of a comprehensive angiographic analysis: Importance of the eccentricity index. Circulation 1992;86:820-827.
4. Appleman YEA, Piek JJ, Strikwerda S, et al. Randomized trial of excimer laser angioplasty vs. balloon angioplasty for treatment of obstructive coronary artery disease. Lancet 1996;347:79-84.
5. Appelman YE, Piek J, Redekop WK, de Feyter PJ, et al. Excimer laser angioplasty versus balloon angioplasty in longer coronary lesions: A multivariate analysis. Circulation 1995;92:I-74.
6. Appleman YE, Birnie E, Piek JJ, de Feyter PJ, et al. Excimer laser angioplasty versus balloon angioplasty in longer coronary lesions: A cost-effectiveness analysis. Circulation 1995;92:I-512.
7. Reifart N, Vandormael M, Krajear M, Gohring S, Preusler W, Schwart F, Storger H, Hofmann M, Klopper J, Muller S, Haase J. Randomized comparison of angioplasty of complex coronary lesions at a single center. Excimer laser, rotational atherectomy, and balloon angioplasty comparison (ERBAC) study. Circulation 1997;96:91-98.

116. Answer: b (false)

Lesions > 10-20 mm were excluded from the early stent experience since the use of multiple stents increased the risk of subacute stent thrombosis. Recent data are much more favorable: Maiello et al.[1] implanted stents in 108 lesions > 20 mm in length (using IVUS to optimize stent deployment). Procedural success was achieved in 93% of patients; stent thrombosis occurred in 1.5% and restenosis occurred in 35%. In another report, 90-day clinical event rates after emergent or elective implantation of the Gianturco-Roubin stent were associated with vessel diameter and stent expansion, but not lesion length. Excellent results were also obtained by Shaknovich et al.[2] in 54 long lesions or dissections. Restenosis may be more common in long lesions.[3-5]

References:
1. Maiello L, Hall P, Nakamura S, et al. Results of stent implantation of diffuse coronary disease assisted by intravascular ultrasound. J Am Coll Cardiol 1995;February Special Issue:156A.
2. Shaknovich A, Moses JW, Undemir C, Cohen NT, et al. Procedural and short-term clinical outcomes in multiple Palmaz-Schatz stents (PSSs) in very long lesions/dissections. Circulation 1995;92:I-535.
3. Hall P, Nakamura S, Maiello L, Blengino S, et al. Factors associated with late angiographic outcome after intravascular ultrasound guided Palmaz-Schatz coronary stent implantation: A multivariate analysis. J Am Coll Cardiol 1995;February Special Issue:36A.
4. Tamura T, Kimura T, Nosaka H, Nobuyoshi M. Predictors of restenosis after Palmaz-Schatz stent implantation. Circulation 1994;90:I-324.
5. Hamasaki N, Nosaka H, et al. Influence of lesion length on late angiographic outcome and restenotic outcome and restenotic process after successful stent implantation. J Am Coll Cardiol 1997;29(Suppl A):239A.

CHRONIC TOTAL OCCLUSION

117. Answer: a, c

With total coronary occlusion, the underlying pathological process is the principal determinant of clinical presentation, presence of collaterals, myocardial viability, and the nature of the coronary obstruction.

Total Coronary Occlusion: Clinical and Pathological Features

	Acute Occlusion	**Chronic Occlusion**
Presentation	Acute MI	Change in anginal status. Angina is usually exertional (collateral insufficiency).
Histopathology	Ruptured fibrous cap overlies soft atheroma; Acute occlusive thrombus is common.	Complex fibrocalcific atherosclerosis. Layered, chronic organized thrombus.
Spontaneous recanalization	Occasional	Rare

Collaterals
    Intracoronary
    Intercoronary
	
	Rare
	Less common
		
		Occasional (bridging collaterals)
		Common

Myocardial viability	Uncommon unless collaterals present.	Common; collaterals sustain viability. May have normal wall motion.
PTCA success	High	Variable; depends on duration and morphology.

118. Answer: b

Compared to PTCA of nontotal occlusions, revascularization rates for chronic total occlusions are disappointingly low. Reported series comprising more than 4400 total coronary occlusions indicate an overall success rate of 69% (range 47-81%). The most common reasons for procedural failure include the inability to cross the occlusion with a guidewire (80%), failure to cross the occlusion with a balloon (15%), and the inability to dilate the stenosis (5%).

119. Answer: a (true)

120. Answer: a,d

Chronic Total Coronary Occlusions: Predictors of PTCA Outcome

Procedural Success	**Procedural Failure**
Functional Occlusion	Total Occlusion
Occlusion age < 12 weeks	Occlusion age > 12 weeks
Length < 15 mm	Length > 15 mm
Tapered Stump	Abrupt Cut-off
No Sidebranch at Point of Occlusion	Sidebranch Present
No Intracoronary Bridging Collaterals	Extensive Bridging Collaterals ("Caput Medusa")

Answers

121. Answer: b (false)

The duration of occlusion may be estimated by time interval between a major ischemic event (Q-wave myocardial infarction, new onset angina, or abrupt worsening in anginal status) and PTCA. Successful revascularization is highest for occlusions < 1 week, intermediate for occlusions 2-12 weeks, and lowest for those > 3 months. Occlusion duration alone should not preclude revascularization since procedural success for occlusions > 6 months old may be as high as 50-75%.[1,2] Small angioplasty series suggested that bridging collaterals was the most important determinant of successful PTCA of chronic total occlusions. However, in a recent large study, Kinoshita et al[3] reported equally high success rates among 109 total occlusions with bridging collaterals and 324 occlusions without bridging collaterals (75% vs. 83%, p = 0.07). The authors attributed the high success rate to operator experience and aggressive use of stiff wires.

References:
1. Safian RD, McCabe CH, Sipperly ME, et al. Initial success and long-term follow-up of percutaneous transluminal coronary angioplasty in chronic total occlusions versus conventional stenoses. Am J Cardiol 1988;61:23G-28G.
2. Shimizu M, Kato O, Otsuji S, et al. Progress in initial outcome of PTCA for complete occlusion. Circulation 1993;88:I-504.
3. Kinoshitaw I, Katoh O, Nariyama J, Otsuji S, et al. Coronary angioplasty of chronic total occlusions with bridging collateral vessels: Immediate and follow-up outcome from a large single-center experience. J Am Coll Cardiol 1995;26:409-15.

122. Answer: a (true)

Although PTCA of a chronic total occlusion is generally considered a "low-risk" procedure, *it is not risk-free!* Several reports have found that major complications occur with equal frequency among total and nontotal occlusions, and the presence of a chronic total occlusion is an independent predictor of acute closure.[1,2] Major complications include acute closure (5-10%), MI (0-2%), emergency CABG (0-3%), and death (0-1%).

References:
1. Tenaglia A, Fortin D, Califf R. Predicting the risk of abrupt closure after angioplasty in an individual patient. J Am Coll Cardiol 1994;24:1004-1011.
2. Ruocco NA, Ring ME, Holubkov R, Jacobs AK. Results of coronary angioplasty of chronic total occlusions (the National Heart, Lung, and Blood Institute 1985-1986 Percutaneous Transluminal Angioplasty Registry). Am J Cardiol 1992;69:69-76.

123. Answer: a, b,

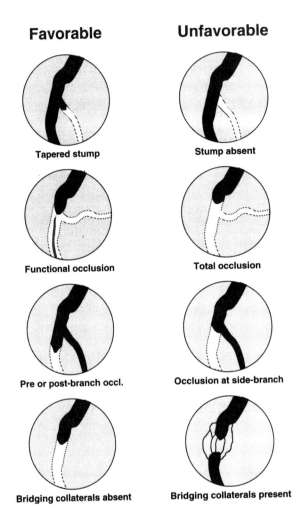

Favorable   **Unfavorable**

Tapered stump   Stump absent

Functional occlusion   Total occlusion

Pre or post-branch occl.   Occlusion at side-branch

Bridging collaterals absent   Bridging collaterals present

Chronic Total Occlusion: Anatomic Descriptors of Procedural Success

124. Answer: a, c

The majority of patients with successful PTCA are asymptomatic at follow-up. In the three largest reports, 76%, 69%, and 66% of patients were asymptomatic 1 year[1] 2 years,[2] and 4 years after PTCA.[3] Absence of symptoms does not exclude restenosis since 40% of patients with restenosis may be free of chest pain.[4] Although data are limited, successful PTCA may improve ventricular relaxation and regional wall motion.[5,6] Global ejection fraction improved in one study,[7] but not in another.[8] Among patients with successfully recanalized occlusions, those with persistent patency and normal flow had better global function and less ventricular dilatation than patients with occluded vessels.[9] Most studies indicate that successful recanalization of a chronic total occlusion reduces the need for CABG by 50-75%. However, PTCA does not appear to improve survival or reduce the incidence of late MI.[3,10-12]

References:
1. Bell MR, Berger PB, Bresnahan JF, Reeder GS. Initial and long-term outcome of 354 patients after coronary balloon angioplasty of total coronary artery occlusions. Circulation 1992;85:1003-1011.
2. Ruocco NA Jr, Ring ME, Holubkov R, et al. Results of coronary angioplasty of chronic total occlusions (the National Heart, Lung, and Blood Institute 1985-1986 Percutaneous Transluminal Angioplasty Registry). Am J Cardiol 1992;69:69-76.
3. Ivanhoe RJ, Weintraub WS, Douglas JS Jr, et al. Percutaneous transluminal coronary angioplasty of chronic total occlusions. Primary success, restenosis, and long-term clinical follow-up. Circulation 1992;85:106-115.
4. Haerer W, Schmidt A, Eggeling T, et al. Angioplasty of chronic total coronary occlusions. Results of a controlled randomized trial. J Am Coll Cardiol 1991;17:113A.
5. Melchior JP, Meier B, Urban P, et al. Percutaneous transluminal coronary angioplasty for chronic total coronary arterial occlusion. Am J Cardiol 1987;59:535-538.
6. Meier B. Total coronary occlusion: A different animal? J Am Coll Cardiol 1991;17:50B.
7. Anderson TJ, Knudtson ML, Roth DL, et al. Improvement in left ventricular function following PTCA of chronic totally occluded arteries. Circulation 1991;84:II-519.
8. Serruys PW, Umans V, Heyndrickx GR, et al. Elective PTCA of totally occluded coronary arteries not associated with acute myocardial infarction; short-term and long-term results. Eur Heart J 1985;6:2-12.
9. Danchin N, Angiol M, Beurrie D, et al. Late recanalization of chronic total coronary occlusion: Maintained vessel patency improves global and regional left ventricular function and avoids remodeling. J Am Coll Cardiol 195;25:345A.
10. Stewart J, Denne L, Bowker T, et al. Percutaneous transluminal coronary angioplasty in chronic coronary artery occlusion. J Am Coll Cardiol 1993;21:1371-1376.
11. Bell MR, Berger PB, Reeder GS, et al. Successful PTCA of chronic total coronary occlusions reduces the need for coronary artery bypass surgery. Circulation 1991;84:II-250.
12. Finci L, Meier B, Fayre J et al. Long-term results of successful and failed angioplasty for chronic total coronary arterial occlusion. Am J Cardiol 1990;66:660.

125. **Answer: a-e**

Observational data suggest that some incremental benefit can be achieved using these devices when a chronic total occlusion cannot be crossed with a conventional PTCA guidewire.[1-6]

References:
1. Haerer W, Schmidt A, Eggeling T, et al. Angioplasty of chronic total coronary occlusions. Results of a controlled randomized trial. J Am Coll Cardiol 1991;17:113A.
2. Freed M, Boatman JE, Siegel N, Safian RD, Grines CL, O'Neill WW. Glidewire treatment of resistant coronary occlusions. Cathet Cardiovasc Diagn 1993;30:201-204.
3. Rees MR, Sivananthan MV, Verma SP. The use of hydrophilic terumo glidewires in the treatment of chronic coronary artery occlusions. Circulation 1991;84:II-519.
4. Hosny A, Lai D, Mancherje C, Lee G. Successful recanalization using a hydrophilic-coated guidewire in total coronary occlusions after unsuccessful PTCA attempts with standard steerable guidewires. J Interven Cardiol 1990;3:225-230.
5. Rees M, Michalis L. Vibrational coronary angioplasty: Challenging chronic total occlusions. Preliminary clinical data. J Am Coll Cardiol 1995;25:368A.
6. Kaltenbach M, Vallbracht C, and Hartmann A. Recanalization of Chronic Coronary Occlusions by Low Speed Rotational Angioplasty (ROTACS). J Interven Cardiol 1991;4:155-165.

126. **Answer: b (false)**

Data from small reports (using different lytic agents and infusion regimens) suggest that prolonged intracoronary thrombolytic infusions may improve the recanalization rate of chronic total coronary occlusions. Among 56 resistant occlusions (combined data from 3 studies),[1-3] a post-lytic improvement in coronary flow and PTCA success was achieved in 63% and 73% of cases, respectively. These finding were corroborated by Zidar et al.[4] in a small randomized trial.

References:
1. Ajluni S, Jones D, Zidar F, Puchrowicz S, Margulis A. Prolonged urokinase infusion for chronic total native coronary occlusions: Clinical, angiographic, and treatment observations. Cath Cardiovas Diagn. 1995;34:106-110.
2. Cecena FA. Urokinase infusion after unsuccessful angioplasty in patients with chronic total occlusion of native coronary arteries. Cath Cardiovasc Diagn. 1993;28:214-218.
3. Vaska KJ, Whitlow PL. Selective tissue plasminogen activator infusion for chronic total occlusions of native coronary arteries failing angioplasty. Circulation

1991;84:II-250.
4. Zidar FJ, Kaplan BM, O'Neill WW, et al. Prospective, randomized trial of prolonged intracoronary urokinase infusion for chronic total occlusions in native coronary arteries. J Am Coll Cardiol 1996;27:1406-12.

CORONARY ARTERY BYPASS GRAFTS

127. Answer: a, c, d

Of the more than 600,000 saphenous vein bypass grafts placed each year, approximately 60-90,000 (10-15%) will be occluded at one year and 300,000 (50%) by 10 years after operation. Among the 10-20% of patients who require re-operation within 10 years, repeat bypass surgery is technically more difficult and has been associated with increased morbidity and mortality compared to the initial operation. The etiology of saphenous vein graft occlusion is dependent on the time interval following bypass surgery:[1,2] In the first month, graft occlusion is almost always due to graft thrombosis from poor surgical technique (suture line stenosis, intraoperative vein trauma) or poor distal run-off. Between 1-12 months, initial hyperplasia is the most common cause. After 1 year, occlusion is caused by graft atherosclerosis, which is indistinguishable from coronary arteriosclerosis. Once graft occlusion occurs, retrograde thrombosis to the aorto-ostial junction is common.

References:
1. Saber RS, Edwards WD, Holmes DR Jr, et al. Balloon angioplasty of aortocoronary saphenous vein bypass grafts: A histopathologic study of six grafts from five patients, with emphasis on restenosis and embolic complications. J Am Coll Cardiol 1988;12:1501-1509.
2. Waller BF, Rothbaum DA, Gorfinkel HJ, et al. Morphologic observations after percutaneous transluminal balloon angioplasty of early and late aortocoronary saphenous vein bypass grafts. J Am Coll Cardiol 1984;4:784-792.

128. Answer: a, b, c

Although PTCA can successfully revascularize approximately 70% of occluded vein grafts, there is a high incidence of distal embolization (10%), late graft occlusion (40-50%), and late cardiac events (event-free survival of 54% and 34% at 1- and 3-years).[1] When distal embolization occurs, ~ 50% are associated with vessel closure and/or CK elevation ≥ 2 times normal.[1] Embolization may present as abrupt cutoff of distal vessels (amenable to repeat dilation or lytics), or may be inferred on the basis of myocardial staining ("blush phenomenon") or no-reflow. This latter manifestation was evident in 29% of occluded vein grafts treated with PTCA, of which 55% had subsequent MI.

Reference:
1. Kahn J, Rutherford B, McConahay D, et al. Initial and long-term outcome of 83 patients after balloon angioplasty of totally occluded bypass grafts. J Am Coll Cardiol 1994;23:1038-1042.

129. Answer: a, b, c, d

Coronary artery bypass surgery (CABG) is a well-established form of revascularization. Despite its ability to relieve angina, and prolong survival in some patients, deficiencies exist: Ischemia recurs in 17% and 63% of patients at 1- and 10-years, respectively, which may be due to new disease in vessels not previously bypassed, progressive disease in native vessels beyond the graft anastomosis, or disease in the bypass conduits themselves. The rate of saphenous vein graft failure is 8% at 1-year, 38% at 5-years and 75% at 10-years.[1] In asymptomatic patients, silent occlusion occurs in 28%, 32%, and 35% of vein grafts at 1-3, 4-6, and 7-11 years after CABG, respectively.[2] Repeat CABG or PTCA is required in 4% of patients at 5-years, 19% of patients 10-years, and 31% of patients 12-years after initial CABG.

References:
1. Campeau L, Enjalbert M, Lesperance J, et al. The relation of risk factors to the development of atherosclerosis in saphenous-vein bypass grafts and the progression of disease in the native circulation. N Engl J of Med 1984;311:1329-1332.
2. White C, Campeau L, Knatterud G, Probstfield J, Investigators atPCCT. Patency of saphaneous vein bypass grafts following elective angiography: Preliminary results from the POST CABG Clinical Trial. J Am Coll Cardiol 1993;21:18A.

130. Answer: a, b, c, f

The risks of repeat CABG are 2- to 4-fold higher than initial CABG, with periprocedural death and MI in 2-5% and 2-8% of patients, respectively.[1-7] Five- and 10-year survival rates are 84-94% and 75%, respectively,[8-15] but 5-year event-free survival (freedom from death, MI, PTCA, or CABG) and angina-free survival are only 64% and 50%, respectively.[9,10] These immediate and long-term results reflect the technical difficulty of reoperation and the frequency of unfavorable patient characteristics. Risk factors for perioperative morbidity and mortality after repeat surgery include left main disease, anginal class III or IV, age > 60 years, diabetes mellitus, ejection fraction < 40%, and incomplete revascularization.[6] Distal embolization causing abrupt vessel cutoff during PTCA occurs in 2-15% of vein grafts > 3 years old, especially in those with soft, friable intraluminal material ("rat-bite" appearance by angiography).[16-20] Independent predictors of distal embolization include diffuse degeneration and large plaque volume, but not thrombus or ulceration.[21] Preliminary data suggest that c7E3 (ReoPro) may lead to 7-fold and 5-fold reductions in distal embolization and non-Q-wave MI during vein graft intervention.[22] The incidence of no-reflow following vein graft intervention is 5-15%, and is more frequent in old (> 3 years) and degenerated grafts.[18,19,23] Abrupt closure complicates 1-2% of vein graft interventions, which is lower than the 2-12% incidence following native vessel intervention.[17,18,24-41] Although coronary artery perforation is a rare complication of balloon angioplasty, the incidence is higher following atherectomy or laser angioplasty.[42,43] Cardiac tamponade is unusual after vein graft perforation due to the extrapericardial course of vein grafts and post-pericardiotomy fibrosis.

References:
1. Reul GJ, Cooley DA, Ott DA, et al. Reoperation for recurrent coronary artery disease. Arch Surg 1979;114:1269-1275.
2. Schaff HV, Orszulak TA, Gersh BJ, et al. The morbidity and mortality of reoperation for coronary artery disease and analysis of late results with use of actuarial estimate of event-free interval. J Thorac Cardiovasc Surg 1983;85:508-515.
3. Foster ED, Fisher LD, Kaiser GC, et al. Comparison of operative mortality and morbidity for initial and repeat coronary artery bypass grafting: The coronary artery surgery study (CASS) registry experience. Ann of Thoracic Surg 1984;38:563-570.
4. Pidgeon J, Brooks N, Magee P, et al. Reoperation for Angina After Previous Aortocoronary Bypass Surgery. Br Heart J 1985;53:269-75.

5. Laird-Meeter K, VanDomBurg R, Vanden Brand MJBM, et al. Incidence, risk, and outcome of reintervention after aortocoronary bypass surgery. Br Heart J 1987;57:427-35.

6. Lytle BW, Loop FD, Cosgrove DM, et al. Fifteen hundred coronary reoperations: results and determinants of early and late survival. J Thorac Cardiovasc Surg 1987;93:847-859.

7. Verheul HA, Moulign AC, Hondema S, et al. Late results of 200 repeat coronary artery bypass operations. Am J of Cardiol 1991;67:24-30.

8. Noyez L, van der Werf T, Janssen D, Klinkenberg T. Early results with bilateral internal mammary artery grafting in coronary reoperations. Am J Cardiol 1992;70:1113-1116.

9. Verheul H, Moulijn A, Hondema S, Schouwink M. Late results of 200 repeat coronary artery bypass operations. Am J Cardiol 1991;67:24-30.

10. Lytle B, Loop F, Cosgrove D, Taylor P. Fifteen hundred coronary reoperations. J Thorac Cardiovasc Surg. 1987;93:847-859.

11. Loop F, Lytle B, Cosgrove D, et al. Reoperation for coronary atherosclerosis. Changing practice in 2509 consecutive patients. Ann Surg 1990;212:378-386.

12. Lamas G, Mudge G, Collins J, et al. Clinical response to coronary artery operation. J Am Coll Cardiol 1986;8:274-279.

13. Pidgeon J, Brook N, MaGee P, Pepper JR. Repoperation of angina after previous aortocoronary bypass surgery. Br Heart J 1985;53:269-275.

14 Foster E, Fisher L, Kaiser G, Meyers W, CASS atPIo. Comparison of operative mortality and morbidity for initial and repeat coronary artery bypass grafting: The CASS Registry Experience. Ann Thorac Surg 1984;38:563-570.

15. Schaff H, Orszulak T, Gersh B, Piehler J. The morbidity and mortality of reoperation for coronary artery disease and analysis of late results with use of actuarial estimate of event-free interval. J Thorac Cardiovasc Surg. 1983;85:508-515.

16. Campeau L, Enjalbert M, Lesperance J, et al. The relation of risk factors to the development of atherosclerosis in saphenous-vein bypass grafts and the progression of disease in the native circulation. N Engl J of Med 1984;311:1329-1332.

17. Dorros G, Lewin RF, Mathiak LM. Coronary angioplasty in patients with prior coronary artery bypass surgery: all prior coronary artery bypass surgery patients and patients more than 5 years after coronary bypass surgery. Cardiol Clin 1989;7:791-803.

18. Platko WP, Hollman J, Whitlow PL, et al. Percutaneous transluminal angioplasty of saphenous vein graft stenosis: long-term follow-up. J Am Coll Cardiol 1989;14:1645-1650.

19. Guzman LA, Villa AE, Whitlow P: New atherectomy devices in the treatment of old saphenous vein grafts: Are the initial results encouraging? Circulation 1992;86:I-780.

20. Altmann D, Popma J, Hong M, et al. CPK-MB elevation after angioplasty of saphenous vein grafts. J Am Coll Cardiol 1993;21:232A.

21. Liu MW, Douglas JS, Lembo NJ, King SBI. Angiographic predictors of a rise in serum creatine kinase (distal embolization) after balloon angioplasty of saphenous vein coronary artery bypass grafts. Am J Cardiol 1993;72:514-517.

22. Challapalli RM, Eisenberg MJ, Sigmon K, Lemberger J. Platelet glycoprotein IIb/IIIa monocional antibody (c7E3) reduces distal embolization during percutaneous intervention of saphenous vein grafts. Circulation 1995;92:I-607.

23. de Feyter PJ, Serruys PW, van den Brand M, Meester H, Beatt K, Surypanyata H. Percutaneous transluminal angioplasty of totally occluded venous bypass grafts: a challenge that should be resisted. Am J Cardiol 1989;64:88-90.

24. Tan K, Henderson R, Sulke N, Cooke R. Percutaneous transluminal coronary angioplasty in patients with prior coronary artery bypass grafting: ten years' experience. Cath Cardiovasc Diagn 1994;31:11-17.

25. Morrison D, Crowley S, Veerakul G, Barbire C, Grover F, Sacks J. Percutaneous transluminal angioplasty of saphenous vein grafts for medically refractory unstable angina. J Am Coll Cardiol 1994;23:1066-1070.

26. Unterberg C, Buchwald A, Wiegand V, Kreuzer H. Coronary angioplasty in patients with previous coronary artery bypass grafting. J Vasc Dis 1992:653-659.

27. Miranda CP, Rutherford BD, McConahay DR, et al. Angioplasty of older saphenous vein grafts continues to be a sound therapeutic option. J Am Coll Cardiol 1992;19, 3:350A.

28. Meester BJ, Samson M, Suryapranata H, et al. Long-term follow-up after attempted angioplasty of saphenous vein grafts: The Thoraxcenter Experience 1981-1988. Eur Heart J 1991;12:648-653.

29. Plokker HWT, Meester BH, Serruys PW. The Dutch experience in percutaneous transluminal angioplasty of narrowed saphenous veins used for aortocoronary arterial bypass. Am J Cardiol 1991;67:361-366.

30. Douglas JS, Weintraub WS, Liberman HA, et al. Update of saphenous graft (SVG) angioplasty: Restenosis and long-term outcome. Circulation 1991; 84: II-249.

31. Jost S, Gulba D, Daniel WG, Amende I. Percutaneous transluminal angioplasty of aortocoronary venous bypass grafts and effect of the caliber of the grafted coronary artery on graft stenosis. Am J Cardiol 1991;68:27-30.

32. Webb JG, Myler RK, Shaw RE, et al. Coronary angioplasty after coronary bypass surgery: Initial results and late outcome in 422 patients. J Am Coll Cardiol 1990;16:812-820.

33. Pinkerton CA, Slack JD, Orr CM, et al. Percutaneous transluminal angioplasty in patients with prior myocardial revascularization surgery. Am J Cardiol 1988;61:15G-22G.

34. Cote GC, Myler RK, Stertzer SH, et al. Percutaneous transluminal angioplasty of stenotic coronary artery bypass grafts: 5 years' experience. J Am Coll Cardiol 1987;9:8-17.

35. Ernst S, van der Feltz T, Ascoop C, et al. Percutaneous transluminal coronary angioplasty in patients with prior coronary artery bypass grafting. J Thorac Cardiovasc Surg 1987;93:268-275.

36. Douglas J, Robinson K, Schlumpf M. Percutaneous transluminal angioplasty in aortocoronary venous graft stenoses: Immediate results and complications. Circulation 1986;74:II-363.

37. Reeder G, Bresnahan J, Holmes DJ, et al. Angioplasty for aortocoronary bypass graft stenosis. Mayo Clin Proc 1986;61:14-19.

38. Corbelli J, Franco I, Hollman J, et al. Percutaneous transluminal coronary angioplasty after previous coronary artery bypass surgery. Am J Cardiol 1985;56:398-403.

39. Gamal M, Bonnier H, Michels R, Heijman J, Stassen E. Percutaneous transluminal angioplasty of stenosed aortocoronary bypass grafts. Br Heart J 1984;52:617-620.

40. Block P, Cowley M, Kaltenbach M, Kent K, Simpson J. Percutaneous angioplasty of stenoses of bypass grafts or of bypass graft anastomotic sites. Am J Cardiol 1984;53:666-668.

41. Douglas JS, Gruentzig AR, King SB, et al. Percutaneous transluminal coronary angioplasty in patients with prior coronary bypass surgery. J Am Colll Cardiol 1983;2:745-754.

42. Ellis SG, Ajluni S, Arnold AZ, Popma JJ, Bittl JA, Eigler NL, Cowley MJ, Raymond RE, Safian RD, Whitlow PL. Increased coronary perforation in the new device era: incidence, classification, management and outcome. Circulation 1994;90:2725-2730

43. Ajluni SC, Glazier S, Blankenship L, O'Neill WW, Safian RD. Perforations after percutaneous coronary interventions: Clinical, angiographic, and theapeutic observations. Cathet Cardiovasc Diagn 1994;32:206-212.

131. Answer: a (4); b (2); c (3); d (1)

132. Answer: b (false)

Many interventionalists believe that older grafts greatly increase the risk of procedural failure and complications. However, several studies suggest that lesion morphology and the presence of degeneration are more important than graft age per se: A recent study of PTCA in grafts > 3 years old reported success in 94%, major complications in 5%, and death in 1.4% — similar to results in grafts < 3 years old.[1] Preliminary studies also suggest that immediate results and complications after DCA or stents are independent of graft age.[2] In contrast, graft age >36 months was associated with lower procedural success, increased complications, and more late cardiac events after TEC.[3] The optimal strategy for old degenerated vein graft lesions is unknown; repeat bypass surgery may be the preferred treatment in some patients.

References:
1. Bredlau CE, Roubin GS, Leimgbruber PP, et Al. In-hospital morbidity and mortality in patients undergoing elective coronary angioplasty. Circulation 72;5:1044-1052.
2. Abdelmeguid A, Ellis S, Whitlow P, et al. Lack of graft age dependency for success of directional coronary atherectomy and Palmaz-Schatz stenting. J Am Coll Cardiol 1993;21:31A.
3. Abdelmeguid A, Ellis S, Whitlow P, et al. Discordant results of extraction atherectomy in old and young saphenous vein grafts: The NACI Experience. J Am Coll Cardiol 1993;21:442A.

133. Answer: a (true)

PTCA of proximal and ostial vein graft lesions have lower success rates (86% vs. 93%) and higher restenosis rates (up to 80%) compared to PTCA of other vein graft sites.

134. Answer: a, b, c

There are limited data on percutaneous revascularization of vein grafts in the setting of acute myocardial infarction.[1,2] These studies suggest a larger burden of thrombus in culprit vein grafts (compared to coronary arteries), which is commonly refractory to intravenous thrombolytic therapy; more effective reperfusion may be achieved by percutaneous techniques (PTCA, TEC, Hydrolyzer, Angiojet) with or without intragraft thrombolytic therapy.[3]

References:
1. Spencer FC. The internal mammary artery: The ideal coronary bypass graft? N Engl J Med 1986;314:50-51.
2. Loop FD, Lytle BW, Cosgrove DM, et al. Influence of internal mammary-artery graft on 10 year survival and other cardiac events. N Engl J Med 1986;314:1-6.
3. Kaplan BM, Larkin T, Safian RD, O'Neill WW, et al. A prospective study of extraction atherectomy in patients with acute myocardial infarction. J Am Coll Cardiol 1996;27:365A.

135. Answer: a, d

The internal mammary artery (IMA) is the conduit of choice for CABG.[1,2] Compared to saphenous vein grafts, IMA grafts demonstrate better flow, less atherosclerosis, and higher 10-year patency rates (95% vs. 25-30%). Despite excellent long-term patency, recurrent ischemia may occur secondary to stenosis in either the IMA or native vessel beyond the anastomosis. PTCA of the IMA can be performed with success rates of 80-100% and a low incidence of abrupt closure, distal embolization, acute MI, and emergency surgery.[3-6] Procedural failures and largely due to failure to cross the lesion with the guidewire or balloon, or inability to reach the stenosis due to vessel tortuosity. Restenosis rates are < 20% and generally lower for lesions at the distal anastomosis compared to the body of the graft.[3] PTCA of the right IMA[7,8] and stenting of both IMA's have also been reported.[9-11]

References:
1. Spencer FC. The internal mammary artery: The ideal coronary bypass graft? N Engl J Med 1986;314:50-51.
2. Loop FD, Lytle BW, Cosgrove DM, et al. Influence of internal mammary-artery graft on 10 year survival and other cardiac events. N Engl J Med 1986;314:1-6.
3. Hearne S, Wilson J, Harrington J, et al. Angiographic and clinical follow-up after internal mammary artery graft angioplasty: A 9-year experience. J Am Coll Cardiol 1995;25:139A.
4. Sketch MH Jr., Quigley PJ, Perez JA et al. Angiographic follow up after internal mammary artery angioplasty. Am J Cardiol 1992;70:401.
5. Popma JJ, Cooke RH, Leon MB et al. Immediate procedural and long-term clinical results in internal mammary artery angioplasty. Am J Cardiol 1992;69:1237
6. Dimas AP, Arora RR, Whitlow PL, et al. Percutaneous transluminal angioplasty involving internal mammary artery grafts. Am Heart J 1991;122:423
7. Steffenin o G, Meier B. Finci L, von Segesser L, Velebit V. Percutaneous transluminal angioplasty of right and left internal mammary artery grafts. Chest 1986;90:849-51
8. Brown RI, Galligan L, Penn IM, Weinstein L. Right internal mammary artery graft angioplasty through a right brachial approach using a new custom guide catheter: a case report. Cathet Cardiovasc Diagn 1992;25:42-5
9. Almagor Y, Thomas J, Colombo A. A balloon expandable stent at the origin of the left internal mammary artery graft: a case report. Cathet Cardiovasc Diagn 1991;24:256-258
10. Bajaj RK, Roubin GS. Intravascular stenting of the right internal mammary artery. Cathet Cardiovasc Diagn 1991; 24:252-255
11. Hadjimiltiades S, Gourassas J, Louridas G, Tsifodimos D. Stenting the distal anastomotic site of the left internal mammary artery graft: a case report. Cathet Cardiovasc Diagn 1994;32:157-161

136. Answer: a, d, e

Coronary artery fistulae are the most common hemodynamically significant coronary anomaly. Fistulae arising from either the left or right coronary arteries are common and over 90% drain into the venous circulation (RV, RA, PA). The majority are asymptomatic until the fifth or sixth decade when symptoms of left ventricular failure occur secondary to the left-to-right shunt. Other complications include angina (resulting from a coronary "steal" syndrome), endocarditis, fistula rupture, and progressive dilatation. Indications for closure include a significant left-to-right shunt (QP/QS >1.5), signs of heart failure, or ischemia. Selected fistulae may be closed surgically or percutaneously using detachable balloons, microcoil embolization, or microparticle embolization.

CORONARY ARTERY SPASM

137. Answer: a (2); b (3); c (1)

Coronary artery spasm at the target lesion has been reported in 1-5% of balloon angioplasty procedures.[1,2] Risk factors include noncalcified lesions, [1,3] possibly eccentric lesions[4] and younger patients, but not variant angina.[5,6] Intravascular ultrasound or angioscopy may be useful in cases where it is difficult to distinguish refractory spasm from severe recoil or dissection. Fortunately, most cases can be successfully treated by intracoronary vasodilators (nitrates and/or calcium blockers) with or without repeat PTCA at low inflation pressures. In contrast, spasm of the distal vessel is common after PTCA and virtually all percutaneous devices; repeat angiograms taken 15-30 minutes after balloon deflation demonstrate a 16-30% reduction in minimal lumen diameter[7,8] and a 28% reduction in cross-sectional area.[9] Treatment consists of nitrates (sublingual, intravenous, or intracoronary), nifedipine (sublingual), and/or diltiazem or verapamil (intravenous or intracoronary). In contrast to epicardial spasm, spasm of the distal microvascular bed rarely response to nitrates; the preferred treatment is intracoronary calcium antagonists.

References:
1. Cowley M, Dorros G, Kelsey S, Van Raden M, Detre K. Acute coronary events associated with percutaneous transluminal coronary angioplasty. Am J Cardiol 1984;53:12C-16C.
2. Holmes DJ, Holubkov R, Vlietstra R, et al. Comparison of complications during percutaneous transluminal coronary angioplasty from 1977 to 1981 and from 1985 to 1986: The National Heart, Lung, and Blood Institute Percutaneous Transluminal Coronary Angioplasty Registry. J Am Coll Cardiol 1988;12:1149-1155.
3. Fitzgerald PJ, Stertzer SH, Hidalgo BO, et al. Plaque characteristics affect lesion and vessel response to coronary rotational atherectomy: An intravascular ultrasound study. J Am Coll Cardiol 1994:March Special Issue:353A.
4. Fischell T, and Bausback K. Effects of luminal eccentricity on spontaneous coronary vasoconstriction after successful percutaneous transluminal coronary angioplasty. Am J Cardiol 1991;68:530-534.
5. Corcos T, David PR, Bourassa MG, et al. Percutaneous transluminal coronary angioplasty for the treatment of variant angina. J Am Coll Cardiol 1985;5:1046-1054.
6. David PR, Waters DD, Scholl M, et al. Percutaneous coronary angioplasty in patients with variant angina. Circulation 1982;66:695-702.
7. Indolfi C, Piscione F, Esposito G, et al. Mechanisms of coronary vasoconstriction after successful single angioplasty of the left anterior descending artery. J Am Coll Cardiol 1993:February Special Issue:340A.
8. Fischell T, Derby G, Tse T, Stadius M. Coronary artery vasoconstriction routinely occurs after percutaneous transluminal coronary angioplasty. A quantitative arteriographic analysis. Circulation 1988;78:1323-1334.
9. Golino P, Piscione F, Benedict CF, et al. Local effect of serotonin released during coronary angioplasty. N Engl J Med 1994;330:523-8.

138. Answer: a (true)

The PTCA site remains susceptible to spasm for several months after the procedure. Ergonovine[1] and acetylcholine [2] can induce vasospasm after PTCA in 15% and 46% of patients, respectively.[1] Spontaneous angina due to spasm may develop in the weeks or months following PTCA.[1,3]

References:
1. Hollman J, Austin GE, Gruentzig AR, et al. Coronary artery spasm at the site of angioplasty in the first two months after successful percutaneous transluminal coronary angioplasty. J Am Coll Cardiol 1983;2:1039-1045.
2. Kirigaya H, Aizawa T, Ogasaware K, et al. Enhanced vasospastic activity to acetylcholine of the coronary arteries undergoing previous balloon angioplasty. J Am Coll Cardiol 1993:February Special Issue:341A.
3. David PR, Waters DD, Scholl M, et al. Percutaneous coronary angioplasty in patients with variant angina. Circulation 1982;66:695-702.

139. Answer: a, b, c, d, e, f

Compared to PTCA, coronary artery spasm after new devices occurs with equal or greater frequency.[1-8] Spasm has been reported in 4 - 36% of Rotablator cases;[5,9-12] in one study, severe spasm resulting in threatened or abrupt occlusion and requiring repeat PTCA or CABG occurred in 12/743 patients (1.6%).[1] Spasm has been reported in 1.2 - 16% of ELCA procedures.[3,4,6-8,13] Independent predictors include smoking (relative risk 2.1), no diabetes (relative risk 2.2), and stenosis severity ≤ 90% (relative risk 1.6). Spasm has also been reported in 0.8 - 1.6% of DCA and 6.6% of holmium-laser cases.[2,8] Most cases of coronary spasm following new devices respond to intracoronary and intravenous nitrates with or without repeat balloon dilatation.

References:
1. Warth D, Leon M, et al. Rotational atherectomy multicenter registry: Acute results, complications and 6-month angiographic follow-up in 709 patients. J Am Coll Cardiol 1994;24:641-648.
2. deMarchena EJ, Mallon SM, et al. Effectiveness of holmium laser-assisted coronary angioplasty. Am J Cardiol 1994;73:117-121.
3. Bittl J, Sanborn T, et al. Clinical success, complications and restenosis rates with excimer laser coronary angioplasty. Am J Cardiol 1992;70:1533-1539.
4. Ghazzal Z, Hearn J, et al. Morphological predictors of acute complications after percutaneous excimer laser coronary angioplasty. Results of a comprehensive angiographic analysis: Importance of the eccentricity index. Circulation 1992;86:820-827.
5. Safian R, Niazi K, et al. Detailed Angiographic Analysis of High-Speed Mechanical Rotational Atherectomy in Human Coronary Arteries. Circulation 1993;88:961-968.
6. Litvack F, Eigler N, et al. Percutaneous excimer laser coronary angioplasty: Results in the first consecutive 3,000 patients. J Am Coll Cardiol 1994;23:323-9.
7. Baumback A, Bittl J, Fleck E, et al. Acute complications of excimer laser coronary angioplasty: A detailed analysis of multicenter results. J Am Coll Cardiol 1994;23:1305-1313.
8. Mehta S, Popma JJ, Margolis JR, et al. Angiographic complications after new device angioplasty in native coronary arteries: A NACI Angiographic Core Laboratory Report. TCT Meeting (Washington DC),February, 1995.
9. Gregorini L, Marco J, Fajadet J, Brunel, P, et al. Urapidil (α 1-sympathetic blocker) attenuates post-rotational ablation "elastic recoil". Circulation 1995;92:I-94.
10. Bertrand M, Lablanche J, Leroy F, Bauters C. Percutaneous transluminal coronary rotary ablation with Rotablator (European experience). Am J Cardiol 1992;69:470-474.
11. Teirstein PS, Warth DC, Haq N, et al. High-speed rotational coronary atherectomy for patients with diffuse coronary artery disease. J Am Coll Cardiol 1991;18:1694-1701.
12. Mehta S, Popma J, Margolis JR, et al. Complications with new angioplasty devices. Are these device specific? J Am Coll Cardiol 1996;27:168A.
13. Initial results of the European Multicenter Registry on Coronary Excimer Laser Angioplasty. European Study Group. Circulation 1991;84:II-362.

140. Answer: b

Coronary artery spasm usually resolves promptly after the administration of intracoronary nitroglycerin (100-300 mcg), but repeated doses may be necessary (up to 2 mg).

141. Answer: b (false)

If intralesional spasm is evident, the guidewire should remain across the lesion to maintain vascular access. If spasm occurs distal to the PTCA site, partial or complete removal of the guidewire may facilitate resolution of spasm.

142. Answer: a (true)

143. Answer: b (false)

A temporary transvenous pacemaker should be readily available. However, since the risk of AV block, bradycardia and hypotension are low, prophylatic insertion is not routinely recommended.

144. Answer: a, d

Intracoronary verapamil (100 mcg/min up to 1.0 - 1.5 mg)[1] or intracoronary diltiazem (0.5-2.5 mg over ≥ 1 min.; total: 5-10 mg)[2] may reverse coronary spasm refractory to intracoronary nitroglycerin.

Answers

Intravenous calcium antagonists, however, do no reliably relieve coronary vasospasm.

References:
1. Babbitt DG, Perry JM, and Forman MB. Intracoronary verapamil for reversal of refractory coronary vasospasm during percutaneous transluminal coronary angioplasty. J Am Coll Cardiol 1988;12:1377-1381.
2. McIvor ME, Undemir C, Lawson J, Reddinger J. Clinical effects and utility of intracoronary diltiazem. Cathet Cardiovasc Diagn. 1995;35:287-291.

145. Answer: a (true)

If intralesional spasm persists despite the use of nitrates, a prolonged (2-5 minute) low-pressure (1-4 atm.) inflation using a balloon matched to the reference segment is frequently successful at "breaking" the spasm. In fact, the vast majority of episodes of spasm respond to nitrates and repeat PTCA.

146. Answer: a (true)

Intracoronary stenting has been used successfully for refractory spasm, but should be reserved for situations in which all other nonoperative alternatives have failed. Most such cases of "refractory" spasm are probably dissections, which should respond to stenting.

147. Answer: a (true)

Emergency bypass surgery is rarely necessary but should be considered for refractory spasm when there is ongoing ischemia, the vessel is suitable for grafting, and all other approaches have been exhausted.

148. Answer: a

PTCA of organic stenosis in patients with variant angina is associated with a high technical success rate; procedural complications, including coronary artery spasm, are no more frequent than during PTCA for other lesions. Recurrent spasm and rest angina are not uncommon following PTCA. Pharmacologic therapy with high-dose nitrates and calcium channel antagonists may reduce their frequency and severity, but restenosis rates approach 50%. Many patients derive symptomatic benefit, although the impact on event-free survival (compared to medical therapy or CABG) has not been evaluated.

DISSECTION AND ABRUPT CLOSURE

149. Answer: a, c, e

Acute closure occurs in 2-11% of elective PTCAs; [1-4] 50-80% occur while the patient is still in the catheterization laboratory.[5-7] Episodes developing outside the angioplasty suite usually occur within the first 6 hours and are rare after 24 hours. In one report, 63% of acute closures occurred within 1 hour, and 84% within 6 hours of the procedure.[8] In another report, 54% occurred within 6 hours, 21% within 6-12 hours, 25% within 12-24 hours, and no cases presented later than 24 hours after PTCA.[6] Acute closure does not appear to be reduced after the primary use of atherectomy or laser devices.[9-15] In CAVEAT-I,[16] abrupt closure was more common after DCA than PTCA (8% vs. 3.8%, p = 0.005), although in CAVEAT-II and CCAT, there was no difference in acute closure between these devices. In contrast to other devices, primary stenting has reduced the incidence of acute closure to < 1%; in the randomized STRESS and BENSTENT trials, vessel closure was 1.5-2 times higher after PTCA. A recent report from the NACI Registry of 2233 native coronaries treated by new devices revealed an acute closure rate of 0% for stents compared to 1.3-8.3% for atherectomy and 7.4% for excimer laser (devices were not matched for lesion morphology).[15]

References:
1. Ramee SR, White CJ, Jain A, et al. Percutaneous coronary angioscopy versus angiography in patients undergoing coronary angioplasty. J Am Coll Caridol 1991;17:125A.
2. Tan K, Sulke N, Taub N, Sowton E. Clinical and lesion morphologic determinants of coronary angioplasty success and complications: Current experience. J Am Coll Cardiol 1995;25:855-65.
3. Van Belle E, Bauters C, Lablanche J-M, McFadden E, Bertrand M. Angiographic determinants of acute outcome after coronary angioplasty: A prospective quantitative coronary angiographic study of 3679 procedures. J Am Coll Cardiol 1994:223A.
4. Lincoff AM, Popma JJ, Ellis SG, Hacker J. Abrupt vessel closure complicating coronary angioplasty: Clinical, angiographic, and therapeutic profile. J Am Coll Cardiol 1992;19:926-935.
5. Ellis S, Roubin G, King S, et al. In-hospital cardiac mortality after acute closure after coronary angioplasty: Analysis of risk factors from 8,207 procedures. J Am Coll Cardiol 1988;11:211-216.
6. de Feyter PJ, van den Brand M, Jaarman G, van Domburg R. Acute coronary artery occlusion during and after percutaneous transluminal coronary angioplasty. Frequency, prediction, and clinical course, management, and follow-up. Circulation 1991;83:927-936.
7. The Bypass Angioplasty Revascularization Investigation (BARI): Five year mortality and morbidity in a randomized study comparing CABG and PTCA in patients with multivessel coronary disease. The BARI Investigators. N Engl J Med (submitted)
8. Simpfendorfer C, Belardi J, Bellamy G, Galan K. Frequency, management and follow-up of patients with acute coronary occlusions after percutaneous transluminal coronary angioplasty. Am J Cardiol 1987;59:267-269.
9. Safian R, Lai S, Buchbinder M, Sanbron T, Sketch M. Incidence and management of abrupt closure after new device interventions. Report from the NACI Registry in 2988 lesions. Circulation 1993;88(Suppl.):I-585.
10. Mehta S, Popma J, Margolis J, et al. Angiographic complications after new device angioplasty in native coronary arteries: A NACI Angiographic Core Laboratory Report. TCT Meeting (Washington DC), February, 1995.
11. Popma J, Topol E, Hinohara T, et al. Abrupt vessel closure after directional coronary atherectomy. J Am Coll Cardiol 1992;19:1372-1379.
12. Warth D, Leon M, O'Neill W, et al. Rotational atherectomy multicenter registry: Acute results, complications and 6-month angiographic follow-up in 709 patients. J Am Coll Cardiol 1994;24:641-648.
13. Litvack F, Eigler N, Margolis J, et al. Percutaneous excimer laser coronary angioplasty: Results in the first consecutive 3,000 patients. J Am Coll Cardiol 1994;23:323-329.
14. Painter J, Popma J, Pichard A, et al. A comparison of early and late clinical outcomes in patients undergoing concentric and directional laser coronary angioplasty. TCT Meeting (Washington DC), February, 1995.
15. Mehta S, Popma J, Margolis JR, et al. Complications with new angioplasty devices. Are these device specific? J Am Coll Cardiol 1996;March Special Issue.
16. Holmes DR, Simpson JB, Berdan LG, et al. Abrupt closure: The CAVEAT I Experience. J Am Coll Cardiol 1995;26:1494-500.

150. Answer: b (false)

The most common cause of acute closure is coronary dissection.

151. Answer: a (true)

Following balloon angioplasty, coronary dissection is detected by angiography in 20-40% of cases,[1-5] and by intravascular ultrasound (IVUS) or angioscopy in 60-80% of cases.[6,7] Non-flow-limiting dissections should be not necessarily be considered a complication, since the mechanism of lumen enlargement for PTCA involves stretching of the vessel wall and cracking of plaque, which are manifest as dissection.

References:
1. Tan K, Sulke N, Taub N, Sowton E. Clinical and lesion morphologic determinants of coronary angioplasty success and complications: Current experience. J Am Coll Cardiol 1995;25:855-65.
2. Hermans WR, Foley DP, Rensing BJ, Rutsch W. Usefulness of quantitative and qualitative angiographic lesion morphology, and clinical characteristics in predicting major adverse cardiac events during and after native coronary balloon angioplasty. Am J Cardiol 1993;72:14-20.
3. Bailey S, Ricci D, Kiesz S, et al. Incidence and clinical impact of dissections after PTCA and stent placement: Results from the Randomized STent REStenosis Study. TCT Meeting (Washington DC), February, 1995.
4. Hermans WR, Rensing BJ, Foley DP, Deckers JW. Therapeutic dissection after successful coronary balloon angioplasty: No influence on restenosis or on clinical outcome in 693 patients. J Am Coll Cardiol 1992;20:767-780.
5. Sharma SK, Israel DH, Kamean JL, Bodian CA. Clinical, angiographic, and procedural determinants of major and minor coronary dissection during angioplasty. Am Heart J 1993;126:39-47.
6. Kovach J, Mintz G, Pichard A, et al. Sequential intravascular ultrasound characterization of the mechanisms of rotational atherectomy and adjunct balloon angioplasty. J Am Coll Cardiol 1993;22:1024-32.
7. den Heijer P, Foley D, Escaned J, Hillege H. Angioscopic versus angiographic detection of intimal dissection and intracoronary thrombus. J Am Coll Cardiol 1994;24:649-654.

152. Answer: a, b, c

In some situations, angiography may suggest the presence of a dissection when none exists; these are important to recognize to avoid unnecessary attempts to repair the "dissection." Simple technical faults, such as weak contrast injections, may cause contrast streaming and give the false impression of an intimal tear; these are readily identified by better injections to clearly opacify the lumen. In addition, deep guide catheter intubation may deform the proximal vessel and suggest the presence of a stenosis or dissection; repositioning the guide will often correct this problem, and intracoronary nitroglycerin (100-200 mcg i.c.) may also be used to relieve associated spasm. Finally, a common angiographic findings is a pseudolesion, which is a segmental shelf-like deformity due to excessive straightening and invagination of the vessel wall, frequently associated with extra support guidewires. These pseudolesions can be very disturbing and easily confused with vessel injury from balloons or other devices. It is important to consider a pseudolesion when a new stenosis develops remote from the target lesion, particularly when heavy-duty guidewires are employed in tortuous vessels or for tracking new interventional devices. Because of the uncertainly created by these pseudolesions, it is generally best to substitute a more flexible guidewire, if possible; if the pseudolesion does not improve or resolve, it may be necessary to completely remove the guidewire to ensure that a real lesion is not present.

53. Answer: b (false)

Angiographic dissection rates vary for different devices, probably reflecting differences in the mechanism of lumen enlargement and the nature of the target lesion.

Angiographic Dissection Rates After Percutaneous Intervention

Modality	Incidence (%)
PTCA[1-5]	20 - 40
ELCA[6-11] DELCA[8] TEC[6]	20 - 30*
Rotablator[6,11-14]	10 - 30
DCA[6,15]	10 - 15
Stent[3,6]	< 10

Abbreviations: DELCA = directional excimer laser coronary angioplasty; TEC = transluminal extraction catheter; DCA = directional coronary atherectomy

* 10-20% when ELCA is performed with the saline infusion technique

References:
1. Tan K, Sulke N, Taub N, Sowton E. Clinical and lesion morphologic determinants of coronary angioplasty success and complications: Current experience. J Am Coll Cardiol 1995;25:855-65.
2. Hermans WR, Foley DP, Rensing BJ, Rutsch W. Usefulness of quantitative and qualitative angiographic lesion morphology, and clinical characteristics in predicting major adverse cardiac events during and after native coronary balloon angioplasty. Am J Cardiol 1993;72:14-20.
3. Bailey S, Ricci D, Kiesz S, et al. Incidence and clinical impact of dissections after PTCA and stent placement: Results from the Randomized STent REStenosis Study. TCT Meeting (Washington DC), February, 1995.
4. Hermans WR, Rensing BJ, Foley DP, Deckers JW. Therapeutic dissection after successful coronary balloon angioplasty: No influence on restenosis or on clinical outcome in 693 patients. J Am Coll Cardiol 1992;20:767-780.
5. Sharma SK, Israel DH, Kamean JL, Bodian CA. Clinical, angiographic, and procedural determinants of major and minor coronary dissection during angioplasty. Am Heart J 1993;126:39-47.
6. Mehta S, Popma J, Margolis J, et al. Angiographic complications after new device angioplasty in native coronary arteries: A NACI Angiographic Core Laboratory Report. TCT Meeting (Washington DC), February, 1995.
7. Litvack F, Eigler N, Margolis J, et al. Percutaneous excimer laser coronary angioplasty: Results in the first consecutive 3,000 patients. J Am Coll Cardiol 1994;23:323-329.
8. Painter J, Popma J, Pichard A, et al. A comparison of early and late clinical outcomes in patients undergoing concentric and directional laser coronary angioplasty. TCT Meeting (Washington DC), February, 1995.
9. Ghazzal Z, Hearn J, Litvack F, et al. Morphological predictors of acute complications after percutaneous excimer laser coronary angioplasty. Results of a comprehensive angiographic analysis: Importance of the eccentricity index. Circulation 1992;86:820-827.
10. Baumbach A, Bittl J, Fleck E, Geschwind H, Sanborn T. Acute complications of excimer laser coronary angioplasty: A detailed analysis of multicenter results. J Am Coll Cardiol 1994;23:1305-1313.
11. Dussaillant G, Popma J, Pichard A, et al. Rotational atherectomy vs. excimer laser angioplasty: A multivariable analysis of early and late procedural outcome. J Am Coll Cardiol 1995;25:330A.
12. Warth D, Leon M, O'Neill W, et al. Rotational atherectomy multicenter registry: Acute results, complications and 6-month angiographic follow-up in 709 patients. J Am Coll Cardiol 1994;24:641-648.
13. Safian R, Niazi K, et al. Detailed Angiographic Analysis of High-Speed Mechanical Rotational Atherectomy in Human Coronary Arteries. Circulation 1993;88: 961-968.
14. Brown D, Giordano F, Buchbinder M. Coronary dissection following rotational atherectomy: Clinical characteristics, angiographic predictors and acute outcomes. J Am Coll Cardiol 1995;25:123A.
15. Hinohara T, Rowe M, Robertson G, et al. Effect of lesion characteristics on outcome of directional coronary atherectomy. J Am Coll Cardiol 1991;17:1112-1120.

154. Answer: b

The saline infusion technique has reduced the incidence of dissection after ELCA; in a randomized trial, patients undergoing ELCA with blood displacement by intracoronary saline had fewer severe dissections compared to conventional ELCA (7% vs. 24%; p = 0.05).[1]

References:
1. Deckelbaum LI, Natarajan MK, Bittl JA, et al. Effect of intracoronary saline infusion on dissection during excimer laser coronary angioplasty: A randomized trial. J Am Coll Cardiol 1995;26:1264-9.

Answers

155. Answer: c, d, e, f

Huber et al.[1] reviewed 691 angioplasties complicated by arterial dissection, to determine whether dissection type, as defined by the NHLBI classification system, had prognostic value for in-hospital complications. Patients with types A and B dissection had an excellent prognosis that did not differ from those without dissection. Compared to type B dissections, those with dissection types C to F experienced lower clinical success rates (38% vs 94%), and a higher rate of acute closure (31% vs 3%), emergency CABG (37% vs 1%), Q-wave MI (13% vs 0%), and elective CABG (12% vs 3%).

References:
1. Huber MS, Mooney JF, Madison J, Mooney MR. Use of a morphologic classification to predict clinical outcome after dissection from coronary angioplasty. Am J Cardiol 1991;68:467.

156. Answer: a, b, c

157. Answer: b, c

Complex dissections are characterized by deep medial tears which may create long or spiral dissections. Dissections frequently occur at the junction between calcified and non-calcified plaque, and may be due to the nonuniform transmission of dilating force across vessel segments of differing elastic properties.[1] Absorption of excimer laser energy produces acoustic shock waves, which may generate a pressure of 100 atm.; this acoustic effect induces vessel trauma, manifested as dissection, abrupt closure, or perforation.[2] Administration of a saline bolus and infusion at time of lasing (saline infusion technique) may attenuate acoustic injury.[3,4]

References:
1. Fitzgerald PJ, Ports TA, Yock PG. Contribution of localized calcium deposits to dissection after angioplasty. An observational study using intravascular ultrasound. Circulation 1992;86:64-70.
2. van Leeuwen T, Meertens J, Velema E, Post M, Borst C. Intraluminal vapor bubble induced by excimer laser pulse causes microsecond arterial dilation and invagination leading to extensive wall damage in the rabbit. Circulation 1993;87:1258.
3. Tcheng J, Wells L, Phillips H, Deckelbaum L, Golobic R. Development of a new technique for reducing pressure pulse generation during 308-nm excimer laser coronary angioplasty. Cathet Cardiovas Diagn. 1995;34:15-22.
4. Deckelbaum LI, Natarajan MK, Bittl JA, et al. Effect of intracoronary saline infusion on dissection during excimer laser coronary angioplasty: randomized trial. J Am Coll Cardiol 1995;26:1264-9.

158. Answer: d

References:
1. Huber M, Mooney J, Madison J, Mooney M. Use of a morphologic classification to predict clinical outcome after dissection from coronary angioplasty. Am J Cardiol 1991;68:467-471.
2. Bell M, Berger PB, Reeder GS, et al. Coronary dissection following PTCA: Predictors of major ischemic complications. Circulation 1991;84:II-130.

159. Answer: b, c

Randomized trials by Talley et al.[1] and Safian et al.[2] suggest that balloon material (compliant vs. noncompliant) has no impact on dissection or clinical outcome. In contrast, use of oversized balloons[3] and gradual (vs. fast) balloon deflation[4,5] appear to increase the risk of dissection. Long balloons for

The Impact of Balloon Angioplasty Technique or Coronary Dissection Rate

Parameter	Effect on Dissection Rate			Comments
	Possible ↑	Possible ↓	None	
Balloon catheter design			✓	Choice of catheter type (over-the-wire, on-the-wire, monorail) based on operator preference.
Balloon material (compliant vs. noncompliant)			✓	Compliant balloons have been associated with higher,[8] equal,[9,10] and lower dissection rates.[11] More recent randomized trials show no difference in clinical outcome.[1,2] High-pressure inflations suing compliant balloons for resistant lesions may cause "dog-boning" and increase the risk of dissection.
Balloon sizing	✓			Most reports indicate that balloon oversizing (balloon-to-artery ratio > 1.2) is a powerful independent predictor of dissection.[3] Attempt to match the balloon diameter to the distal reference segment (balloon-to-artery ratio + 1.0).
Inflation pressure (high vs. low)			✓	Studies are small or retrospective. Most operators begin with low-pressure inflations and reserve high-pressure inflations for significant residual stenosis. Inflations exceeding rated burst pressure increase the risk of balloon rupture and vessel dissection. High-pressure inflations using compliant balloons may result in overstretching and dissection.
Duration of inflation (long vs. short)		✓		Randomized studies comparing 3 inflations at 1 min. vs. 4-5 min. demonstrated fewer and less severe dissections with prolonged inflations.[12] Whether multiple short inflations are comparable to fewer long inflations is unknown.
Inflation speed (slow vs. fast)		✓		Two randomized studies reported fewer dissections with gradual inflations,[13,14] while no effect was seen in another.[15] Studies also suggest a benefit for gradual, prolonged inflations.[16,17]
Oscillating inflations		✓		Nonrandomized study reported major dissections in 0.3% of lesions using this technique.[18] When combined with gradual balloon deflation, more dissections occurred.[4]

Answers

Parameter	Effect on Dissection Rate			Comments
	Possible ↑	**Possible ↓**	**None**	
Deflation speed (slow vs. fast)	✓			Gradual deflation resulted more of major dissections in two randomized trials.[19,20]
Predilatation		✓		Nonrandomized study reported major dissections in only 1.3% of patients,[21] while no effect was seen in a small randomized study.[22] Use of a dual-balloon catheter (distal balloon to predilate, proximal balloon for final dilatation) resulted in a low dissection rate.[23]
Long balloon for long lesions		✓		
Noncompliant long-balloon of angulated lesions		✓		
Noncompliant balloon for calcified lesions		✓		
Tapered balloon for tapered lesions		✓		

References:

1. Talley JD, Blankenship S, Spokojny WA, Anderson HV, et al. Does the type of balloon material used in elective PTCA make a difference in clinical complications? Results from the CRAC study. Circulation 1995;92:I-74.
2. Safian RD, Hoffmann MA, Almany S, et al. Comparison of coronary angioplasty with compliant and noncompliant balloons (The Angioplasty Compliance Trial). Am J Cardiol 1995;76:518-520.
3. Sharma SK, Israel DH, Kamean JL, Bodian CA. Clinical, angiographic, and procedural determinants of major and minor coronary dissection during angioplasty. Am Heart J 1993;126:39-47.
4. Blankenship J, Ford A, Henry S, Frey C. Coronary dissection resulting from angioplasty with slow oscillating vs. rapid inflation and slow vs. rapid deflation. Cath Cardiovasc Diagn. 1995;34:202-209.
5. Foster C, Teskey R, Kells C, et al. Does the speed of balloon deflation affect the complication rate of coronary angioplasty. J Am Coll Cardiol 1993;21:290A. 26.
6. Zidar JP, Tenaglia AN, Jackman JD, et al. Improved acute results for PTCA of long coronary lesions using long angioplasty balloon catheters. J Am Coll Cardiol 1992;19:34A.
7. Brymer JF, Khaja F, and Kraft L. Angioplasty of long or tandem coronary artery lesions using a new longer balloon dilatation catheter: A comparative study. Cathet and Cardiovasc Diagn 1991;23:84-88.
8. Berry K, Drew T, McKendall G, et al. Balloon material as a risk factor for coronary angioplasty procedural complications. Circulation 1991;84:II-130.
9. Mooney MR, Fishman-Mooney J, Longe TF, Brandenburg RO. Effect of balloon material on coronary angioplasty. Am J Cardiol 1992;69:1481-1482.
10. Raymenants E, Bhandari S, Stammen F, De Scheerder I, Desmet W, Piessens J. Effects of angioplasty balloon material and lesion characteristics on the incidence of coronary dissection in 2150 dilated lesions. J Am Coll Cardiol 1993;21:291A.
11. Hermans WR, Rensing BJ, Foley DP, Deckers JW. Therapeutic dissection after successful coronary balloon angioplasty: No influence on restenosis or on clinical outcome in 693 patients. J Am Coll Cardiol 1992;20:767-780.
12. Cribier A, Elchaninoff H, Chan C, et al. Comparative effects of long (> 12 min) versus standard (<3 min) sequential balloon inflations in PTCA. Preliminary results of a prospective randomized study: Immediate results and restenosis rates. J Am Coll Cardiol 1994;23:58A.
13. Remetz MS, Cabin HS, McConnell S, Cleman M. Gradual balloon inflation protocol reduces arterial damage following percutaneous transluminal coronary angioplasty. J Am Coll Cardiol 1988;11:131A.
14. Ilia R, Cabin H, McConnell S. et al. Coronary angioplasty with gradual versus rapid balloon inflation. Cathet Cardiovasc Diagn 1993;29:199-202.
15. Bansal A, Choksi N, Levein AB, et al. Determinants of arterial dissection after PTCA: lesion type versus inflation rate. J Am Coll Cardiol 1989;13:229A.
16. Tenaglia AN, Quigley PJ, Kereiakes DJ, et al. Coronary angioplasty performed with a gradual and prolonged inflation using a perfusion balloon catheter: procedural success and restenosis rate. Am Heart J 1992;124:585-589.
17. Farcot JC, Berland J, Stix A, et al. Gradual, low-pressure and prolonged (10 minutes) protected inflations decreased complications and improved results of proximal LAD angioplasty. Eur Heart J 1991;12:263.
18. Shawl F, Dougherty K, Hoff S. Does inflation strategy influence acute outcome and long-term results. Circulation 1993;88:I-587.
19. Blankenship J, Ford A, Henry S, Frey C. Coronary dissection resulting from angioplasty with slow oscillating vs. rapid inflation and slow vs. rapid deflation. Cath Cardiovasc Diagn. 1995;34:202-209.
20. Foster C, Teskey R, Kells C, et al. Does the speed of balloon deflation affect the complication rate of coronary angioplasty. J Am Coll Cardiol 1993;21:290A.
21. Banka V, Kochar G, Maniet A, Voci G. Progressive coronary dilation: An angioplasty technique that creates controlled arterial injury and reduces complications. Am Heart J 1993;125:61-71.
22. McKeever LS, O'Donnell MJ, Stamato NJ, et al. The effect of predilatation on coronary angioplasty-induced vessel wall injury. Am Heart J 1991;122:1515-1518.

23. Banka VS, Fail PS, Kochar GS, Maniet AR.   Dual-balloon progressive coronary dilatation catheter: design and initial clinical experience. Am Heart J. 1994;127:430-435.

160. Answer: a, b

Severe coronary artery dissections increase the risk of ischemic complications (death, MI, emergency CABG) more than 5-fold.[1-4] In the STRESS trial, the presence of a dissection resulted in lower procedural success (75% vs. 92%) and higher in-hospital ischemic events (15% vs. 3%).[2] The majority of dissections that do not result in acute ischemic complications disappear with time.[5,6] Follow-up angiography indicates that 4-16% of dissections disappear within 24 hours, and 63-93% by 3-6 months.[6-8] While small earlier studies suggested a lower incidence of restenosis with dissection, large recent reports indicate that dissection has no impact on restenosis rates.[6,8,9]

References:
1. Warth D, Leon M, O'Neill W, et al. Rotational atherectomy multicenter registry: Acute results, complications and 6-month angiographic follow-up in 709 patients. J Am Coll Cardiol 1994;24:641-648.
2. Bailey S, Ricci D, Kiesz S, et al. Incidence and clinical impact of dissections after PTCA and stent placement: Results from the Randomized STent REStenosis Study. TCT Meeting (Washington DC), February, 1995.
3. Bredlau CE, Roubin GS, Leimgruber PP, Douglas JS. In-hospital morbidity and mortality in patients undergoing elective coronary angioplasty. Circulation 1985;72:1044-1052. 71.
4. Foley D, Hermans W, Rensing B, Serruys P. Predictability of major adverse cardiac events after balloon angioplasty from clinical data and quantitative and qualitative angiographic analysis. J Am Coll Cardiol 1993;21:339A.
5. Nobuyhshi M, Kimura T, Nosaka H, et al. Restenosis after successful percutaneous transluminal coronary angioplasty: Serial angiographic follow-up of 229 patients. J Am Coll Cardiol 1988;12:616-623.
6. Cappelletti A, Margonato A, Berna G, Chierchia S. Spontaneous evolution of nonocclusive coronary dissection after PTCA: A 6-month angiographic follow-up study. J Am Coll Cardiol 1995;25:345A.
7. Popma J, Topol E, Hinohara T, et al. Abrupt vessel closure after directional coronary atherectomy. J Am Coll Cardiol 1992;19:1372-1379.
8. Savage M, Dischman D, Bailey S, et al. Vascular remodeling of balloon-induced intimal dissection: Long-term angiographic assessment. J Am Coll Cardiol 1995;25:139A.
9. Hermans WR, Rensing BJ, Foley DP, Deckers JW. Therapeutic dissection after successful coronary balloon angioplasty: No influence on restenosis or on clinical outcome in 693 patients. J Am Coll Cardiol 1992;20:767-780.

161. Answer: e

Of the many clinical, angiographic, and procedural variables reported to increase the risk of acute closure, the most powerful predictor is the presence of a complex dissection (relative risk ~ 6).[1]

References:
1. Tenaglia A, Fortin D, Califf R. Predicting the risk of abrupt closure after angioplasty in an individual patient. J Am Coll Cardiol 1994;24:1004-1011.

162. Answer: c

Clinical and angiographic variables have been used to identify patients at increased risk of cardiac death after acute closure. The most powerful predictor of mortality is the jeopardy score, which estimates net ventricular dysfunction and correlates with mortality if acute closure occurs (see Table).[1]

Answers

Systolic Blood Pressure and Risk of Death Following Acute Closure: Correlation With the Jeopardy Score[1]

Jeopardy Score*	Systolic Blood Pressure (mmHg)		Jeopardy Score*	Mortality (%)
	Men	Women		
≤ 2.0	113 ± 20	109 ± 15	≤ 2.0	2.3
2.5-3.0	117 ± 13	81 ± 24	2.5-3.0	10.0
3.5-4.5	96 ± 7	65 ± 4	3.5-5.0	11.5
5.0-6.0	75 ± 5	68 ± 13	5.5-6.0	33.3

References:
1. Ellis SG, Myler RK, King SB, Douglas JS. Causes and correlates of death after unsupported coronary angioplasty: Implications for use of angioplasty and advanced support techniques in high-risk settings. Am J Cardiol 1991;68:1447-1451.

163. Answer: a (true)

Preprocedural aspirin has been shown to reduce the incidence of acute coronary occlusion by 50-75%.[1] Although the optimal dose and timing are unknown, equivalent reductions in ischemic complications were seen for patients randomly assigned to low-dose (80 mg/day) or high-dose (1500 mg/day) therapy.[2]

References:
1. Barnathan E, Schwartz J, Taylor L, et al. Aspirin and dipyridamole in the prevention of acute coronary thrombosis complicating coronary angioplasty. Circulation 1987;76:125-134.
2. Mufson L, Black A, Roubin G, et al. Randomized trial of aspirin in PTCA: Effect of high versus low dose aspirin on major complications and restenosis. J Am Coll Cardiol 1988;11:236A.

164. Answer: b (false)

In the EPIC trial,[1] 2099 patients undergoing PTCA for unstable angina, acute MI, or high-risk lesion morphology were randomized to one of 3 treatment arms: bolus and maintenance infusion of ReoPro (bolus 0.25 mg/kg; infusion of 10 mcg/min x 12 hrs.); bolus dose only; or placebo. Aspirin and heparin were given in conventional doses. Patients receiving the bolus + infusion had a 35% reduction in major ischemic complications (12.8% to 8.3%; p = 0.008) and fewer repeat revascularizations (i.e., clinical restenosis). Angiographic restenosis rates were not determined.

References:
1. The EPIC Investigors. Use of a monoclonal antibody directed against the platelet glycoprotein IIb/IIIa receptor in high risk coronary angioplasty. N Engl J Med 1994;330:956-61.

165. Answer: a (true)

In the EPILOG trial,[1] the combined endpoint of death or MI (CPK 3x normal) at 30-days was lower in patients receiving ReoPro plus low-dose heparin compared to those receiving standard-dose heparin without ReoPro (2.6% vs. 8.2%; p < 0.01); this benefit was observed without an increase in major bleeding (1.8% vs. 3.1% for heparin only group; p = NS).

References:
1. Lincoff AM, Tcheng JE, et al. Abciximab (c7E3 Fab, ReoPro) with reduced heparin dosing during coronary intervention: Final results of the EPILOG trial. J Am Coll Cardiol 1997;29(Suppl A):187A.

166. Answer: b (false)

Conventional bolus dosing of 10,000 units of heparin results in suboptimal prolongation of the activated clotting time (ACT) in 5% of patients with stable angina and 15% of patients with unstable angina.[1]

References:
1. Ogilby JD, Kopelman HA, Klein LW, et al. Adequate heparinization during PTCA: Assessment using activated clotting time. J Am Coll Cardiol 1988;11:237A.

167. Answer: b (false)

Adjunctive thrombolytic therapy with intracoronary urokinase (250,000-500,000 units over 5-15 min.) or tPA (20 mg over 1-3 min.) is reserved for situations where definite residual thrombus is identified; routine lytic therapy for abrupt closure caused by dissection may prevent adherence of the intimal flap to the underlying vessel wall and is not recommended.[1]

References:
1. Spielberg C, Schnitzer L, Linderer T, et al. Influence of catheter technology and adjunct medication on acute complications in percutaneous coronary angioplasty. Cathet Cardiovasc Diagn 1990;21:72-76.

168. Answer: b (false)

In vessels ≥ 3.0 mm, focal dissections or simple plaque separations are best managed by stenting, which has proven to be more effective than prolonged perfusion balloon inflations.

Prolonged Perfusion Balloon (PPB) Inflations vs. Stenting for Acute Closure

Series	Design	Stent	N	Results
Ricci[1]	Randomized TASC II trial	-	22 PPB 22 Stent	Stent with greater success (91% vs. 46%), able to salvage 83% of PB failures, and lower restenosis (22% vs. 50%). CABG avoided in 91%; stent thrombosis resulting in MI in 11%.
deMuinck[2]	Retrospective, non-randomized	PSS	61 PPB 36 Stent	Stent with less residual stenosis, better restoration of normal flow (94% vs. 70%), less emergency CABG (0% vs. 21%), and more subacute thrombosis (22% vs. 0%). No difference in acute closure, restenosis, or event-free survival at 3-month.

Answers

Series	Design	Stent	N	Results
Barberis[3]	Retrospective	PSS	36 PPB 37 Stent	Stent with greater success (95% vs. 72%), more subacute thrombosis (13% vs. 0%); able to salvage 90% of PB failures.
Lincoff[4]	Matched case-control	GRS	61 PPB* 61 Stent	Stent with less residual stenosis (26% vs. 49%), better restoration of TIMI 3 flow (97% vs. 72%), and reduced need for emergency surgery (9% vs. 27%) for patients with acute closure. No clinical benefit for stenting patients with threatened closure (i.e., dissection with normal flow).

Abbreviations: GRS = Gianturco-Roubin Stent, PSS = Palmaz-Schatz Stent; TASC = Trial of Angioplasty versus Stents in Canada
- = Not reported
* Prolonged inflations ± perfusion balloon

References:
1. Ricci HR, Ray S, Buller CE, O'Neill B, et al. Six month follow-up of patients randomized to prolonged inflation of stent for abrupt occlusion during PTCA—Clinical and angiographic data: TASC II. Circulation 1995;92:I-475.
2. de Muinck E, den Heijer P, van Dijk R. Autoperfusion balloon versus stent for acute or threatened closure during percutaneous transluminal coronary angioplasty. Am J Cardiol 1994;74:1002-1005.
3. Barberis P, Marsico F, De Servi S, et al. Treatment of failed PTCA with perfusion balloon versus intracoronary stent: A short-term follow-up. J Am Coll Cardiol 1994:136A.
4. Lincoff M, Topol E, Chapekis A, et al. Intracoronary stenting compared with conventional therapy for abrupt vessel closure complicating coronary angioplasty: A matched case-control study. J Am Coll Cardiol 1993;21:866-875.

169. Answer: a, b

To minimize the risk of perforation during bailout DCA, a slightly undersized AtheroCath is chosen, oriented away from the angiographically normal vessel wall, and inflated at low inflation pressures (10-20 psi).

170. Answer: a, c, d, e

Bailout DCA of acute closure should be avoided when a dissection is present and is > 10 mm, is associated with periadventitial dye staining, or occurs on a severely angulated vessel segment; when the vessel diameter is < 3 mm; when there is moderate-to-severe tortuosity and/or heavy lesion calcium; or when there is a large amount of untreated clot.

171. Answer: a (true)

172. Answer: b (false)

The treatment of more extensive non-flow-limiting dissections is controversial. In a matched case-control study, stenting failed to confer a clinical benefit over conventional therapy and resulted in more transfusions and a longer hospital stay.[1] Nevertheless, the majority of interventionalists stent non-flow-limiting dissections with high-risk features (residual stenosis $\geq$ 30%, dissection length $\geq$ 15 mm).

References:
1. Lincoff M, Topol E, Chapekis A, et al. Intracoronary stenting compared with conventional therapy for abrupt vessel closure complicating coronary angioplasty: A matched case-control study. J Am Coll Cardiol 1993;21:866-875.

173. Answer: b (false)

Coronary artery dissection is a much more common cause of abrupt closure after PTCA than primary vessel thrombosis.

174. Answer: a (true)

In contrast to PTCA, primary thrombosis may account for $\geq$ 50% of abrupt closures after DCA.[1,2]

References:
1. Popma J, Topol E, Hinohara T, et al. Abrupt vessel closure after directional coronary atherectomy. J Am Coll Cardiol 1992;19:1372-1379.
2. Carrozza J, Baim J. Complications of directional coronary atherectomy: Incidence, causes, and management. Am J Cardiol 1993;72:47E-54E.

175. Answer: a, c, d, e, f

For thrombotic acute closure, PTCA with lytics, new devices, and antiplatelet agents may be of value. TEC atherectomy has been used to aspirate thrombus, but is contraindicated in vessels < 3.0 mm when a dissection is present. When used in conjunction with intracoronary thrombolysis, DCA may effectively excise small amounts of clot. ELCA may desiccate thrombus but is not usually considered a first-line rescue device, and the Rotablator is contraindicated due to the risk of distal embolization. Other devices such as the Hydrolyzer and Angiojet are under investigation, and may be potentially useful. Other measures include the use of a continuous overnight superselective infusion of urokinase (80,000 units per hour through an end-hole infusion wire just proximal to the clot, and 40,000 units per hour through the guiding catheter).[1] In a small observational report, ReoPro (0.25 mg/kg IV bolus followed by a 12-hr infusion of 10 mcg/min) was given to 16 patients who developed intracoronary thrombus in response to PTCA, 4 of whom failed intracoronary urokinase. ReoPro decreased thrombus, improved flow, and was well-tolerated. All 16 cases underwent successful repeat PTCA without in-hospital ischemic complications.[2]

References:
1. Chapekis A, George B, Candela R. Rapid thrombus dissolution by continuous infusion of urokinase through an intracoronary perfusion wire prior to and following PTCA: Results in native coronaries and patent saphenous vein grafts. Cathet Cardiovasc Diagn 1991;23:89-92.
2. Muhlestein JB, Gomez, MA, Karagounis LA, Anderson JL. "Rescue ReoPro": Acute utilization of abciximab for the dissolution of coronary thrombus developing as a complication of coronary angioplasty. Circulation 1995;92:I-607.

No-Reflow

176. Answer: b (false)

No-reflow is defined angiographically as an acute reduction in coronary flow (TIMI grade 0-1) in the absence of dissection, thrombus, spasm, or high-grade residual stenosis at the original target lesion.

177. Answer: a, c, d

No-reflow is more common after mechanical revascularization of thrombus-containing lesions (i.e., acute MI) and degenerated vein grafts containing friable debris. Among new devices, no-reflow is highest after Rotablator atherectomy (1.2-9.0%), correlates with total burr activation time,[1-3] and is reversible in > 60% of episodes; the frequent response to intracoronary calcium antagonists is strongly suggestive of microvascular spasm.[4]

References:
1. Safian RD, Niazi KA, Strzelecki M, et al. Detailed angiographic analysis of high-speed mechanical rotational atherectomy in human coronary arteries. Circulation 1993;88:961-968.
2. Ellis SG, Popma JJ, Buchbinder M, et al. Relation of clinical presentation, stenosis morphology, and operator technique to the procedural results of rotational atherectomy and rotational atherectomy-facilitated angioplasty. Circulation 1994;89:882-892.
3. Warth DC, Leon MB, O'Neill W, et al. Rotational atherectomy multicenter registry: Acute results, complications and 6-month angiographic follow-up in 709 patients. J Am Coll Cardiol 1994;24:641-8.
4. Abbo KM, Dooris M, Glazier S, et al. No-reflow after percutaneous coronary intervention: Clinical and angiographic characteristics, treatment and outcome. Am J Cardiol 1995;75:778-782.

178. Answer: b (false)

In the catheterization laboratory, no-reflow usually manifests as ECG changes and chest pain.[1] However, depending on the myocardial territory, baseline ventricular function, and the presence of other coronary artery disease, no-reflow may be clinically silent, or induce a spectrum of ischemic manifestations including conduction disturbances, hypotension, myocardial infarction, cardiogenic shock, and death.[1-3]

References:
1. Abbo KM, Dooris M, Glazier S, et al. No-reflow after percutaneous coronary intervention: Clinical and angiographic characteristics, treatment and outcome. Am J Cardiol 1995;75:778-782.
2. Kitazume H, Iwama T, Kubo H, et al. No-reflow phenomenon during percutaneous transluminal coronary angioplasty. Am Heart J 1988;116:211-215.
3. Piana RN, Paik GY, Moscucci M, et al. Incidence and treatment of no-reflow after percutaneous coronary intervention. Circulation 1994;89:2514-2518.

179. Answer: a (true)

In one study, no-reflow was associated with a 10-fold higher incidence of death (15%) and myocardial infarction (31%) compared to patients without no-reflow (even after excluding patients who presented with acute MI).[1]

References:
1. Abbo KM, Dooris M, Glazier S, et al. No-reflow after percutaneous coronary intervention: Clinical and angiographic characteristics, treatment and outcome. Am J Cardiol 1995;75:778-782.

180. Answer: a, d

In heavily calcified lesions, Rotablator ablation may liberate large amounts of microparticles leading to no-reflow. Techniques to minimize complications include initial use of a 1.5 mm burr; further incremental steps in burr size of 0.25-0.5 mm; ablation runs $\leq$ 30 seconds; and extended (occasionally several minutes) intervals between runs until hemodynamic dysfunction, ECG changes, and symptoms resolve. A fall in platform speed > 5000 RPM increases the risk of microparticulate embolization and no-reflow.

181. Answer: a, b

The most recent and important advance in the treatment of no-reflow is the use of intracoronary calcium antagonists. Intracoronary nitrates are much less effective, but may reverse superimposed spasm and are routinely administered. There are no data to support the use of β-blockers, and since obstruction to coronary flow occurs at the level of the capillary, CABG is not beneficial.

182. Answer: b (false)

Hypotension caused by no-reflow is not a contraindication to intracoronary calcium blockers — adjunctive therapy with pressures, inotropes, and IABP should be used as needed to support the systemic circulation while the calcium blocker is administered.

CORONARY ARTERY PERFORATION

183. Answer: b

Coronary artery perforation is a rare but important complication of percutaneous revascularization. Angiographic perforation has been reported in 0.1% of lesions treated with PTCA and 0.5-3.0% of lesions treated with Rotablator, DCA, TEC, or ELCA.[1-7]

References:
1. Ajuni SC, Glazier S, Blankenship L, et al. Perforations after percutaneous coronary interventions: clinical, angiographic, and therapeutic observations. Cath Cardiovasc Diagn. 1994;32:206-212.
2. Ellis SG, Ajluni S, Arnold AZ, et al. Increased coronary perforation in the new device era. Incidence, classification, management, and outcome. Circulation

Answers

1994;90:2725-2730.

3. Flood RD, Popma JJ, Chuang, Ya Chien, et al. Incidence, angiographic predictors, and clinical significance of coronary perforation occurring after new device angioplasty. J Am Coll Cardiol 1994;23:301A.

4. Lansky A, Popma JJ, Baim DS, et al. Angiographic outcome after new devices saphenous vein graft Angioplasty. Abstract from Transcatheter Cardiovascular Therapeutics, 1995.

5. Bittl JA, Ryan TJ, Keaney JF, et al. Coronary artery perforation during excimer laser coronary angioplasty. J Am Coll Cardiol 1993;21:1158-1165.

6. Holmes DR, Reeder GS, Ghazzai ZM, et al. Coronary perforation after excimer laser coronary angioplasty: the excimer laser coronary angioplasty registry experience. J Am Coll Cardiol 1994;23:330-335.

7. Cowley MJ, Dorros G, and Kelsey SF. Acute coronary events associated with percutaneous transluminal coronary angioplasty. Am J Cardiol 1984;53:12C-16C.

184. Answer: All except b

During PTCA, perforation may occur as a consequence of guidewire advancement, balloon advancement, balloon inflation, or balloon rupture.[1-7]

References:

1. Saffitz JE, Rose TE, Oaks JB, et al. Coronary arterial rupture during coronary angioplasty. Am J Cardiol 1983;51:902-904.

2. Kimbiris DM, Iskandrian AS, Goel I, et al. Transluminal coronary angioplasty complicated by coronary artery perforation. Cathet Cardiovasc Diagn 1982;8:481-487.

3. Iannone LA and Iannone DP. Iatrogenic left coronary artery fistula-to-left ventricle following PTCA: A previously unreported complication with nonsurgical treatment. Am Heart J 1990;120:1215-1217.

4. Cherry S and Vandormael M. Rupture of a coronary artery and hemorrhage into the ventricular cavity during coronary angioplasty. Am Heart J 1990;113:386-388.

5. Teirstein PS and Hartzler GO. Nonoperative management of aortocoronary saphenous vein graft rupture during percutaneous transluminal coronary angioplasty. Am J Cardiol 1987;60:377-378.

6. Meier B. Benign coronary perforation during percutaneous transluminal coronary angioplasty. Br Heart J 1985;54:33-35.

7. Grollier G, Bories H, Commeau P, et al. Coronary artery perforation during coronary angioplasty. Clin Cardiol 1986;9:27-29.

185. Answer: a, b, c, g

Since PTCA results in dissection and stretching of the vessel wall, oversized balloons (balloon/artery ratio >1.2) may extend these dissections through the adventitia, resulting in vessel perforation. Balloon rupture, particularly those associated with pinhole leaks (as opposed to longitudinal tears), may create high-pressure jets that increase the risk of dissection and/or perforation. Devices that alter the integrity of the vascular wall may also lead to perforation by tissue removal (TEC, DCA), pulverization (Rotablator), or ablation (ELCA).[1-6] Oversized devices, especially when used to treat bifurcation lesions and lesions located in severely angulated vessel segments, substantially increase the risk of perforation. Intracoronary stenting can also lead to perforation from the use of stiff guidewires or oversized compliant (for stent delivery) or high-pressure balloons (for optimal stent expansion), or from subintimal passage of the stent into a vessel with severe dissection.[7] Regardless of the device, the risk of perforation is increased when complex lesion morphology is present (e.g., chronic total occlusion, vessel bifurcation, severe tortuosity or angulation).[6,7]

References:

1. Ajuni SC, Glazier S, Blankenship L, et al. Perforations after percutaneous coronary interventions: clinical, angiographic, and therapeutic observations. Cath Cardiovasc Diagn. 1994;32:206-212.

2. Ellis SG, Ajluni S, Arnold AZ, et al. Increased coronary perforation in the new device era. Incidence, classification, management, and outcome. Circulation 1994;90:2725-2730.

3. Flood RD, Popma JJ, Chuang, Ya Chien, et al. Incidence, angiographic predictors, and clinical significance of coronary perforation occurring after new device angioplasty. J Am Coll Cardiol 1994;23:301A.

4. Lansky A, Popma JJ, Baim DS, et al. Angiographic outcome after new devices saphenous vein graft Angioplasty. Abstract from Transcatheter Cardiovascular Therapeutics, 1995.

5. Bittl JA, Ryan TJ, Keaney JF, et al. Coronary artery perforation during excimer laser coronary angioplasty. J Am Coll Cardiol 1993;21:1158-1165.
6. Holmes DR, Reeder GS, Ghazzai ZM, et al. Coronary perforation after.
7. Benzuly K, Safian RD. Coronary artery perforation: an unreported complication after stenting. Cathet Cardiovasc Diagn (in-press).

186. Answer: a (true)

References:
1. Ajuni SC, Glazier S, Blankenship L, et al. Perforations after percutaneous coronary interventions: clinical, angiographic, and therapeutic observations. Cath Cardiovasc Diagn. 1994;32:206-212.

187. Answer: a (true)

While bypass graft perforation may result in chest wall or mediastinal hemorrhage, cardiac tamponade is unusual due to partial pericardiectomy during bypass surgery, the subsequent development of pericardial adhesions, and the location of most bypass grafts outside the pericardium.[1,2]

References:
1. Ajuni SC, Glazier S, Blankenship L, et al. Perforations after percutaneous coronary interventions: clinical, angiographic, and therapeutic observations. Cath Cardiovasc Diagn. 1994;32:206-212.
2. Teirstein PS and Hartzler GO. Nonoperative management of aortocoronary saphenous vein graft rupture during percutaneous transluminal coronary angioplasty. Am J Cardiol 1987;60:377-378.

188. Answer: b

In some studies, oversized devices (device-to-artery ratio ≥ 0.8 for TEC, ELCA and Rotablator; balloon-to-artery ratio >1.2 for PTCA) were important correlates of angiographic perforation.[1,2] Therefore, high-risk lesions (e.g., bifurcations, angulated stenoses, total occlusion) are best approached using balloon-to-artery ratios of 1.0 for PTCA, and device-to-artery ratio of 0.5-0.6 for lasers, TEC, and Rotablator. When these latter devices are used, it may be prudent to achieve further lumen enlargement by adjunctive PTCA (balloon-to-artery ratio = 1) rather than upsizing to a larger device.

References:
1. Ajuni SC, Glazier S, Blankenship L, et al. Perforations after percutaneous coronary interventions: clinical, angiographic, and therapeutic observations. Cath Cardiovasc Diagn. 1994;32:206-212.
2. Bittl JA, Ryan TJ, Keaney JF, et al. Coronary artery perforation during excimer laser coronary angioplasty. J Am Coll Cardiol 1993;21:1158-1165.

189. Answer: b (false)

In general, guidewire perforations rarely result in adverse sequelae.[1] In contrast, perforations caused by balloons, atherectomy devices, or lasers may result in hemopericardium and hemodynamic collapse.[1,2]

References:
1. Ajuni SC, Glazier S, Blankenship L, et al. Perforations after percutaneous coronary interventions: clinical, angiographic, and therapeutic observations. Cath Cardiovasc Diagn. 1994;32:206-212.

2. Ellis SG, Ajluni S, Arnold AZ, et al. Increased coronary perforation in the new device era. Incidence, classification, management, and outcome. Circulation 1994;90:2725-2730.

190. Answer: d

Regardless of the cause, initial management should focus on sealing the perforation nonoperatively and stabilizing the patient hemodynamically. The cardiac surgeons should be notified immediately and the operating room prepared for possible emergency. A balloon (balloon-to-artery ratio = 0.9-1.0) should be immediately positioned at the site of contrast extravasation and inflated to 2-6 atm for at least 10 minutes. If sealing is incomplete, a second low-pressure inflation should be performed for 15-45 minutes, using a perfusion balloon catheter whenever possible to prevent distal myocardial ischemia. Additional heparin should not be given. Echocardiography should be performed at the first sign of perforation, if possible. If pericardial hemorrhage is evident, immediate pericardiocentesis is performed. If hemodynamic collapse occurs secondary to perforation, pericardiocentesis should not be delayed for any reason. As nonoperative attempts proceed to treat the perforation, the pericardiocentesis needle should be exchanged for a multiple-side-hole catheter, allowing continuous aspiration and monitoring of pericardial blood. Initial efforts to seal the perforation should occur while the patient remains fully anticoagulated (to prevent vessel thrombosis). However, some interventionalists recommend immediate administration of protamine to reverse the effects of systemic heparinization when free perforation occurs after atherectomy or laser devices. If contrast extravasation persists despite prolonged balloon inflations, incremental doses of protamine should be administered (25-50mg intravenously over 10-30 minutes) while repeat balloon inflations are attempted. Vessel closure may be an acceptable alternative to pericardial hemorrhage if bypass surgery is not feasible or if perforation occurs in a small sidebranch. If the perforation is large, associated with severe ischemia, or if hemodynamic instability or perforation persists despite nonoperative measures, emergency surgery should be performed to control hemorrhage, repair the perforation or ligate the vessel, and bypass all vessels containing significant stenoses. If possible, a perfusion balloon catheter should be positioned and inflated at low pressure while the operating room is being prepared; intermittent flushing of the central lumen with heparinized saline will prevent clotting and ensure antegrade blood flow. Operative management may be required in 30-40% of patients who develop perforation.[1-4]

References:
1. Ajuni SC, Glazier S, Blankenship L, et al. Perforations after percutaneous coronary interventions: clinical, angiographic, and therapeutic observations. Cath Cardiovasc Diagn. 1994;32:206-212.
2. Ellis SG, Ajluni S, Arnold AZ, et al. Increased coronary perforation in the new device era. Incidence, classification, management, and outcome. Circulation 1994;90:2725-2730.
3. Bittl JA, Ryan TJ, Keaney JF, et al. Coronary artery perforation during excimer laser coronary angioplasty. J Am Coll Cardiol 1993;21:1158-1165.
4. Holmes DR, Reeder GS, Ghazzai ZM, et al. Coronary perforation after excimer laser coronary angioplasty: the excimer laser coronary angioplasty registry experience. J Am Coll Cardiol 1994;23:330-335.

191. Answer: b (false)

Prolonged balloon inflations (and pericardiocentesis if needed) successfully seal 60-70% of vessel perforations without the need for surgery;[1-4] operative management is required in 30-40% of cases.

References:
1. Ajuni SC, Glazier S, Blankenship L, et al. Perforations after percutaneous coronary interventions: clinical, angiographic, and therapeutic observations. Cath Cardiovasc Diagn. 1994;32:206-212.
2. Ellis SG, Ajluni S, Arnold AZ, et al. Increased coronary perforation in the new device era. Incidence, classification, management, and outcome. Circulation 1994;90:2725-2730.
3. Bittl JA, Ryan TJ, Keaney JF, et al. Coronary artery perforation during excimer laser coronary angioplasty. J Am Coll Cardiol 1993;21:1158-1165.
4. Holmes DR, Reeder GS, Ghazzai ZM, et al. Coronary perforation after excimer laser coronary angioplasty: the excimer laser coronary angioplasty registry experience. J Am Coll Cardiol 1994;23:330-335.

192. Answer: c

Indications for emergency surgery following coronary intervention include refractory acute occlusion or dissection of a major coronary artery, coronary perforation with refractory pericardial tamponade, and occlusion of the left main coronary artery. CABG is not beneficial for no-reflow, since the epicardial coronary artery is widely patent and the obstruction to coronary flow is at the capillary level.

RESTENOSIS

193. Answer: a (true)

Restenosis rates vary widely depending on the definition.[1]

Angiographic Definition of Restenosis

EMORY	Diameter stenosis ≥ 50% at follow-up.
NHLBI I	An increase in diameter stenosis ≥ 30% at follow-up (compared to immediately after intervention).
NHLBI II	Residual stenosis < 50% after PTCA increasing to diameter stenosis ≥ 70% at follow-up.
NHLBI III	An increase in diameter stenosis at follow-up to within 10% of the diameter stenosis before PTCA.
NHLBI IV	A > 50% loss of the initial gain achieved after PTCA
THORAXCENTER IIA	≥ 0.72 mm lumen loss at follow-up.

Abbreviations: NHLBI = National Heart, Lung, and Blood Institute

References:
1. Beatt KJ, Serruys PW, Renseing BJ, Hugenoltz PG. Restenosis after coronary angioplasty: New standards for clinical studies. J Am Coll Cardiol 1990;15:491-498.

194. Answer: a (4); b (1); c (3)

195. Answer: b, c

An important advance in the analysis of restenosis comes from expressing the relationship between lumen diameter at baseline, immediately after intervention, and during follow-up in terms of *acute gain* and *late loss*. Acute gain, defined as the difference in lumen diameter before and immediately after intervention, is due to plaque removal and/or arterial expansion. Late loss, defined as the difference in lumen diameter after intervention and at follow-up,[1] reflects the net effects of intimal hyperplasia, elastic recoil, and vascular remodeling.[2] The *loss index* is the numerical description of this relationship, and is defined as late loss divided by acute gain;[3] a typical loss index is 0.5.

References:
1. Kuntz R, Safian R, Levine M, Reis G, Diver D, Baim D. Novel approach to the analysis of restenosis after the use of three new coronary devices. J Am Coll Cardiol 1992;19:1493-1499.
2. Gordon PC, Gibson M, Cohen DJ, Carrozza J, Kuntz R, Baim D. Mechanisms of restenosis and redilation within coronary stents-quantitative angiographic assessment. J Am Coll Cardiol 1993;21:1166-1174.
3. Guidance for the Submission of Research and Marketing Applications for Interventional Cardiology Devices: PTCA Catheters, Atherectomy Catheters, Lasers, Intravascular Stents. Interventional Cardiology Devices Branch, Division of Cardiovascular, Respiratory and Neurology Devices, Office of Device Evaluation, US Food and Drug Administration, May 1993:29.

196. Answer: a, c

Restenosis was originally thought to be caused solely by intimal hyperplasia. Data now support the notion that restenosis is a complex process consisting of various degrees of elastic recoil, intimal thickening, and vascular remodeling. Elastic recoil is defined as the difference between inflated balloon diameter and minimal lumen diameter upon balloon deflation. The degree of elastic recoil depends on plastic changes in the atherosclerotic plaque and elastic characteristics of the arterial wall. Most elastic recoil occurs within 30 minutes after balloon deflation (but may occur up to 24 hours), can result in a 50% decrease in cross-sectional area,[1] and is more common after PTCA of eccentric and ostial lesions. Elastic recoil is greatest after PTCA, intermediate after DCA, and lowest after stenting. Angiographic analysis suggests that early recoil is associated with a higher incidence of restenosis;[2,3] elimination of elastic recoil may explain the reduction in angiographic restenosis and repeat revascularization after stenting.[4] Intimal thickening is a generalized response to vessel injury caused by PTCA and other devices. Atherectomy specimens support the proliferative nature of restenosis; de novo lesions are usually hypocellular, whereas restenotic lesions are typically hyperplastic.[5,6] Experimental studies[7,8] and serial intravascular ultrasound imaging in human[9] demonstrate a "constriction" or shrinkage of the vessel and loss in luminal diameter after coronary intervention (arterial remodeling). The ability of stents to virtually eliminate late arterial remodeling is an important factor in the ability of stents to reduce restenosis.

References:
1. Rensing BJ, Hermans WRM, Beatt KJ, et al. Quantitative angiographic assessment of elastic recoil after percutaneous transluminal coronary angiography. Am J Cardiol 1990;66:1039-1044.
2. Rodriguez A, Lassileau M, Santaera O, et al. Early decreases in minimal luminal diameter after PTCA are associated with higher incidence of late restenosis. J Am Coll Cardiol 1993;21:34A.
3. LaBlanche JM on behalf of the FACT Investigators. Recoil twenty-four hours after coronary angioplasty: A computerized angiographic study. J Am Coll Cardiol 1993;21:34A.

4. Rodriguez A, Santaera O, Larribau M, et al. Coronary stenting decreases restenosis in lesions with early loss in luminal diameter 24 hours after successful PTCA. Circulation 1995;91:1397-1402.
5. Johnson DE, Hinohara T, Selmon MR, Braden LJ. Primary peripheral arterial stenoses and restenoses excised by transluminal atherectomy: A histopathologic study. J Am Coll Cardiol 1990;15:419-425.
6. Garratt K, Edwards W, Kaufmann U, Vlietstra R, Holmes D. Differential histopathology of primary atherosclerotic and restenotic lesions in coronary arteries and saphenous vein bypass grafts: Analysis of tissue obtained from 73 patients by directional atherectomy. J Am Coll Cardiol 1991;17:442-448.
7. Post M, Borst C, Kuntz R. The relative importance of arterial remodeling compared with intimal hyperplasia in lumen renarrowing after balloon angioplasty (A study in the normal rabbit and the hypercholesterolemic Yucatan micropig). Circulation 1994;89:2816-2821.
8. Lafont A, Guzman L, PLW. Restenosis after experimental angioplasty. Intimal, medial and adventitial changes associated with constrictive remodeling. Circ Res 1995;76:996-1002.
9. Mintz G, Kovach J, Javier S, Ditrano C, Leon M. Geometric remodeling is the predominant mechanism of late lumen loss after coronary angioplasty. Circulation Am Coll Cardiol 1988;12:616-623.

197. Answer: b (false)

Restenosis after PTCA is uncommon in the first month, plateaus within 3-6 months, and is unusual after 12 months.[1,2]

References:
1. Serruys PW, Luijten HE, Beatt KJ, et al. Incidence of restenosis after successful coronary angioplasty: a time-related phenomenon. A quantitative angiographic study in 342 consecutive patients at 1, 2, 3, and 4 months. Circulation 1988;77:361-371.
2. Nobuyoshi M, Kimura T, Nosaka H, Mioka S. Restenosis after successful percutaneous transluminal coronary angioplasty: Serial angiographic follow-up of 229 patients. J Am Coll Cardiol 1988;12:616-623.

198. Answer: b (false)

The time course of restenosis after atherectomy, laser, and stenting is similar to PTCA, but several angiographic studies have shown a further increase in minimal lumen diameter between 6 months and 3 years after stent implantation, suggesting that 6-month angiography may *underestimate* the benefit of stenting.[1-3]

References:
1. Kimura T, Yokoi H, Tamura T, Nakagawa Y, Nosaka H, Nobuyoshi M. Three years clinical and quantitative angiographic follow-up after the Palmaz-Schatz coronary stent implantation. J Am Coll Cardiol 1995;25:375A.
2. Hermiller J, Fry E, Peters T, et al. Late lesion regression within the Gianturco-Roubin Flex stent. J Am Coll Cardiol 1995;25`:375A.
3. Kimura T, Nosaka H, Yokoi H, Iwabuchi M. Serial angiographic follow-up after Palmaz-Schatz stent implantation: Comparison with onventional balloon angioplasty. J Am Coll Cardiol 1993;21:1557-1563.

199. Answer: a

Important studies by Kuntz and colleagues,[1-3] and results from the CAVEAT-I[4] and STRESS trials,[5] indicate an inverse relationship between post-procedural lumen diameter and restenosis (i.e., "bigger is better"). Neither PTCA-induced dissection[6-8] nor deep wall excision[9,10] after DCA appear to affect restenosis rates.

References:
1. Kuntz R, Safian R, Levine M, Reis G, Diver D, Baim D. Novel approach to the analysis of restenosis after the use of three new coronary devices. J Am Coll Cardiol 1992;19:1493-1499.
2. Kuntz RE, Gibson CM, Nobuyoshi M, Baim DS. Generalized model of restenosis after conventional balloon angioplasty, stenting and directional atherectomy. J Am Coll Cardiol 1993;21:15-25.
3. Kuntz R, Safian R, Carrozza J, Fishman R, Mansour M, Baim D. The importance of acute luminal diameter in determining restenosis after coronary atherectomy or stenting. Circulation 1992;86:1827-1835.
4. Topol E, Leya F, Pinkerton C, et al. A comparison of directional atherectomy with coronary angioplasty in patients with coronary artery disease. N Engl J Med 1993;329:221-227.

5. Fishman D, Leon M, Baim D. A randomized comparison of coronary stent placement and balloon angioplasty in the treatment of coronary artery disease. N Engl J Med 1994;331:496-501.
6. Hermans WR, Rensing BJ, Foley DP, Deckers JW. Therapeutic dissection after successful coronary balloon angioplasty: No influence on restenosis or on clinical outcome in 693 patients. J Am Coll Cardiol 1992;20:767-780.
7. Cappelletti A, Margonato A, Berna G, Chierchia S. Spontaneous evolution of nonocclusive coronary dissection after PTCA: A 6-month angiographic follow-up study. J Am Coll Cardiol 1995;25:345A.
8. Savage M, Dischman D, Bailey S, et al. Vascular remodeling of balloon-induced intimal dissection: Long-term angiographic assessment. J Am Coll Cardiol 1995;25:139A.
9. Kuntz RE, Hinohara T, Safian RD, et al. Restenosis after directional coronary atherectomy: Effects of luminal diameter and deep wall excision. Circulation 1992;86:1394-1399.
10. Holmes DR, Garratt KN, Isner JM, et al. Effect of subintimal resection on initial outcome and restenosis for native coronary lesions an saphenous vein graft disease treated by directional coronary atherectomy: A report from the CAVEAT I and II investigators. J Am Coll Cardiol 1996;28:645-651.

200. Answer: a, c, e

Certain clinical, angiographic, and procedural variables have been identified as risk factors for restenosis.[1-15]

Risk Factors for Primary Restenosis

	YES*	MAYBE	NO**
CLINICAL			
Variant angina	X		
Recent onset angina (<2-6	X		
mos)	X		
Unstable angina	X		
IDDM	X		
Chronic dialysis		X	
Tobacco use (continued)		X	
Primary PTCA in AMI		X	
Hypercholesterolemia		X	
Male gender			X
Previous MI			X
Hypertension			X
Age			X
Previous Restenosis			
ANGIOGRAPHIC			
Long lesion (>20mm)	X		
Multivessel/Multilesional+	X		
SVG (proximal & body	X		
lesions)	X		
Chronic total occlusion	X		
Collaterals to dilated vessel	X		
Ostial stenosis	X		
Angulation (>45° angle)		X	
LAD stenosis			X
Eccentricity			X
Calcification			X
Bifurcation lesion			X
Thrombus			X
Proximal location			X
LIMA			
SVG (distal anastomosis)			

	YES*	MAYBE	NO**
PROCEDURAL			
Pressure gradient > 20mmHg	X		
Residual stenosis > 30%	X		
No dissection present			X
Balloon inflation variables			
Number of inflations			X
Inflation time			X
Maximum inflation			X
pressure			X
Balloon material			X
Inflation technique			

*   Majority of studies demonstrate an association

** Majority of studies fail to find an association

+   Although multivessel/multilesional PTCA leads to an increased probability that at least one lesion will restenoses when compared to single lesion PTCA, the overall rate is lower than predicted based on cumulative probabilities.

References:

1. Carrozza JR, Kuntz RE, Fishman RF, Baim DS. Restenosis after arterial injury caused by coronary stenting in patients with diabetes mellitus. Ann Intern Med. 1993;118(5):344-349.
2. Simons M, Leclerc G, Safian RD, Isner JM. Relation between activated smooth-muscle cells in coronary artery lesions and restenosis after atherectomy. N Engl J Med 1993;328:608-613.
3. Kuntz RE, Hinohara T, Robertson GC, et al. Influence of vessel selection on the observed restenosis rate after endoluminal stenting or directional coronary atherectomy. Am J Cardiol 1992;70:1101-1108.
4. Hirshfeld JW, Schwartz JS, Jugo R, et al. Restenosis after coronary angioplasty: A multivariate statistical model to relate lesion and procedure variables to restenosis. J Am Coll Cardiol 1991;18:647-656.
5. Hermans WR, Rensing BJ, Kelder JC, et al. Postangioplasty restenosis rate between segments of the major coronary arteries. Am J Cardiol 1992;194-200.
6. Violaris A, Melkert R, Serruys P. Influence of serum cholesterol and cholesterol subfractions on restenosis after successful coronary angioplasty. A quantitative angiographic analysis of 3336 lesions. Circulation 1994;90:2267-2279.
7. Fishman RF, Kuntz RE, Carrozza JP, Miller MJ, et al. Long-term results of directional coronary atherectomy: Predictors of restenosis. J Am Coll Cardiol 1992;20:1101-1110.
8. Williams DO, Gruentzig A, Kent K, Detre K, Kelsey S, To T. Efficacy of repeat percutaneous transluminal coronary angioplasty for coronary restenosis. Am J Cardiol 1984;53:32C-35C.
9. Dimas AP, Grigera F, Arora RR, et al. Repeat coronary angioplasty as treatment for restenosis. J Am Coll Cardiol 1992;19:1310-1314.
10. Meier B, King SBI, Gruentzig AR. Repeat coronary angioplasty. J Am Coll Cardiol 1984;4:463-466.
11. Moscucci M, Piana R, Kuntz R, Kugelmass A, et al. The effect of prior coronary restenosis on the risk of subsequent restenosis after stent placement or directional atherectomy. Am J Cardiol 1994;73:1147-1153.
12. Glazier J, Varricchione T, Ryan T. Factors predicting recurrent restenosis after percutaneous transluminal coronary balloon angioplasty. Am J Cardiol 1989;63:902-905.
13. Quigley P, Hlatky M, Hinohara T. Repeat percutaneous transluminal coronary angioplasty and predictors of recurrent restenosis. Am J Cardiol 1989;63:409-413.
14. Hinohara T, Robertson G, Selmon M, et al. Restenosis after directional coronary atherectomy. J Am Coll Cardiol 1992;20:623-632.
15. Teirstein P, Hoover C, Ligon R. Repeat coronary angioplasty: Efficacy of a third angioplasty for a second restenosis. J Am Coll Cardiol 1989;13:291-296.

201. Answer: d

Over the last decade, there have been numerous clinical trials of fish oil, corticosteroids, cytostatic agents, calcium channel blockers, lipid lowering agents, ACE inhibitors, low molecular weight heparin, high-dose vitamin E, and somatostatin analogues; only calcium channel blockers and fish oil appear to have some beneficial effects on restenosis.[1] Two recent randomized trials suggest that c7E3 (platelet GP receptor IIb/IIa inhibitor) and angiopeptin (somatostain analog) significantly decrease clinical restenosis;[2] however, follow-up angiography was not performed in the EPIC trial of c7E3, and there was no difference in angiographic restenosis in the angiopeptin trial. Trials in which clinical but not angiographic restenosis was reduced, suggest that plaque stabilization ("passivation") may decrease clinical events without directly impacting intimal proliferation. The Palmaz-Schatz stent is the only device that has been shown to reduce the incidence of angiographic restenosis compared to PTCA; randomized trials (STRESS, BENESTENT) have conclusively demonstrated a decrease in restenosis for de novo lesions in native coronary arteries. Unpublished data from the Balloon vs. Optimal Atherectomy Trial (BOAT) suggest that optimal DCA results in less restenosis than PTCA.

References:
1. Haulages WB, Ohman ME and Califf RM. Restenosis: the clinical issues. In Topol EJ (ed). Textbook of Interventional Cardiology, 2nd Edition, Philadelphia, WB Saunders Company, 1993; 415-435.
2. Topol E, Califf R, Weisman H, et al. Randomized trial of coronary intervention with antibody against platelet IIb/IIIa integrin for reduction of clinical restenosis: results at six months. Lancet 1994;343:881-86.
3. Emanuelsson H, Beatt K, Bagger J. Long-term effects of angiopeptine treatment in coronary angioplasty. Reduction of clinical events but not of angiographic restenosis. European Angiopeptin Study Group. Circulation 1995;91:1689-1696.

202. Answer: a, b, c, d

Recurrent symptoms have a low positive predictive value for restenosis; in contrast, absence of symptoms in previously symptomatic patients is good evidence for the absence of restenosis (i.e., good negative predictive value).[1] While exercise testing without perfusion imaging can provide useful information about symptomatic status, functional capacity, and the presence of myocardial ischemia, it has low sensitivity for detecting restenosis.[1-3] Stress testing using thallium-201 scintigraphy has better sensitivity (for detection) and specificity (for exclusion) and is often used to evaluate patients with symptoms suggestive of restenosis. Exercise radionuclide angiography has an even better ability to exclude restenosis after a negative test, but only 40% of patients with positive tests have restenosis. Finally, the sensitivity and specificity of exercise and dobutamine echocardiography appear to be similar to thallium-201 scintigraphy.[2] Functional testing performed within 4 weeks of PTCA is frequently associated with false positive results,[4] which may be due to local vasoconstriction, myocardial stunning, or hibernating myocardium.

References:
1. Bengston J, Mark D, Honan M. Detection of restenosis after elective percutaneous transluminal angioplasty using the exercise treadmill test. Am J Cardiol 1990;65:28-34.
2. Hecht H, DeBord L, Shaw R. Usefulness of supine bicycle stress echocardiography for the detection of restenosis after percutaneous transluminal coronary angioplasty. Am J Cardiol 1993;71:293-296.
3. Pfisterer M, Rickenbacher P, Klowski W, Muller-Brand J. Silent ischemia after percutaneous transluminal coronary angioplasty: Incidence and prognostic significance. J Am Coll Cardiol 1993;22:1446-1454.
4. Manyari D, Knudtson M, Kloiber R. Sequential thallium-201 myocardial perfusion studies after successful percutaneous transluminal coronary angioplasty: delayed resolution of exercise-induced scintigraphic abnormalities. Circulation 1988;77:86-95.

203. Answer: b (false)

Routine early (< 6 months) noninvasive testing is not recommended in all patients. However, if the dilated vessel supplies a large amount of viable myocardium, an exercise test may be performed at 4-6 weeks; repeat angiography is reasonable for a markedly positive test regardless of symptomatic status.[1] If the dilated vessel supplies a small area, asymptomatic individuals may be followed clinically; a stress test is recommended for recurrent angina and repeat cardiac catheterization may be performed for either recurrent angina or a positive stress test. Some interventionalists perform an exercise test at 4-6 months after PTCA to screen for restenosis particularly in patients who were asymptomatic before PTCA or who had large caliber target vessels.

References:
1. Miller D, Verani M. Current status of myocardial perfusion imaging after percutaneous transluminal coronary angioplasty. J Am Coll Cardiol 1994;24:260-266.

204. Answer: a (true)

Repeat PTCA can be performed with high success (> 95%) and low complications rates (< 3-5%),[1-3] and is frequently the procedure of choice for restenosis after PTCA or stenting.[4]

References:
1. Williams DO, Gruentzig A, Kent K, Detre K, Kelsey S, To T. Efficacy of repeat percutaneous transluminal coronary angioplasty for coronary restenosis. Am J Cardiol 1984;53:32C-35C.
2. Dimas AP, Grigera F, Arora RR, et al. Repeat coronary angioplasty as treatment for restenosis. J Am Coll Cardiol 1992;19:1310-1314.
3. Meier B, King SBI, Gruentzig AR. Repeat coronary angioplasty. J Am Coll Cardiol 1984;4:463-466.
4. Baim D, Levine M, Leon M, Levine S, Ellis S, Schatz R. Management of restenosis within the Palmaz-Schatz coronary stent (the U.S. multicenter experience). Am J Cardiol 1993;71:364-366.

MEDICAL AND PERIPHERAL COMPLICATIONS

205. Answer: a, c

Depending upon the etiology, PTCA-induced renal insufficiency may be transient and quickly respond to medical measures or may progress to oliguria renal failure with volume overload, electrolyte and acid-base disturbances, and frank uremia. The most common manifestations include decreasing urine output and a rising serum creatinine in the first 3-5 days after PTCA. The most common cause of renal insufficiency in the post-PTCA patient is dye-induced tubular injury, with or without superimposed hypovolemia (NPO status, dye-induced diuresis, procedural blood loss). Less common causes include prerenal azotemia from PTCA-induced myocardial ischemia and LV dysfunction, renal ischemia from angiotensin converting enzyme inhibitors, athero- or thromboembolism, aortic dissection, a malpositioned intra-aortic balloon pump, and post-renal obstruction from prostatism or anticholinergic drugs. Dye-induced renal dysfunction is the most common cause of renal insufficiency in the PTCA patient. Defined as a rise in serum creatinine

>25% within 48 hrs of exposure, the incidence of dye-induced renal dysfunction varies from <1% in normal patients to approximately 50% in the highest risk groups.[1-3]

References:
1. Porter GA. Experimental contrast-associated nephropathy and its clinical implications. Am J Cardiol 1990;66:18F-22F.
2. Cronin RE. Renal failure following radiologic procedures. Am J Med Sci 1989;298:342-356.
3. Porter GA. Contrast-associated nephropathy. Am J Cardiol 1989;64:22E-26E.

206. Answer: d, e

Patients with pre-existing renal insufficiency (especially when due to diabetic nephropathy) are are increased risk for dye-induced nephrotoxicity. Other risk factors for renal dysfunction in high-risk patients include large contrast load, baseline hypovolemia, and impaired left ventricular function.

207. Answer: b

Once renal dysfunction develops, creatinine levels generally peak at 3-5 days and remain elevated for 1-2 weeks.[1,2] Oliguria occurs in 30% of patients. Although recovery is most common, some patients develop irreversible renal failure requiring temporary or permanent dialysis.

References:
1. Porter GA. Contrast-associated nephropathy. Am J Cardiol 1989;64:22E-26E.
2. Manske CL, Sprafka JM, Strong JT, et al. Contrast nephropathy in azotemic diabetic patients undergoing coronary angiography. Am J Med 1990;89(5):615-620.

208. Answer: b (false)

Nonionic contrast agents are associated with less volume overload than ionic agents, but do not decrease the risk of contrast nephropathy.[1,2]

References:
1. Davidson CJ, Hiatky M, Morris KG, et al. Cardiovascular and renal toxicity of a nonionic radiographic contrast agent after cardiac catheterization. A prospective trial. Ann Intern Med 1989;110:119-124.
2. Jeunikar AM, Finnie KJ, Dennis B, et al. Nephrotoxicity of high-and-low-osmolality contrast media. Nephron 1988;48:300-305.

209. Answer: a, b, d

In the post-PTCA patient with decreasing urine output and/or a rising serum creatinine, vigorous post-procedure hydration (100-150cc of crystalloid x 6-12 hrs; 1-2 L of water PO) help to maintain a stable blood pressure and urine output, thus facilitating excretion of contrast. A helpful "rule of thumb" is to match urine output with IV fluids during the first 8-10 hrs post-procedure. If the urine output falls below 40-60cc/hr, intravenous fluids are increased (may give 200cc boluses of normal saline in those without evidence of congestive heart failure). If the patient is felt to have adequate intravascular volume, especially in the presence of baseline LV dysfunction or renal insufficiency, furosemide (20-80mg IV over 1-2 minutes) will frequently relieve the prerenal state. Loop diuretics have an advantage over other diuretics because they are effective in patients with reduced glomerular filtration rate (GFR). Metolazone, a thiazide-like diuretic, is also effective in patients with reduced GFR. For severe oliguria, the combination of these agents has the theoretical advantage over either agent alone because it results in sequential nephron blockade. Dopamine may add some additional benefit and is commonly added in low doses ($5\mu g/Kg/min$ IV) for patients with severe oliguria. Right heart catheterization and hemodynamic monitoring should be considered in all cases of oliguria or anuria when the volume status is in question. On occasion, retroperitoneal or GI bleeding, or bladder obstruction (particularly in males with prostatic enlargement) may first manifest as diminished urine output. These conditions must be excluded early, since they are readily reversible and their treatment is different from that of contrast nephropathy.

210. Answer: a, c

Despite excellent overall tolerance, contrast media can result in undesirable reactions, ranging from mild nausea to life-threatening anaphylaxis; overall mortality attributable to contrast agents in coronary angiography is 4-23 deaths per million patients.[1,2] Patients with a previous history of an adverse dye reaction are at highest risk for a subsequent severe reaction; previous anaphylaxis carries a recurrence rate of 40% without premedication.[3] Asthmatics, especially those with nasal polyps, represent another high-risk group (6-9 fold risk compared to non-asthmatics).[4] Other predisposing conditions include dehydration, systemic illness, preexisting cardiac disease, and certain ethnic groups.[1,2] Transient ventricular dysfunction and hypotension have been ascribed to the hyperosmolar content and calcium-binding properties, and are more common following administration of high osmolar agents. In a large study of 337,647 patients, the five most frequent symptoms following intravenous contrast administration (nausea, urticaria, itching, heat sensation, vomiting) were reduced by low osmolar contrast agents.[5] Low osmolar contrast media also result in less patient discomfort during internal mammary artery and peripheral angiography. Routine use of non-ionic contrast media should be avoided in patients with acute ischemic syndromes undergoing percutaneous intervention. In-vitro and in-vivo studies have demonstrated that ionic contrast has anticoagulant and antiplatelet activities (prolongation of PTT and clotting time; inhibition of platelet aggregation and degranulation; and reduced time to thrombolysis) compared to non-ionic contrast. In prospective trials, ionic contrast was associated with fewer complications than nonionic contrast after PTCA.[6-8] In one trial, ionic contrast reduced the risk of in-lab abrupt closure,[6] and in others, ionic contrast was associated with less no-reflow and recurrent ischemia.[8,9] The EPIC trial demonstrated less abrupt closure, Q-wave MI and death with ionic contrast compared to non-ionic contrast in patients with recent MI, unstable angina, or high-risk lesion morphology.[10]

References:
1. Ansell G, Tweedie MCK, West CR, et al. The current status of reactions to intravenous contrast media. Invest Radiol 1980;15:532-539.
2. Bilazarian SD, Mittal S, Mills RM. Recognizing the extrarenal hazards of intravascular contrast agents. J Crit Illness 1991;6:859-869.
3. Lasser EC, et al. Pre-Treatment with corticosteroids to alleviate reactions to intravenous contrast material. N Engl J Med 1987;317:845-849.
4. Lang DM, Alpern MB, Visintainer PF, et al. Increased risk for Anaphylactoid reaction from contrast media in Patients on β-adrenergic blockers or with asthma. Ann Intern Med 1991;115:270-276.
5. Katayama H, Yamaguchi K, Kozuka T, et al. Adverse reactions to ionic and nonionic contrast media. Radiology 1990;175:621-628.
6. Weaver WD, Goldberg S, Feldman RL, et al. Non-ionic contrast during high risk PTCA is associated with subsequent ischemic events. Circulation 1996;94:I-249.
7. Piessens, et al. Effects of an ionic versus a nonionic low osmolar contrast agent on the thrombotic complications of coronary angioplasty. Cathet Cardiovasc

Answers

Diagn 1993;28:99-105.

8. Grines CL, Zidar F, Jones D, et al. A randomized trial of ionic vs. nonionic contrast in myocardial infarction or unstable angina patients undergoing coronary angioplasty. Circulation 1993;88:1886.

9. Grines CL, Schreiber TL, Savas V, et al. A randomized trial of low osmolar ionic versus nonionic contrast media in patients with myocardial infarction or unstable angina undergoing PTCA. J Am Coll Cardiol 1996;27:1381-6.

10. Aguirre FV, Topol EJ, Donohue TJ, et al. Impact on ionic and non-ionic contrast media on post-PTCA ischemic complications: results from the EPIC trial. J Am Coll Cardiol 1995;March, Special Issue:8A.

211. Answer: a (True)

Pretreatment with corticosteroids decreases the risk of contrast reactions: Pretreatment less than 12 hours before expose had no difference in adverse reactions compared to untreated patients.[1] Thus, the timing of steroid administration is important for achieving prophylaxis against adverse events.

References:

1. Lasser EC, Berry CC, Talner LB, et al. Pretreatment with corticosteroids to alleviate reactions to intravenous contrast material. N Engl J Med 1987;317:845-9.

212. Answer: a, c, d

Contrast Reactions: Presentation, Onset, and Treatment

Type	Presentation	Onset	Treatment
Minor	Nausea, burning sensation, flushing, mild urticaria without hives, minor bradycardia or vasovagal episodes.	Usually occur within minutes of exposure	Requires intervention infrequently. Treatment is supportive, including observation and cool compresses; oral benadryl and atropine (0.5-1.0 mg IV) are occasionally needed.
Moderate	Persistent nausea with vomiting, anaphylactoid reaction (urticaria with hives and tongue swelling), bradycardia or vasovagal episodes that persist or produce hypotension.	Usually occur within minutes to hours of exposure.	Usually requires intervention. Treatment includes IV fluids, Benadryl (50 mg IV), steroids (e.g. hydrocortisone 100 mg IV), centrally-acting antiemetics (e.g., Compazine 2 mg IV followed by a 25 mg rectal suppository), and atropine (0.5-2.0 mg for bradycardia or vasovagal reactions). Anaphylactoid reactions are also treated with epinephrine (0.1-0.5 cc of a 1:1,000 dilution subcutaneously every 5-15 minutes as necessary).
Severe	Anaphylaxis (bronchospasm, laryngeal edema and/or profound hypotension).	May occur immediately with a single contrast injection.	Life-threatening and requires aggressive attention. Epinephrine (1-5cc of a 1:10,000 solution via IV or ET tube every 5 min as needed), steroids (e.g., hydrocortisone 100mg IV followed by solumedrol 125 mg IV), Benadryl (50 mg IV), and possible intubation. Bronchodilator treatments (e.g., Albuterol aerosol 2.5 mg nebulized mist every 1-2 hrs) might be of benefit.

213. Answer: a

214. Answer: d

215. Answer: a, c, d, e, f

It is the practice of most vascular surgeons to repair all AV fistulas shortly after the diagnosis is made. Complications of delaying surgical repair include accelerated atherosclerosis, increased cardiac output, and worsening of distal extremity swelling and tenderness. Surgical repair involves division or excision of the fistula, and occasionally synthetic grafting of the involved vessels. Ultrasound guided compression repair is being used with increasing frequency, but current experience is limited. One small series reported a success rate of 67% (6/9).[1] The need for repair of a pseudoaneurysm is dependent on size, expansion and whether the patient requires long-term anticoagulation. Pseudoaneurysms less than 3cm in size can often be easily compressed without surgery. A follow-up ultrasound 1-2 weeks after initial diagnosis often demonstrates spontaneous thrombosis and obviates the need for surgical repair. However, spontaneous thrombosis is less likely to occur when the pseudoaneurysm is ≥3cm in size on initial ultrasound evaluation. When the defect persists beyond two weeks or expands, the risk of femoral artery rupture necessitates correction. Ultrasound-guided compression is commonly used with success related to the anticoagulation status and a pseudoaneurysm that can be readily visualized and compressed. Among patients not receiving anticoagulation, high success rates have been reported (92%-98%), with lower success rates (54%-86%) in those receiving anticoagulation.[1-4] There have been no randomized trials comparing ultrasound compression to surgical repair, but it seems reasonable to first attempt this noninvasive approach in patients with favorable anatomy prior to surgical repair. Symptoms following arterial occlusion include the sudden onset of severe pain or numbness, cyanosis, pallor, absence of a distal pulse, and a cool extremity. Systemic heparization and urgent thrombectomy are recommended. Most guidewire induced peripheral arterial perforations are benign and result in insignificant blood loss. Most will undergo spontaneous closure but rarely, pseudoaneurysm formation may occur. After confirmation of retroperitoneal hematoma, cessation of heparin and removal of arterial catheters with prolonged compression of the involved vessel is mandatory. The majority of retroperitoneal bleeds will stop spontaneously. Although many patients may require a blood transfusion, most are hemodynamically stable. However, continued decline in hematocrit, signs of volume depletion, or hemodynamic instability despite reversal of anticoagulants indicate that hematoma expansion is likely and surgical exploration may be warranted. The clinician makes a diagnosis of atheroembolic disease primarily from the history and physical exam. Blue-toe syndrome or livedo reticularis involving the extremities and trunk may be the cardinal manifestation of peripheral microemboli.

References:
1. Schaub F, Theiss W. Heinz M, et al. New Aspects in ultrasound-guided compression repair of post catheterization femoral artery injuries. Circulation 1994;90:1861-5.
2. Moote JJ, Hilborn MD, Harris KA, et al. Postarteriographic femoral pseudoaneurysms: treatment with ultrasound-guided compression. Annals of Vascular Surgery 1994;8:325-31.
3. Cox GS, Young JR, Gray BR, et al. Ultrasound-guided compression repair of postcatheterization pseudoaneurysms: results of treatment in one hundred cases. J Vascular Surg 1994;19:683-6.
4. Chatterjee T, Do-Dai D, Kaufmann U, et al. Ultrasound-guided compression repair for treatment of femoral artery pseudoaneurysm. Cathet & Cardiovasc Diagn 1996;38:335.

ADJUNCTIVE PHARMACOTHERAPY

216. Answer: a (true)

Demerol is contraindicated in patients who have received monoamine oxidase (MAO) inhibitors within 14 days due to unpredictable and potentially fatal reactions; these can manifest either as respiratory depression, hypotension and coma, or as paradoxical agitation, seizures, hypertension and hyperpyrexia. Severe reactions should be treated with IV hydrocortisone (100-250 mg IV); when hypertension and hyperpyrexia coexist, chlorpromazine (25 mg IV Q 6-8 hrs) may be of additional value.

217. Answer: a (true)

Although aspirin inhibits the thromboxane A_2-mediated platelet aggregation, it does not prevent platelet aggregation caused by thrombin, catecholamines, ADP, serotonin, or shear-stress. Thrombin generation and platelet activation may persist in some patients despite "adequate" aspirin and heparin therapy[1] but is difficult to detect in routine clinical settings such as PTCA and unstable angina.

References:
1. Chronos NA, Patel D, Sigwart U, et al. Intracoronary activation of human platelets following balloon angioplasty despite aspirin and heparin: a flow cytometric study. Circulation 1994;90:I-181.

218. Answer: a, b

Ticlopidine is a more potent antiplatelet agent than aspirin whose primary mechanism of action appears to be inhibition of ADP-mediated fibrinogen binding to the platelet GP IIb/IIIa receptor.[1,2] Ticlopidine also inhibits platelet aggregation in response to collagen, thrombin, and shear-stress,[3] and may enhance the antiaggregatory effects of prostacyclin[4] and promote deaggregation of thrombin-activated platelets.[5,6] Ticlopidine (250 mg BID) should be administered for at least 3 days prior to the procedure to maximize its antiplatelet effect. Some data suggest that an oral loading of 500 mg PO BID for 48 hours may expedite the onset of antiplatelet effect,[7] which may confer some benefit in emergency situations. After ticlopidine is stopped, the antiplatelet effects gradually resolve over 1-2 weeks.[6] The most serious side effect of ticlopidine is neutropenia, which occurs in 1-2% of patients after 4 weeks of use and is almost always reversible;[8,9] complete blood counts are therefore recommended every 2-4 weeks during the first few months of therapy. Nausea, vomiting, and diarrhea are common and can be minimized by the administration of ticlopidine with food; skin rash and elevated transaminases are rare. Long-term administration of ticlopidine lowers plasma fibrinogen and increases cholesterol.

References:
1. Di Minno G, Cerbone AM, Mattioli PL. Turco S, et al. Functionally thrombasthenic state in normal platelets following the administration of ticlopidine. J Clin Intest 1985;75:328-338.
2. Maffrand JP, Herbert JM. Effect of clopidogrel and ticlopidine on the binding of [^{3}H]-2 Methyl-Thio-ADP to RAT platelets. Thromb Haemost 1993;69:637.

3. Cattaneo M, Lombardi R, Bettega D et al. Shear-induced platelet aggregation is potentiated by desmopressin and inhibited by Ticlopidine. Arteriosclerosis and Thrombosis 1993;13:393-397.

4. Dembinska-Kiec A, Virgolini I, Rauscha F, et al. Ticlopidine and platelet function in healthy volunteer, Thrombosis Research 1992;65:559-570.

5. Cattaneo M, Akkawat B, Kinlough-Rathbone RL, et al. Ticlopidine facilitates the deaggregation of human platelets aggravated by thrombin. Thrombosis and Hemostasis 1994,71:91-94.

6. Heptinstall S, May JA, Glenn JR, Sanderson HM, et al. Effects of Ticlopidine administered to healthy volunteers on platelet function in whole blood. Thrombosis and Haemostasis 1995;74:1310-5.

7. Khurana S, Westley S, Mattson J, Safian RD. Is it possible to expedite the antiplatelet effect of Ticlopidine? 1996 Transcatheter Therapeutics (TCT-VIII) meeting Washington Hospital, Washington D.C. J Inv. Card. 1996;8:65.

8. Russo RJ, Stevens K, Norman S et al. Ticlopidine administration after stent placement: Frequency of adverse reactions. J Am Coll Cardiol 1997;(Suppl A):353A.

9. Szto G, Lewis S, Punamiya K, et al. Incidence of neutropenia/fatal thrombocytopenia associated with one month of ticlopidine therapy post coronary stenting. J Am Coll Cardiol 1997;(Suppl A):353A.

219. Answer: b, c, d

ReoPro is a potent inhibitor of the platelet glycoprotein IIb/IIIa receptor, the final common mediator of platelet aggregation in response to all possible agonists. ReoPro (abciximab) has now been tested in several large-scale, placebo-controlled randomized trials. In the EPIC trial (Evaluation of c7E3 Fab in the Prevention of Ischemic Complications),[1] 2099 patients undergoing PTCA or atherectomy for unstable angina, acute MI, or high-risk coronary lesion morphology were randomized to receive bolus + maintenance infusion of ReoPro, bolus dose only, or placebo; all patients were also treated with aspirin (325 mg QD) and IV heparin during and for ≥ 12 hours after the procedure. Compared to placebo, patients receiving ReoPro bolus + infusion had 35% and 23% reductions in ischemic endpoints at 30-days and 6-months, respectively (Table 1); these benefits were observed in all patient subgroups. In addition, ReoPro reduced the need for target vessel repeat revascularization at 6 months, and reduced the incidence of non-Q-wave MI after atherectomy by 71%.[2] In the EPILOG trial,[3] patients undergoing elective PTCA randomized to ReoPro (and low- or standard-dose heparin) had a lower incidence of death or MI (CPK 3x normal) at 30-days compared to placebo (plus standard-dose heparin) (Table 2). This benefit was observed without an increase in major bleeding events (1.8% vs. 3.1% for placebo + heparin group; p = NS). Because of these results, the main trial was stopped prematurely in December 1995. Enrollment was also stopped prematurely in the European CAPTURE trial (ReoPro vs. conventional medical therapy 18-24 hrs. prior to PTCA for unstable angina) due to a significant reduction in the combined endpoint of death, MI, or urgent reintervention in ReoPro-treated patients at 30-days (10.8% vs. 16.4% for placebo).[4]

Table 1. EPIC Trial: 30-Day and 6-Month Outcomes

Event	Placebo[1] (n=696)	ReoPro Bolus[2] (n=695)	ReoPro Bolus + infusion[3] (n=708)
	Number of patients (%)		
30-DAY ENDPOINT*	89 (12.8)	79 (11.4)	59 (8.3)[+]
Components of 30-d endpoint			
Death	12 (1.7)	9 (1.3)	12 (1.7)
Acute MI in survivors	60 (8.6)	43 (6.2)	37 (5.2)
Urgent intervention	54 (7.8)	44 (6.4)	28 (4.0)

Event	Placebo[1] (n=696)	ReoPro	
		Bolus[2] (n=695)	Bolus + infusion[3] (n=708)
6-MONTH ENDPOINT**	241 (35.1)	224 (32.6)	189 (27.0)[+]
Components of 6-mo. endpoint			
Death	23 (3.4)	18 (2.6)	22 (3.1)
MI	72 (10.5)	55 (8.0)	48 (6.9)
Repeat TLR	141 (20.9)	133 (19.7)	99 (14.4)[+]
CABG	74 (10.9)	67 (9.9)	65 (9.4)

Abbreviations: MI = myocardial infarction, TLR = target lesion revascularization, CABG = coronary artery bypass grafting

* Death from any cause, nonfatal MI, CABG or repeat percutaneous intervention for acute ischemia, insertion of a stent for procedural failure, placement of an IABP to relieve refractory ischemia.

** Death, nonfatal MI, or need for PTCA or CABG.

\+ p < 0.01 compared to placebo

1. Bolus + infusion of placebo.
2. 0.25 mg/kg 10-60 minutes prior to intervention.
3. 0.25 mg/kg 10-60 minutes prior to intervention followed by an infusion of 10 mcg/min for 12 hours.

Table 2. EPILOG Trial[3]

Event rate at 30-days (%)	Placebo + standard heparin[1] (n=939)	ReoPro + low-dose heparin[2] (n=935)	ReoPro + standard heparin (n=918)
Composite	11.7	5.2*	5.4*
Death	0.8	0.3	0.4
MI	8.7	3.7*	3.8*
Death or MI	9.1	3.8*	4.2*
Urgent Revasc	5.2	1.6*	2.3*
Major Bleed	3.1	2.0	3.5
Transfusion	3.9	2.4	3.8

* p < 0.001 compared to placebo (plus standard heparin) group

1. Standard heparin: 100 u/kg bolus, ACT ≥ 300 sec
2. ReoPro (0.25 mg/kg 10-60 min. prior to intervention followed by an infusion of 10 mcg/min for 12 hrs.) plus low-dose heparin (70 u/kg bolus, ACT ≥ 200 sec)

References:
1. The EPIC Investigators. Use of a monoclonal antibody directed against the platelet glycoprotein IIb/IIIa receptor in high-risk coronary angioplasty. N Engl J Med 1994;330:956-61.
2. Simoons M. The CAPTURE study, as presented at the 45th Annual Session of the American College of Cardiology in Orlando, Florida, USA, 1996.
3. The EPILOG Investigators. Placelet glycoprotein IIb/IIIa receptor blockade and low-dose heparin during percutaneous coronary revascularization. N Engl J Med 1997;336:1689-96.
4. Lefkovits J, Blankenship JC, Anderson K, et al. Increased risk of non-Q-wave MI after directional atherectomy is platelet dependent: Evidence from the EPIC trial. J Am Coll Cardiol 1996;28:849.

220. Answer: a (true)

Intravenous heparin is always employed during PTCA and reduces the risk of abrupt closure. In the cath lab, heparin effect is measured by the activated clotting time (ACT), which is the time for whole blood to form a firm, grossly-apparent clot in response to a potent procoagulant (kaolin or diatomaceous earth). The ACT may be measured by the HemoTec or HemoChron devices.[29] The HemoTec ACT (HemoTec, Inc., Englewood, Colorado) uses kaolin to activate clotting and optically senses the "drop time" of a mechanical plunger. The HemoChron ACT (Interventional Technidyne Corp., Edison, New Jersey) uses diatomaceous earth (4% Celite) in a pre-warmed rotating glass tube to activate clotting; a magnet placed at the bottom of the tube is displaced when the clot achieves a certain degree of "firmness." A "therapeutic" ACT depends on which system is used: For the same heparin concentration, a higher ACT is obtained using the HemoChron compared to the HemoTec system. The ACT provides a relatively crude estimate of heparin effect;[2] ACT varies when arterial or venous blood is sampled.[1]

References:
1. Rath B, Bennett DH. Monitoring the effect of heparin by measurement of activated clotting time during and after percutaneous transluminal coronary angioplasty. Br Heart J. 1990;63:18-21.
2. Dougherty KG, Gaos CM, Bush HS, Leachman R, Ferguson JJ. Activated clotting times and activated partial thromboplastin times in patients undergoing coronary angioplasty who receive bolus doses of heparin. Catheterization and Cardiovascular Diagnosis 1992;26:260-263.

221. Answer: a, b, c

Heparin must bind with antithrombin III to exert its anticoagulant effect (i.e., catalyze the inactivation of thrombin and activated factor Xa). Despite its clinical efficacy, heparin's antithrombotic activity is limited by its: 1) inability to inactivate clot-bound thrombin;[2]) neutralization by platelet factor IV from platelet-rich thrombi; and 3) inactivation by fibrin II monomers, which are formed by the action of thrombin on fibrinogen. Accordingly, "therapeutic" concentrations of heparin, even when supplemented by intracoronary antithrombin III,[2] may not prevent propagation of thrombus.[3]

References:
1. Chesebro JH, Badimon L, Fuster V. Importance of antithrombin therapy during coronary angioplasty. J Am Coll Cardiol 1991;17:96B-100B.
2. Schachinger V, Allert M, Kasper W et al. Adjuvant intracoronary infusion of antithrombin III during PTCA: Results of a prospective, randomized trial. Circulation 1994;90:2258-2266.
3. Mabin TA, Holmes DR Jr., Smith HC et al. Intracoronary thrombus: Role in coronary occlusion complicating PTCA. J Am Coll Cardiol 1985;3:198-202.

222. Answer: a, b, c, d, e

The incidence, time course, and clinical features of heparin-induced thrombocytopenia (HIT) and the more ominous heparin-associated thrombotic thrombocytopenia (HATT)[1] are shown in the Table. Platelet transfusions should be avoided in the setting of heparin-induced thrombocytopenia because of the risk of thrombotic complications. An infusion of the prostacyclin analog Iloprost (Berlex Laboratories), titrated to eliminate in-vitro heparin-induced platelet activation (infusion rates of 10 - 48 ng/kg/min), was successful in preventing a recurrence in 11 patients with confirmed HATT requiring a rechallenge with heparin during cardiovascular surgery.[1,2] Anticoagulation with defibrinating viper venoms like Ancrod or Reptilase, and with the heparinoid Org 10172, has also been performed when such patients require anticoagulation.[2] Low molecular weight heparin, which may reduce[3,4] but not eliminate[5] the risk of HIT, is also contraindicated in patients with a prior history of HATT.

Answers

Features of Heparin-Induced Thrombocytopenia[1,4,6,7]

	Heparin-Induced Thrombocytopenia	
	Type I	**Type II (Heparin-associated thrombotic thrombocytopenia; HATT)**
Incidence	10%	Rare
Mechanism	Direct platelet aggregating effect of heparin	Autoantibody (IgG or IgM) directed against platelet factor IV-heparin complex
Onset	Early (1-5 days)	Late (> 5 days); may occur sooner if prior heparin exposure
Platelet count	50,000/mm³ - 150,000 mm³	< 50,000/mm³
Duration	Transient; often improves even if heparin is continued	Requires discontinuation of ALL heparin; gradual recovery in platelet count over 1-5 days in most patients
Clinical course	Benign	Refractory venous and arterial thromboses and thromboembolism; may be fatal

References:
1. Becker PS, Miller VT. Heparin-induced thrombocytopenia. Stroke 1989;20:1449-1459.
2. Kappa J, Fisher C, Todd B, Stenach N, Bell P, Campbell F, Ellison N, Addonizio VP. Intraoperative management of patients with heparin-induced thrombocytopenia. Ann Thorac Surg 1990;49:714-23.
3. Warkentin TE, Levine MN, Hirsh J, Horsewood P, et al. Heparin-induced thrombocytopenia in patients treated with low-molecular-weight heparin or unfractionated heparin. N Engl J Med 1995;332:1330-5.
4. Aster RH. Heparin-induced thrombocytopenia and thrombosis. New Engl J Med 332:1374.
5.. Eichinger S, Kyrle PA, Brenner B, et al. Thrombocytopenia associated with low-molecular-weight heparin. Lancet 1991;1:1425-6.
6. Warkentin TE, Hayward CPM, Boshkov LK, Santos AV, et al. Sera from patients with heparin-induced thrombocytopenia generate platelet-derived microparticles with procoagulant activity: An explanation for the thrombotic complications of heparin-induced thrombocytopenia. Blood 1994;84:3691-3699.
7. Amiral J, Bridey F, Wolf M, et al. Antibodies to macromolecular platelet factor 4-heparin complexes in heparin-induced thrombocytopenia: a study of 44 cases. Thromb Haemost 1995;73:21-8.

223. **Answer: a, b**

Hirudin, the naturally occurring anti-thrombin isolated from leech saliva, is an extremely potent and specific inhibitor of thrombin.[1,2] Unlike heparin, hirudin does not require Antithrombin III for its anticoagulant effect; in addition, hirudin forms a highly stable noncovalent complex with *circulating and clot-bound thrombin*, and is not inhibited by platelet factor 4. In one report, hirulog was as effective as heparin in decreasing ischemic complications, and was associated with less bleeding (3.8% vs 9.8%; p < 0.001);[3] in addition, hirulog was associated with fewer ischemic complications than heparin for high-risk patients with post-infarct angina (9.1% vs. 14.2%; p=0.04). In the Hirudin European Trial versus Heparin in the Prevention of Restenosis after PTCA (HELVETICA),[4] 1141 patients undergoing PTCA for unstable angina were randomized to heparin or one of two hirudin regimens (all hirudin-treated patients received an intraprocedural dose of 40 mg followed by an IV infusion for 24 hrs; these patients were then randomized to subcutaneous hirudin or placebo for 72 hrs.). Hirudin reduced early ischemic events, but failed to decrease restenosis. A higher incidence of intracranial hemorrhage was noted in 3 different trials of hirudin and thrombolytics (GUSTO IIa,[5] TIMI 9A,[6] HIT-III[7]); current studies are attempting to define the optimal dose, timing, and route of administration of these agents.

Referenes:
1. Lefkovits J, Topol E. Direct thrombin inhibitors in cardiovascular medicine. Circulation 1994;90:1522-1536.
2. Heras M, Cheseboro JH, Webster MWI et al. Hirudin, heparin, and placebo during deep arterial injury in the pig: the in vivo role of thrombin in platelet-

mediated thrombosis. Circulation 1990;82:1476-1484.

3. Bittl JA, Strony J, Brinker JA, Ahmed WH, et al. Treatment with bivalirudin (Hirulog) as compared with heparin during coronary angioplasty for unstable or post-infarction angina. N Engl J Med 1995;333:764-9.
4. Serruys PW, Herrman JPR, Simon R, Rutsch W, Bode C, et al. A Comparison of Hirudin with heparin in the prevention of restenosis after coronary angioplasty. N Engl J Med 1995;333:757-63.
5. The Global Use of Strategies to Open Occluded Coronary Arteries (GUSTO) IIa Investigators. Randomized trial of intravenous heparin versus recominant hirudin for acute coronary syndromes. Circulation 1994;90:1631-1637.
6. Antman EM, for the TIMI 9A Investigators. Hirudin in acute myocardial infarction, Safety report from the thrombolysis and thrombin inhibition in myocardial infarction (TIMI) 9A trial. Circulation 1994;90:1624-1630.
7. Neuhaus KL, Essen R.v, Tebbe U, Jessel A, Heinrichs H, Mäurer W, et al. Safety Observations from the pilot phase of the randomized r-Hirudin for improvement of thrombolysis (HIT-III) study. Circulation 1994;90:1638-1642.

CORONARY STENTS

224. Answer: b

The Wallstent consists of an interwoven mesh of 16 stainless steel wire filaments; a specially designed stent delivery system permits release of the stent within the target lesion, followed by continued expansion of the stent until an equilibrium is achieved between the elastic constraint of the vessel wall and the dilating force of the stent. Stents are selected to achieve diameters 0.5 mm larger than the size of the adjacent reference segment.[1] The second generation Wallstent shortens by only 25% after deployment.

References:

1. Serruys PW, Strauss BH, Beatt KJ, et al. Angiographic follow-up after placement of a self-expanding coronary artery stent. N Engl J Med 1991 324:13.

225. Answer: d

The SciMed Radius stent is a new self-expanding stent made of nitinol wire. Advantages of the stent include its ease of deployment and shortening <5% after deployment. Clinical trials began in 1996. Two balloon-expandable stainless steel stents are currently approved for use in the United States: the Gianturco-Roubin stent and Palmaz-Schatz stent. A newer Cook stent (GR-II) has added radial strength, enhanced trackability, and decreased thrombogenicity; new flatwire stent construction, lower profile, expanded diameters up to 5 mm, and stent length of 40 mm are added features. Other stainless steel stents include the MultiLink stent (Advanced Cardiovascular Systems, Inc., Santa Clara, CA), which consists of a stainless-steel cylinder with laser-etched overlapping loops and bridges. The MicroStent (Arterial Vascular Engineering, Santa Rosa, CA) has been widely used in Europe and may have unique characteristics which permit its application to small vessels and complex, tortuous anatomy. One or more stents can be crimped on a balloon to treat a wide range of lesion lengths. The Nir stent (SciMed, Inc., Minneapolis, MN) entered clinical trials in 1996 and has become one of the most popular stents in Europe.

226. Answer: d

The Wiktor stent consists of a single strand of tantalum wire wrapped around an angioplasty balloon in a U-shaped configuration; advantages of this stent include its flexibility and radiopacity.[1] In contrast, use of thermal memory of stents in the coronary circulation is complex because of the need for refrigeration before insertion, and the risk of premature expansion in the guiding catheter before delivery.[2]

References:
1. Buchwald A, Unterberg C, Werner G, et al. Initial clinical results with the Wiktor stent: A new balloon-expandable coronary stent. Clin Cardiol 1991;14:374.
2. Cragg A, Lund G, Rysavy J, et al. Nonsurgical placement of arterial endoprostheses: A new technique using nitinol wire. Radiol 1983;147:261.

227. Answers: a (1); b (2); c (3); d (4); e (5); f (6)

228. Answer: b (false)

Although experimental studies in animals suggest that tantalum and Nitinol may be less thrombogenic than stainless steel, further studies in humans are necessary.

229. Answer: b (false)

The tendency for thrombosis can be minimized by using highly polished, ultra-pure grades of stainless steel, by minimizing the metal surface area of the stent, and possibly by thrombo-resistant coatings. At present, all stent patients require antiplatelet medications to prevent stent thrombosis.

230. Answer: a

Of the balloon-expandable stents, the least flexible is the Palmaz-Schatz stent. The flexibility of the Gianturco-Roubin, Wiktor, Microstent, Nir stent, and Wallstent is excellent.

231. Answer: b (false)

The ability to visualize the stent by fluoroscopy is dependent on the stent material and design, as well as the X-ray equipment. Optimal stent placement is highly dependent on the ability to visualize the stent; it is not sufficient to rely on balloon markers since the stent-balloon relationship may change slightly during advancement. Furthermore, most stents vary in length from 15-20 mm, mandating precise placement in long tubular lesions or in severe occlusive dissections.

232. Answer: a (true)

The radiopacity of tantalum stents (e.g., Wiktor stent) is superior to stainless steel stents (Palmaz-Schatz, Gianturco-Roubin, AVE stents).

233. Answer: b (false)

Biliary stents are easier to visualize than Palmaz-Schatz coronary stents because of enhanced metal density. Heparin-coating on the new Palmaz-Schatz coronary stent may decrease its thrombogenicity, but has no impact on radiopacity.

234. Answer: b (false)

Many balloon-expandable stents permit expansion from 3.0-5.0 mm in diameter depending on the final size of the balloon used to dilate the stent. At larger diameters, many stents lose their shape and radial strength.

235. Answer: b (false)

Biliary stents permit expansion from 4.0-9.0 mm; they should not be used in smaller vessels because of the increased metal density and the potential risk of thrombosis at diameters < 4 mm.

236. Answer: c

In addition to the length of the lesion and the visibility of the stent, the ability to completely cover the lesion is dependent on the stent surface area, which varies from 7-20% for most stents. However, there may be a relationship between the amount of metal surface area and the tendency toward thrombus formation, which may account for the higher rates of acute and subacute thrombosis with the original Wallstent compared to balloon-expandable stents.[1] On the other hand, stents with inadequate surface area may have insufficient radial strength; consequences include the inability to withstand elastic recoil of the arterial wall, and inadequate scaffolding of severe dissection flaps (or tufts of damaged plaque and endothelium protruding through the stent struts into the lumen), facilitating thrombus formation and/or restenosis.[2] In some cases, multiple overlapping stents are needed to prevent recoil, which increases the metal surface area and may increase the risk of thrombosis and/or restenosis. Clearly, the ideal stent has not yet been developed; the relative merits of each stent design await further investigation.

References:
1. Serruys PW, Strauss BH, Beatt KJ, et al. Angiographic follow-up after placement of a self-expanding coronary-artery stent. N Engl J Med 1991 324:13.
2. den Heijer P, van Dijk R, Twisk SP, Lie K. Early stent occlusion is not always caused by thrombosis. Cathet Cardiovasc Diagn. 1993;29:136-140.

Answers

237. Answer: b (false)

To facilitate placement of self-expanding stents, target lesions should be pretreated with conventional PTCA or debulking devices such as atherectomy or lasers.

238. Answer: b (false)

The selected Wallstent should be 0.5 mm larger than the diameter of the adjacent normal reference segment; to ensure proper embedding in the arterial wall, the stent may be smoothed by further balloon inflations. Stent oversizing may be necessary to prevent stent embolization, resist elastic recoil, and attenuate the impact of late intimal hyperplasia.[1]

References:
1. Ozaki Y, Keane D, Ruygrok P, vd Giessen W, de Feyter P. Six-month clinical and angiographic follow-up of the new less shortening Wallstent in native coronary arteries. Circulation 1995;92:I-79.

239. Answer: c

Predilation with a conventional angioplasty balloon is recommended prior to insertion of all balloon-expandable stents. To minimize the risk of unwanted dissection during planned stenting, the vessel may be slightly underdilated with a balloon measuring 0.5 mm less than the reference diameter. Besides facilitating stent insertion, predilation can confirm that the balloon (and therefore the stent) can be fully inflated, and will also allow the operator to visualize the "shoulders" of the original lesion, thereby facilitating complete coverage by the stent. The inability to fully dilate a rigid stenosis with a high-pressure balloon is a contraindication to stenting, unless atherectomy increases lesion compliance and facilitates full balloon expansion.

240. Answer: d

In situations where a stent cannot be delivered because of proximal vessel tortuosity, techniques to enhance success include the use of guiding catheters that enhance coaxial alignment and optimize backup support; heavy duty or extra support guidewires to facilitate stent advancement; and the "buddy wire" approach to straighten tortuous segments. The "buddy" wire approach relies on the use of double extra-support of heavy duty wires to straighten the vessel; once the stent delivery system is in position across the target lesion, remove the buddy wire; do not deploy the stent until the buddy wire has been removed. Jack-hammering the stent is rarely successful, and can result in vessel injury or premature stent delivery.

241. Answer: c

The delivery system for the Gianturco-Roubin stent does not include a delivery sheath.

242. Answer: a

Recent experience suggests that post-stent angioplasty should be performed using high-pressure balloons matched to the normal reference diameter (balloon/artery ratio = 1.0-1.1) and inflated to 14-20 ATM;[1] intravascular ultrasound may be valuable for determining the actual reference vessel diameter and for confirming ideal stent apposition to the vessel wall.[2] Data from the MUSCAT trial suggest that predilation, stent deployment, and adjunctive PTCA can be achieved with a single balloon.[3] Failure to utilize high-pressure angioplasty will frequently result in suboptimal stent deployment, even when the angiographic result is excellent. Inflation pressures of 12-16 ATM are associated with less stent thrombosis than inflation pressures < 12 ATM. Some studies suggest that inflation pressures > 16 ATM may be associated with more late revascularization procedures,[4,5] while others do not.[6,7]

References:
1. Colombo A, Hall P, Martini G. Ultrasound-guided coronary stenting without anticoagulation. In: Current Review of Interventional Cardiology, Second Edition. Topol EJ, Serruys PW (eds). Current Medicine, Philadelphia, PA. 1995, pg. 115.
2. Kiemeneij F, Laarman G, Slagboom T. Mode of deployment of coronary Palmaz-Schatz stents after implantation with the stent delivery system: An intravascular ultrasound study. Am Heart J 1995;129:638-644.
3. Mudra H, Regar E, Wener F, Rothman MftMI. A focal high pressure dilatation of Palmaz-Schatz stents can safely achieve maximal stent expansion using a single balloon catheter approach. First results from the MUSCAT Trial. Circulation 1995;92:I-280.
4. Waksman R, Shen Y, Ghazzal Z, et al. Optimal balloon inflation pressures for stent deployment and correlates of stent thrombosis and in-stent restenosis. Circulation 1996;94:I-258.
5. Svage MP, Fischman DL, Douglas JS, et al. The dark side of high pressure stent deployment. J Am Coll Cardiol 1997;29(Suppl A):368A.
6. Goldberg SL, Colombo A, DiMario C, et al. Does the use of aggressive stent dilatation lead to more late loss and restenosis? J Am Coll Cardiol 1997;29(Suppl A):368A.
7. Akiyama T, DiMario C, Reimers B, et al. Does high-pressure stent expansion induce more restenosis? J Am Coll Cardiol 1997;29(Suppl A):368A.

243. Answer: c

Most operators use the percutaneous femoral artery approach for stent implantation. Recently, several centers have started using the percutaneous radial artery approach, even in patients who are fully anticoagulated at the time of intervention. Advantages of this technique are primarily related to patient comfort, reduction in bleeding and vascular complications, and a potential reduction in hospital stay; in addition, radial artery stent implants may be performed on an outpatient basis.[1-4] Delivery of biliary stents requires 8- or 9-French guiding catheters, and delivery of the Palmaz-Schatz SDS (stent delivery system) requires an 8F guiding catheter; these stents are not routinely deployed via the radial approach.

References:
1. Kiemeneij F, Laarman GJ, Slagboom T, Stella P. Transradial Palmaz-Schatz coronary stenting on an outpatient basis: Results of a prospective pilot study. J Inv Cardiol 1995;7:5A-11A.
2. Kiemeneij F, Laarman GJ. Transradial artery Palmaz-Schatz coronary stent implantation: Results of a single center feasibility study. Am Heart J 1995;130:14-21.
3. Kiemeneij F, Laarman GJ, Slagboom T. Percutaneous transradial coronary Palmaz-Schatz stent implantation, guided by intravascular ultrasound. Cathet Cardiovasc Diagn. 1995;34:133-136.
4. Kiemeneij F, Laarman G, Slagboom T, van der Wieken R. Transradial coronary stenting in outpatients. Circulation 1995;92:I-535.

244. Answer: e

The Wiktor stent is constructed of tantalum.

Answers

245. Answer: d

The metal surface area for the radius stent is approximately 20%, but is 10-15% for the Wallstent, Palmaz-Schatz coronary stent, the MultiLink stent, and the Microstent.

246. Answer: a, d

A rigid lesion should not be stented unless pretreatment allows full balloon expansion. Strategies for preparing a rigid lesion for stenting include Rotablator,[1,2] directional atherectomy, and high-pressure or force-focused PTCA.

References:
1. Carstens JS, Buchbinder M. Rotastenting: Latest clinical update including technique and results. J Interv Cardiol 1997;10:3:237-239.
2. Moussa I, DiMario C, Moses J, et al. Coronary stenting after rotational atherectomy in calcified and complex lesions. Angiographic and clinical follow-up results. Circulation 1997;96:128-136.

247. Answer: a

If the Palmaz-Schatz stent delivery system will not cross the target lesion, this problem will never be solved by retracting the delivery balloon inside the delivery sheath. The delivery sheath is not tapered, and the abrupt transition at the tip of the sheath can cause potential vascular injury. The "stentless" delivery sheath technique is performed as follows: Remove the stent delivery balloon (and stent) from the delivery sheath and replace it with a low-profile 0.014-inch-compatible balloon catheter; advance the low-profile balloon/delivery sheath across the lesion. Once the delivery sheath is positioned distal to the target lesion, exchange the low-profile balloon for the stent delivery balloon (and stent). Retract the delivery sheath and deploy the stent.

248. Answer: a, c, e

Management of sidebranch occlusion after stenting is relatively straight forward. In some cases, sidebranch patency is restored spontaneously or after administration of nitroglycerin. If clinically indicated, virtually any flexible guidewire can be used to access the sidebranch, and low-profile balloons with mean burst presences >10 ATM[1] are recommended, to reduce the chance of balloon rupture or entrapment after dilating the branch. In some cases, predilation of an ostial sidebranch stenosis may facilitate sidebranch patency after stenting. Finally, high-pressure adjunctive PTCA should always be performed after stent deployment to ensure proper stent expansion, and may "re-orient" the origin of an occluded sidebranch and facilitate passage of the guidewire.

References:
1. Guarneri E, Sklar M, Russo R, Claire D, Schatz R, Teirstein P. Escape from Stent Jail: An in vitro model. Circulation 1995;92:I-688.

249. Answer: a, d

250. Answer: b, d

Generally, high-pressure adjunctive PTCA is recommended to ensure ideal stent deployment, even if the angiographic result appears excellent. After loss of guidewire position, it is virtually impossible to steer the guidewire to avoid passage beneath the stent struts; a flexible wire with a large J-tip should be "prolapsed" across the stented segment.

251. Answer: a, c, d

252. Answer: c, f

When stenting an aorto-ostial lesion, coaxial alignment of the guiding catheter is crucial; use of an aggressive guide is discouraged because it may impede the operator's ability to adequately cover the ostium. Ideally, the proximal edge of the stent should reside 1-2 mm in the aorta. It is important to adequately debulk and/or expand the ostium to ensure successful stent delivery; useful adjunctive techniques include high-pressure balloons, Rotablator, and extra-support guidewires.

253. Answer: a, b, c, d, e

Rupture of the stent deployment balloon indicates inadequate stent expansion; further inflations with noncompliant balloon(s) are recommended to ensure ideal deployment, unless there is antecedent coronary artery perforation.

254. Answer: a, e

When using the Palmaz-Schatz stent delivery system, it may sometimes be necessary to remove the undeployed stent. In such situations, the entire delivery system can be removed if the stent is inside the delivery sheath. However, if the delivery sheath has been retracted and the stent is completely "uncovered," the stent should be retracted up to but not inside the guide, followed by removal en-bloc of the entire system, leaving the guidewire in place. Other maneuvers are unreliable and can potentially lead to stent embolization.

255. Answer: a, b

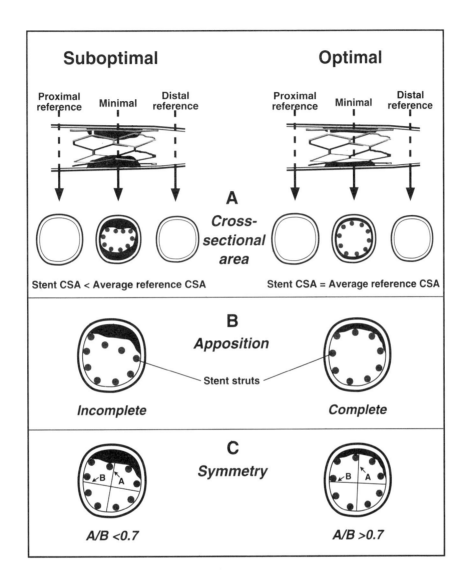

Optimal Stent Deployment: IVUS Criteria

A. Cross-sectional area index > 0.8: The ratio of stent minimal CSA (average CSA proximal and distal to stent).
B. Apposition: Maximum gap < 0.1 mm between stent strut (or coil) and underlying wall.
C. Symmetry index > 0.7: The ratio of the stent minor axis (A) to stent major axis (B).

256. Answer: a, b

Indications for Stenting
Definite
Abrupt closure
Threatened closure
Focal, de novo lesions in native vessel ≥ 3mm
Probable
SVG (focal or tubular lesions)
Possible
SVG (degenerated)
Bifurcation lesions
Aorto-ostial lesions
Restenotic lesions
Vessels < 3mm
Chronic total occlusion
Lesions > 20mm
Contraindications
Gross thrombus

257. Answer: b (false)

The overall incidence of abrupt closure after PTCA is 4-12%; standard methods to reverse abrupt closure (repeat balloon inflations, vasodilators, thrombolytic agents) may reduce the need for emergency surgery to ≤ 2%. In the randomized Trial of Angioplasty and Stents in Canada (TASC-II) and in several observational series, primary stenting was more effective than prolonged balloon inflations for failed PTCA.[1-4]

References:
1. Penn I, Ricci D, Brown R, et al. Randomized study of stenting versus prolonged balloon dilatation in failed angioplasty (PTCA): Preliminary data from the trial of Angioplasty and Stents in Canada (T.A.S.C. II). Circulation 1993;88:I-601.
2. Ricci D, Buller C, O'Neill B, et al. Coronary stent vs. prolonged perfusion balloon for failed coronary angioplasty. A randomized trial. Circulation 1994;90:I-651.
3. Ray S, Penn I, Ricci D, et al. Mechanism of benefit of stenting in failed PTCA. Final results from the trial of Angioplasty and Stents in Canada (TASC II). J Am Coll Cardiol 1995;25:156A.
4. Ricci D, Ray S, Buller C, et al. Six month followup of patients randomized to prolonged inflation or stent for abrupt occlusion during PTCA-clinical and angiographic data: TASC II. Circulation 1995;92:I-475.

258. Answer: b

Despite the success of stents for reversing abrupt closure, there is still significant patient morbidity, including stent thrombosis (0-32%), myocardial infarction (2-16%), emergency bypass surgery (0-16.5%), and death (0-10%). Although unplanned use of stents is associated with a higher incidence of adverse in-hospital events and lower procedural success compared to planned elective stenting, most adverse events relate to abrupt closure *prior* to stenting, rather than stent failure per se.[1] Many dissections leading to abrupt closure exceed 20 mm in length but can be managed by multiple tandem stents;[2-4] focal dissections (10-15 mm) are ideally suited for placement of a single stent.

References:
1. Carrozza J, George C, Curry C. Palmaz-Schatz stenting for non-elective indications: Report from the new approaches to coronary intervention (NACI) Registry. Circulation 1995;92:I-86.
2. Gordon P, Gibson M, Cohen D, Carrozza J, Kuntz R, Baim D. Mechanisms of restenosis and redilation within coronary stents-quantitative angiographic assessment. J Am Coll Cardiol 1993;21:1166-1174.
3. Hermiller J, Fry E, Peters T, Orr C, Van Tassel J, Pinkerton C. Multiple Gianturco-Roubin stent for long dissections causing acute and threatened coronary artery closure. J Am Coll Cardiol 1994;23:73A.
4. Sankardas M, Garrahy J, McEniery PT. Sequential implantation of dissimilar tandem stents for long dissections complicating percutaneous transluminal coronary angioplasty. Cathet Cardiovasc Diagn. 1995;34:155-158.

259. Answer: b (false)

Although a minority of abrupt closures are due to thrombosis, these might be managed better by other methods, such as thrombolytic therapy, extraction devices, PTCA, perfusion balloon angioplasty, or local drug delivery. Stenting in the setting of a large untreated thrombus is relatively contraindicated due to the risk of further thrombus formation, but could be considered if thrombus can be removed or dissolved.

260. Answer: a, c

The risk of MI is nearly 3-fold higher when stents are used for established abrupt closure than for threatened abrupt closure.[1] Since delayed stenting appears to be associated with an increased risk of ischemic complications, early (pre-operative) stenting for threatened closure may be indicated. However, other studies suggest that stenting for threatened abrupt closure was not better than conventional therapy without stenting.[2,3] There appears to be no difference in major ischemic complications, vascular injury, or late outcome when Gianturco-Roubin stents are implanted for failed PTCA with moderate dissection compared to failed PTCA with severe dissection;[4] preliminary data suggest that emergency stenting after failed PTCA is less costly than emergency CABG, resulting in a cost-savings of 17%.[5] Although temporary stenting with the Flow Support Catheter has been shown to stabilize dissection and avoid the need for a permanent implant,[6] this device was withdrawn from the market. A heat-activated recoverable temporary stent (HARTS) is also under investigation for treatment of failed PTCA.[7]

References:
1. Agrawal S, Liu M, Hearn J, et al. Can preemptive stenting improve the outcome of acute closure? J Am Coll Cardiol 1993;21:291A.

2. Lincoff M, Topol E, Chapekis A, et al. Intracoronary stenting compared with conventional therapy for abrupt vessel closure complicating coronary angioplasty: A matched case-control study. J Am Coll Cardiol 1993;21:866-875.
3. Stauffer JC, Eeckhout E, Goy JJ, et al. Major dissection during coronary angioplasty: Outcome using prolonged balloon inflation versus coronary stenting. J Invas Cardiol 1995;7:221-227.
4. Garratt K, Voorhees W, Bell M, et al. Complications related to intracoronary stents placed for moderate and severe dissections: Cook FlexStent Registry report. J Am Coll Cardiol 1994;23:102A.
5. Pilon C, Foley JB, Penn I, Brown R. A costing study of coronary stenting in failed angioplasty. J Am Coll Cardiol 1994;23:73A.
6. Gaspard P, Didier B, Lienhart Y, et al. Emergency temporary stenting should be preferred to permanent stenting for abrupt closure during coronary angioplasty. J Am Coll Cardiol 1994;23:103A.
7. Mahrer J, Eigler N, Khorsandi M, et al. Development of the Heat Activated Recoverable Temporary Stent (HARTS) with a slotted-tube design for coronary application. J Am Coll Cardiol 1994;23:103A.

261. Answer: b (false)

Current data indicate that stenting can be performed with high (>95%) success and low complication rates (< 5%) despite the presence of high-risk clinical and anatomical factors.[1-14] In addition, randomized and observational studies demonstrate that stenting results in a large, smooth lumen and a lower incidence of restenosis compared to PTCA, regardless of baseline lesion morphology.

References:
1. Hall P, Nakamura S, Maiello L, et al. Clinical and angiographic outcome after Palmaz-Schatz stent implantation guided by intravascular ultrasound. J Inv Cardiol 1995;7:12A-22A.
2. Morice M-C. Advances in post stenting medication protocol. J Inv Cardiol 1995;7:32A-35A.
3. Colombo A, Maiello L, Nakamura S, et al. Preliminary experience of coronary stenting with the MicroStent. J Am Coll Cardiol 1995;25:239A.
4. Hamasaki N, Nosaka H, Nobuyoshi M. Initial experience of Cordis stent implantation. J Am Coll Cardiol 1995;25:239A.
5. Karouny E, Khalife K, Monassier J-P, et al. Clinical experience with Medtronic Wiktor stent implantation: A report from the French Multicenter Registry. J Am Coll Cardiol 1995;25:239A.
6. Savage M, Fischman D, Schatz R, et al. Long-term angiographic and clinical outcome after implantation of a balloon-expandable stent in the native coronary circulation. J Am Coll Cardiol 1994;24:1207-1212.
7. Popma J, Colombo A, Chuang YC, et al. Late angiographic outcome after ultrasound-guided stent deployment in native coronary arteries using adjunct high pressure balloon dilatation. Circulation 1994;90:I-612.
8. Webb J, Abel J, Allard M, Carere R, Evans E, Dodek A. AVE Microstent: Initial human experience. Circulation 1994;90:I-612.
9. de Jaegere P, Serruys P, Bertrand M, et al. Angiographic predictors of recurrence of restenosis after Wiktor stent implantation in native coronary arteries. Am J Cardiol 1993;72:165-.
10. Carrozza J, Kuntz R, Levine M, et al. Angiographic and clinical outcome of intracoronary stenting: Immediate and long-term results from a large single-center experience. J Am Coll Cardiol1992;20:328-337.
11. Strauss B, Serruys P, et al. Quantitative angiographic follow-up of the coronary Wallstent in native vessels and bypass grafts (European experience--March 1986 to March 1990). Am J Cardiol 1992;69:475-481.
12. Dawkins K, Emanuelson H, wine VdG, et al. Preliminary results of a European multicenter feasability and safety registry of an innovative stent: The West Study. Circulation 1995;92:I-280.
13. Chevalier B, Royer T, Glatt B, Diab N, Rosenblatt E. Preliminary experience of coronary stenting with the MicroStent. Circulation 1995;92:I-409.
14. Goy J, Eeckhout G, Stauffer J-C, Vogt P. Stenting of the right coronary artery for de novo stenoses. A comparison of the Wiktor and the Palmaz-Schatz stents. Circulation 1995;92:I-536.

262. Answer: a, b, d

The favorable impact of stenting on restenosis relates to its ability to achieve superior lumen enlargement (final diameter stenosis < 10%), to minimize elastic recoil (usually < 8%[1]), and to virtually eliminate arterial remodeling.[2-6] PTCA vs. stent trials suggest *more* intimal proliferation after stenting, but this was more than offset by its other beneficial effects.[7]

References:
1. Fernandez-Ortiz A, Goicolea J, Perez-Vizcaynio M, et al. Is coronary stent recoil different for Gianturco-Roubin and Palmaz-Schatz stent? Circulation 1995;92:I-94.
2. de Jaegere P, Serruys P, van Es G, et al. Recoil following Wiktor stent implantation for restenotic lesions of coronary arteries. Cathet Cardiovasc Diagn 1994;32:147-156.
3. Rodriguez A, Santaera O, Larribau M, et al. Coronary stenting decreases restenosis in lesions with early loss in luminal diameter 24 hours after successful

Answers

PTCA. Circulation 1995;91:1397-1402.

4. Penn I, Ricci D, Almond D, et al. Coronary artery stenting reduces restenosis: Final results from the Trial of Angioplasty and Stents in Canada (TASC) I. Circulation 1995;92:I-279.
5. Mintz G, Pichard A, Kent K, et al. Endovascular stents reduce restenosis by eliminating geometric arterial remodeling: A serial intravascular ultrasound study. J Am Coll Cardiol 1995;25:36A.
6. Serruys PQW, Azar AJ, Sigwart U, et al. Long-term follow-up of "stent-like" ($\leq$ 30% diameter stenosis post) angioplasty: A case for provisional stenting. J Am Coll Cardiology 1996;27:15A.
7. Masotti M, Serra A, Fernandez-Aviles F, et al. Stent vs Angioplasty Restenosis Trial (START). Angiographic results at six month follow-up. Circulation 1996;94:i-685.

263. Answer: b (false)

Recently, two multicenter randomized trials compared immediate and long-term results of elective Palmaz-Schatz stenting vs. PTCA in de novo lesions in native coronary arteries;[1,2] both studies confirmed that stenting resulted in better lumen enlargement, higher procedural success, lower restenosis rates, fewer repeat procedures, and better event-free survival. Similar findings were reported in isolated stenoses in the proximal LAD.[3]

References:

1. Fischman DL, Leon MB, Baim DS, Schatz RA, et al. A randomized comparison of coronary stent placement and balloon angioplasty in the treatment of coronary artery disease. N Engl J Med 1994;331:496-501.
2. Serruys P, de Jaegere P, Kiemeneij F, et al. A comparison of balloon expandable stent implantation with balloon angioplasty in patients with coronary artery disease. N Engl J Med 1994;331:489-495.
3. Versaci F, Gaspardone A, Tomai F, et al. A comparison of coronary artery stenting with angioplasty for isolated stenosis of the proximal left anterior descending coronary artery. N Eng J Med 1997;336:817-822.

264. Answer: b (false)

In the Benestent trial, the relative benefits of stenting were preserved at 1 year: The need for target lesion revascularization was 10% in the stent group and 21% in the PTCA group.[1] Elective stenting of de novo lesions resulted in less restenosis compared to restenotic lesions (14% vs. 39%).[2]

References:

1. Macaya C, Serruys PW, Ruygrok P, et al. Continued benefit of coronary stenting vs. balloon angioplasty: One-year clinical follow-up of Benestent trial. J Am Coll Cardiol 1996;27:255-61.
2. Savage M, Fischman D, Schatz R, et al. Long-term angiographic and clinical outcome after implantation of a balloon-expandable stent in the native coronary circulation. J Am Coll Cardiol 1994;24:1207-1212.

265. Answer: b (false)

The time course of restenosis is similar to PTCA,[1,2] but several angiographic studies suggest that in-stent minimal lumen diameter improves between 6 months and 3 years after implantation; 6 month angiography may actually *underestimate* the long-term benefit of stenting.[3-5] In one study, 85% of target vessel revascularization procedures were performed within 12 months, whereas 15% were performed between 1-3 years after stenting.[6]

References:

1. Kastrati A, Schomig A, Dietz R, Neumann F-J. Time course of restenosis during the first year after emergency coronary stenting. Circulation 1993;87:1498-1505.
2. Kimura T, Nosaka H, Yokoi H, Iwabuchi M, Nobuyoshi M. Serial angiographic follow-up after Palmaz-Schatz stent implantation: Comparison with conventional balloon angioplasty. J Am Coll Cardiol 1993;21:1557-1163.

3. Kimura T, Yokoi H, Tamura T, Nakagawa Y, Nosaka H, Nobuyoshi M. Three years clinical and quantitative angiographic follow-up after the Palmaz-Schatz coronary stent implantation. J Am Coll Cardiol 1995;25:375A.
4. Hermiller J, Fry E, Peters T, et al. Late lesion regression within the Gianturco-Roubin Flex stent. J Am Coll Cardiol 1995;25:375A.
5. Hermiller JB, Fry ET, Peters TF, et al. Late coronary artery stenosis regression within the Gianturco-Roubin intracoronary stent. Am J Cardiol 1996;77:247-51.
6. Klugherz BD, DeAngelo DL, Kim BK, et al. Three-year clinical follow-up after Palmaz-Schatz stenting. J Am Coll Cardiol 1996;27:1185-91.

266. Answer: a (true)

Recurrent ischemia beyond 6-12 months after Gianturco-Roubin or Palmaz-Schatz stenting is virtually always due to progressive disease in a nonstented vessel.[1]

References:
1. Laham RJ, Carrozza JP, Berger JP, et al. Long-term (4-6 year) outcome of Palmaz-Schatz stenting: Paucity of late clinical stent-related problems. J Am Coll Cardiol 1996;28:820-6.

267. Answer: a, b, d, e, f

Results of Multicenter Randomized Trials of PTCA and Palmaz-Schatz Stent[1,2]

	STRESS (n=407)		BENESTENT (n=516)	
	PTCA	**Stent**	**PTCA**	**Stent**
In-hospital results				
Procedural Success (%)	89.6	96.1**	91	92.7
Final DS (%)	35	19*	33	22*
All ischemic events (%)	7.9	5.9	6.2	6.9
Death	1.5	0	0	0
Q-MI/nQMI	3/2	2.9/1.5	0.8/2.3	1.9/1.5
CABG/PTCA	4/1	2/2	3.9/1.2	3.1/0.4
Bleeding/Vascular (%)	4	7.3	3.1	13.5*
Vessel occlusion (%)+	10.2	3.4	6.2	3.5
LOS (day)	2.8	5.8*	3.1	8.5*
6 Month Follow-up (%)				
Angiographic restenosis	42	31**	32	22*
Ischemic events	23	17	24	14
TLR	22	14**	27	18**
EFS	72	78**	60	70**

Abbreviations: STRESS = Stent Restenosis Study; BENESTENT = Belgium-Netherlands Stent Trial; DS = diameter stenosis; nQMI = non-Q-wave myocardial infarction; CABG = emergency coronary artery bypass surgery; LOS = length of stay; TLR = target lesion revascularization; EFS = event-free survival.
* p < 0.001; ** p < 0.005
\+ vessel occlusion due to abrupt closure (PTCA group) or stent thrombosis (stent group)

References:
1. Fischman DL, Leon MB, Baim DS, Schatz RA, et al. A randomized comparison of coronary stent placement and balloon angioplasty in the treatment of coronary artery disease. N Engl J Med 1994;331:496-501.
2. Serruys P, de Jaegere P, Kiemeneij F, et al. A comparison of balloon expandable stent implantation with balloon angioplasty in patients with coronary artery disease. N Engl J Med 1994;331:489-495.

268. Answer: a, b, c, d, e

There appears to be a higher incidence of stent restenosis under the following conditions: Multiple stents, vessel diameter < 3.0 mm, restenotic lesions, lesion length > 10 mm, and post-stent residual stenosis > 10%.[1-3]

References:
1. Ali N, Lowry R, Tawa C, et al. Predictors of restenosis after Gianturco-Roubin coronary stent deployment. Analysis of 135 consecutive patients from a single center. J Am Coll Cardiol 1994;23:71A.
2. Ellis S, Savage M, Dischman D, Baim D, Leon M, Goldberg S. Restenosis after placement of Palmaz-Schatz stents in native coronary arteries. Initial results of a multicenter experience. Circulation 1992;86:1836-1844.
3. Baim D, Levine M, Leon M, Levine S, Ellis S, Schatz R. Management of restenosis within the Palmaz-Schatz coronary stent (the U.S. multicenter experience). Am J Cardiol 1993;71:364-366.

269. Answer: b (false)

In one report, angiographic patterns of stent restenosis included diffuse in-stent restenosis (33%), focal restenosis at the edges of the stent (26%), and focal in-stent restenosis involving the articulation (33%) or the body of the stent (8%);[1] focal in-stent restenosis of the body of the stent was identified in 17% of stent restenosis in another study.[2]

References:
1. Yokol H, Kimura T, Nobuyoshi M. Palmaz-Schatz coronary stent restenosis: Pattern and management. J Am Coll Cardiol 1994;23:117A.
2. Ikari Y, Hara K, Tamura T, Saeki F, Tamaguchi T. Luminal lost and site of restenosis after Palmaz-Schatz coronary stent implantation. Am J Cardiol 1995;76:117-120.

270. Answer: d, e, f

Treatment of in-stent restenosis is relatively straightforward. Conventional PTCA has been applied most commonly;[1-3] success rates generally exceed 90%, although recurrent restenosis occurs in 50%.[2] PTCA generally results in compression and extrusion of intimal tissue rather than stent-expansion.[1] Rotablator atherectomy should not be used with coil stents due to the risk of burr entrapment; its use for in-stent restenosis of Palmaz-Schatz stents is under investigation. ELCA and DCA[4] have also been used, but offer no clear advantage over PTCA. In the multicenter Palmaz-Schatz stent registry, stent restenosis was managed by medical therapy (3%), CABG (13.6%), and re-PTCA (40%). There is probably no need for additional antiplatelet therapy after PTCA for stent restenosis.

References:
1. Gordon P, Gibson M, Cohen D, Carrozza J, Kuntz R, Baim D. Mechanisms of restenosis and redilation within coronary stents-quantitative angiographic assessment. J Am Coll Cardiol 1993;21:1166-1174.
2. Baim D, Levine M, Leon M, Levine S, Ellis S, Schatz R. Management of restenosis within the Palmaz-Schatz coronary stent (the U.S. multicenter experience). Am J Cardiol 1993;71:364-366.
3. Macander P, Roubin G, Agrawal S, Cannon A, Dean L, Baxley W. Balloon angioplasty for treatment of in-stent restenosis: Feasibility, safety, and efficacy.

Cathet Cardiovasc Diagn. 1994;32:125-131.

4. Pathan A, Butte A, Harrell L, et al. Directional coronary atherectomy is superior to PTCA for the treatment of Palmaz-Schatz stent restenosis. J Am Coll Cardiol 1997;29 (Suppl A):68A.

5. Reimers B, Mouss I, Akiyama T, et al. Long-term clinical follow-up after successful repeat percutaneous intervention for stent restenosis. J Am Coll Cardiol 1997;30:186-192.

271. Answer: a

In general, intravascular stents offer the best opportunity for immediate enlargement of the vascular lumen, particularly in large vessels. Acute and long-term results suggest that stents may be the treatment of choice for focal or tubular lesions in nondegenerated vein grafts. Although virtually all stents have been implanted in saphenous vein grafts, the largest experience is with the Palmaz-Schatz coronary stent and the Palmaz-Schatz biliary stent:[1-14] Numerous studies suggest that successful stent delivery can be accomplished in 95-100% of lesions, with a low incidence of stent thrombosis (0-3.4%), emergency CABG (0-2.8%), myocardial infarction (0-4.3%), and death (0-2%). Restenosis rates after Palmaz-Schatz stenting range between 17-35%, but the need for repeat intervention may be as low as 4.9% when "optimal stenting" is employed.[21] In the multicenter prospective randomized trial of PTCA vs. Palmaz-Schatz coronary stents in vein grafts (SAVED), preliminary data suggest that stenting achieves superior immediate lumen enlargement (final diameter stenosis 12% vs. 33%, p <0.001), higher procedural success (96% vs. 85%, p <0.05), and a lower incidence of emergency CABG (0% vs. 6.7%, p <0.05);[15] preliminary follow-up data suggest similar total- and event-free survival at 3 months, but complete 6-month angiographic and clinical outcomes are pending.[16] In contrast to PTCA, stenting of vein grafts does not appear to be influenced by graft age;[22] acute and long-term results were similar for vein grafts less than or greater than 4 years of age.[17] However, similar to PTCA, 2-year event-free survival after vein graft stenting is only 55%; this attrition in late outcome is due to increasing mortality, recurrent ischemia, and unfavorable clinical characteristics of many patients treated with previous CABG.[18,19] Stenting of the internal mammary bypass graft is also feasible,[20] but data are limited.

Results of Stents in Saphenous Vein Bypass Grafts

Series	Stent	No. Lesion	Success (%)	SAT (%)	D/MI/CABG (%)	VSR /XF*	RS (%)
Wong[2] (1995)	PSS	624	98.8	1.4	1.7 / 0.3 / 0.9	8.0 / 6.3	30
Rechavia[3] (1995)	PSS, Biliary	29	100	0	0 / 0 / 0	3.4 / 6.8	-
Wong[4] (1995)	PSS, Biliary	205	95.3	1.7	1.3 / 0.9 / 0.4	15.9 / 25	-
Piana[5] (1994)	PSS, Biliary	200	98.5	0.6	0.6 / 0 / 0	8.5 / 14.0	17
Eeckhout[6] (1994)	Wallstent, Wiktor	58	100		2 / 0 / 2	14	25

Answers

Series	Stent	No. Lesion	Success (%)	SAT (%)	D/MI/CABG (%)	VSR /XF*	RS (%)
Keane[7] (1994)	New Wallstent	29	97	3.4	0 / 0 / 0	3.4 / 6.8	32
Fenton[8] (1994)	PSS	209	98.5	0.5	0.4/ 0 / 0	17.2 / 12	34
Leon[9] (1993)	PSS	589	97	1.4	1.7 / 0.3 / 0.9	7.5 / 15.5	30
Fortuna[10] (1993)	Wiktor	101	90	2	1 / 3 / 1	-	-
Pomerantz[11] (1992)	PSS	84	99	0	0 / 0 / 0	5	25
Bilodeau[12] (1992)	GRS	37	-	-	0 / 2.5 / 0	-	35
Strauss[1] (1992)	Wallstent	145	-	8	-	-	39
deScheerder[13] (1992)	New Wallstent	69	100	10	1.4 / 4.3 / 2.8	33	47
Urban[14] (1989)	Wallstent	14	100	0	0 / 0 / 0	7.7 / 7.7	20

Abbreviations: VSR = vascular surgical repair; XF = blood transfusion; SAT = subacute thrombosis, D = death; MI = myocardial infarction; CABG = emergency coronary artery bypass surgery; RS = restenosis
* Single numbers indicate combined incidence of vascular repair and/or blood transfusion.

References:
1. Strauss B, Serruys P, Bertrand M, et al. Quantitative angiographic follow-up of the coronary Wallstent in native vessels and bypass grafts (European experience--March 1986 to March 1990). Am J Cardiol 1992;69:475-481.
2. Wong SC, Baim D, Schatz R, et al. Immediate results and late outcomes after stent implantation in saphenous vein graft lesions: The multicenter U.S. Palmaz-Schatz Stent Experience. J Am Coll Cardiol 1995;26:704-712.
3. Rechavia E, Litvack F, Macko G, Eigler N. Stent implantation of saphenous vein graft aorto-ostial lesions in patients with unstable ischemic syndromes: Immediate angiographic results and long-term clinical outcome. J Am Coll Cardiol 1995;25:866-870.
4. Wong SC, Popma J, Pichard A, Kent K. Comparison of clinical and angiographic outcomes after saphenous vein grafts angioplasty using coronary versus "biliary" tubular slotted stents. Circulation 1995;91:339-350.
5. Piana R, Moscucci M, Cohen D, et al. Palmaz-Schatz stenting for treatment of focal vein graft stenosis: Immediate results and long-term outcome. J Am Coll Cardiol 1994;23:1296-304.
6. Eeckhout E, Goy J, Stauffer J, Vogt P, Kappenberger L. Endoluminal stenting of narrowed saphenous vein grafts: Long-term clinical and angiographic follow-up. Cathet Cardiovasc Diagn 1994;32:139-146.
7. Keane D, Buis B, Reifart N, Plokker TH. Clinical and angiographic outcome following implantation of the new less shortening Wallstent in aortocoronary vein grafts: Introduction of a second generation stent in the clinical arena. J Interven Cardiol 1994;7:557-564.
8. Fenton S, Fischman D, Savage M, et al. Long-term angiographic and clinical outcome after implantation of balloon-expandable stents in aortocoronary saphenous vein grafts. Am J Cardiol 1994;74:1187-1191.
9. Leon MB, Wong SC, Pichard A. Balloon expandable stent implantation in saphenous vein grafts. In Hermann HC, Hisrschfeld JW (Eds). Clinical use of the Palmaz-Schatz Intracoronary Stent. Futura Publishing Company Inc. 1993; 111-121.
10. Fortuna R, Heuser R, Garratt K, Schwartz R, M B. Intracoronary stent: experience in the first 101 vein graft patients. J Am Coll Cardiol 1993;26:I-308.
11. Pomerantz R, Kuntz R, Carrozza J, et al. Acute and long-term outcome of narrowed saphenous venous grafts treated by endoluminal stenting and directional atherectomy. Am J Cardiol 1992;70:161-167.
12. Bilodeau L, Iyer S, Cannon A, et al. Flexible coil stent (Cook, Inc) in saphenous vein grafts: Clinical and angiographic follow-up. J Am Coll Cardiol 1992;19:264A.
13. de Scheerder I, Strauss B, de Feyter P, et al. Stenting of venous bypass grafts: A new treatment modality for patients who are poor candidates for reintervention. Am Heart J 1992;123:1046-1054.
14. Urban P, Sigwart U, Golf S, Kaufmann U. Intravascular stenting for stenosis of aortocoronary venous bypass grafts. J Am Coll Cardiol 1989;13:1085-1091.
15. Savage M, Douglas J, Fischman D, et al. Coronary stents versus balloon angioplasty for aorto-coronary saphenous vein bypass graft disease: Interim results of a randomized trial. J Am Coll Cardiol 1995;25:79A.

16. Douglas JS, Savage MP, Bailey S, Bailey R, et al. Randomized trial of coronary stent and balloon angioplasty in the treatment of saphaneous vein graft stenosis. J Am Coll Cardiology 1996;27:178A.
17. Wong SC, Chuang Y, Hong M, et al. Stent placement is safe and effective in the treatment of older (>4 years) saphenous vein graft lesions. J Am Coll Cardiol 1995;25:79A.
18. Sketch M, Wong C, Chuang Y, et al. Progressive deterioration in late (2-year) clinical outcomes after stent implantation in saphenous vein grafts: The Multicenter JJIS experience. J Am Coll Cardiol 1995;25:79A.
19. Wong SC, Chuang Y, Popma J, et al. Comparative analysis of long term clinical outcomes after native coronary versus saphaneous vein graft stent implantation. J Am Coll Cardiol 1995;25:198A.
20. Hadjimiltiades S, Gourassas J, Louridas G, Tsifodimos D. Stenting the distal anastomotic site of the left internal mammary artery graft: A case report. Cathet Cardiovasc Diagn. 1994;32:157-161.
21. Abhyankar A, Bernstein L, Harris PH, et al. Reintervention and clinical events after saphenous vein graft angioplasty. A comparison of optimal PTCA vs. stenting. Circulation 1996;94 (Suppl A):I-686.
22. Brener SJ, Ellis SG, Apperson-Hansen C, Leon MB, Topol EJ. Comparison of stenting and balloon angioplasty for narrowings in aortocoronary saphenous vein conduits in place for more than 5 years. Am J Cardiol 1997;79:13-18.

272. Answer: b, c, d, e

The ideal intervention for degenerated vein grafts is unknown. Some operators recommend TEC atherectomy followed by immediate stent implantation to achieve definitive lumen enlargement and reduce restenosis.[1] Others recommend a strategy of initial TEC followed by 1-2 months of oral warfarin and staged stent implantation; compared to immediate stenting, this deferred stent strategy resulted in less distal embolization (10.7% vs. 22.7%) and fewer in-hospital ischemic complications (0% vs. 11.4%), but silent total occlusion occurred in 15%.[2] Reconstruction of occluded vein grafts is feasible with coronary or peripheral Wallstents.[3] In some cases, intragraft urokinase may facilitate stenting; in one report, procedural success was achieved in 93.3%, with stent thrombosis in 6.7%, Q-wave MI in 3.3%, and serious vascular injury in 16.7%.[4] Because of a relatively high incidence of no-reflow and late graft occlusion, re-do surgery, medical, and feasibility of native vessel revascularization should be strongly considered; PTCA alone should virtually never be performed in degenerated vein grafts.

References:
1. Kaplan BM, Safian RD, Grines CL, Goldstein JA, et al. Usefulness of adjunctive angioscopy and extraction atherectomy before stent implantation in high-risk aortocoronary saphenous vein grafts. Am J Cardiol 1995;76:822-824.
2. Hong M, Pichard A, Kent K, et al. Assessing a strategy of stand-alone extraction atherectomy followed by staged stent placement in degenerated saphenous vein graft lesions. J Am Coll Cardiol 1995;25:394A.
3. Kelly PA, Kurbaan AS. Total endovascular reconstruction of occluded Saphenous vein grafts using coronary or peripheral Wallstents. Circulation 1996;94 (Suppl A):I-258.
4. Denardo SJ, Morris NB, Rocha-Singh KJ, Curtis GP, et al. Safety and efficacy of extended urokinase infusion plus stent deployment for treatment of obstructed, older saphenous vein grafts. Am J Cardiol 1995;76:776-780.

273. Answer: d, e

Experimental data have shown that flow into nondiseased sidebranches is well-preserved after stent placement, and several angiographic studies suggest a low incidence of sidebranch occlusion. Nevertheless, stents should be used cautiously in patients with stenoses involving significant sidebranches. While sidebranches may still be accessible by PTCA after Gianturco-Roubin and other coil stent implantation, there may be a greater chance of balloon entrapment in the struts of slotted tubular stents (e.g., Palmaz-Schatz).[1] However, occluded sidebranches can be successfully retrieved by PTCA through 86% of Palmaz-Schatz stents and 75% of Gianturco-Roubin stents.[2] Important considerations include the likelihood of immediate and future revascularization of the sidebranch, the size of the sidebranch, and the amount of myocardium served by that branch. In general, jeopardy of acute marginal branches of the right coronary artery, small diagonal branches of the LAD, and small obtuse marginal branches of the left circumflex do not represent significant contraindications to stent placement. In some anatomically suitable vessels, these are now several reports of "kissing" articulated and disarticulated stents or T-stenting; these techniques are technically demanding and should be reserved for experienced stent operators.[3-6]

References:
1. Guarneri E, Sklar M, Russo R, Claire D, Schatz R, Teirstein P. Escape from Stent Jail: An in vitro model. Circulation 1995;92:I-688.
2. Caputo RP, Chafizedeh ER, Stoler RC, et al. "Stent Jail"— A minimum security prison. Am J Cardiol 1996 (in-press).
3. Nakamura S, Hall P, Maiello L, Colombo A. Techniques of Palmaz-Schatz stent deployment in lesions with a large side branch. Cathet Cardiovas Diagnos 1995;34:353-361.
4. Colombo A, Gaglione A, Nakamura S. "Kissing" stents for bifurcational coronary lesion. Cathet Cardiovas Diag. 1993;30:327-330.
5. Colombo A, Maiello L, Itoh A, Hall P, et al. Coronary stenting of bifurcation lesions immediate and follow-up results. J Am Coll Cardiology 1996;27:277A.
6. Carrie D, Elbaz M, Mebarkia M, ct al. "T" shaped stent placement: A technique for the treatment of coronary bifurcation lesions. J Am Coll Cardiol 1997;29:16A.

274. Answer: c

PTCA of aorto-ostial lesions is frequently suboptimal because of the elasticity and rigidity of the aorta; final diameter stenoses > 50% are common. Stent implantation in the aorto-ostial location is technically challenging because of difficulties seating the guiding catheter, obtaining adequate images to optimize stent placement, ensuring proper stent position to adequately cover the entire lesion (i.e., the proximal end of the stent must be flared in the aorta), and stent migration or embolization. For calcified aorta-ostial lesions, stents should probably be avoided because of the risk of incomplete stent expansion, unless pretreatment with Rotablator and/or high-pressure balloons allows full balloon inflation before stenting. Intravascular ultrasound may be valuable in aorto-ostial lesions to assess the degree and depth of calcification, to ensure adequate stent sizing, and to confirm complete stent apposition and lesion coverage. In several small observational studies, stents have been successfully implanted in > 95% of ostial lesions; restenosis rates range from 15% (for native vessels) to 62% (for vein grafts).[1-7,9-11] In a small randomized study of PTCA and Wiktor stents in ostial RCA lesions, stents resulted in better lumen enlargement, but there was no difference in early or late outcome.[8] Unprotected origin lesions of the LAD or left circumflex may be difficult to stent since proper lesion coverage requires positioning the stent in the distal left main.

Results of Stenting for Ostial Lesions

Series	Stent	Morphology	N	Success (%)	SAT (%)	Comments
Colombo[9] (1996)	PSS, GRS, Wiktor	ostial	35	100	-	ARS (23%)
Rechavia[1] (1995)	PSS	ostial	29	100	-	CRS (15%)
Rocha-Singh[3] (1995)	PSS	ostial	41	100	10	Death (7.3%)

Series	Stent	Morphology	N	Success (%)	SAT (%)	Comments
Wong[5] (1994)	PSS	ostial SVG	104	97	-	Coronary & biliary stents; death (1%), CABG (1%), ARS (62%)
Fenton[6] (1994)	PSS	ostial SVG	20	-	-	ARS (60%)

Abbreviations: ARS = angiographic restenosis; CRS = clinical restenosis; SAT - subacute thrombosis; DS = diameter stenosis; PSS = Palmaz-Schatz stent; GRS = Gianturco-Roubin stent; Wall; Wallstent; - = not reported; CTO = chronic total occlusion; TLR = target lesion revascularization; EFS = event-free survival; * Reocclusion 22% and restenosis 61% for PTCA; ** Reocclusion 35% and restenosis 68% for PTCA; *** Reocclusion 35% and restenosis 68% for PTCA; + Randomized study of stents vs. PTCA; for PTCA: ARS (33%), TLR (29%)

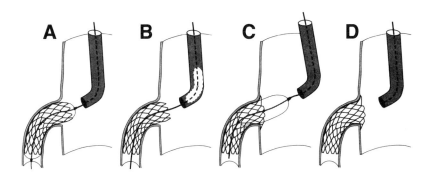

Aorto-Ostial Lesions: Stent Technique

A.   Position the stent-delivery balloon so 1-2 mm of stent extends into the aorta. The guide must be retracted 1-2 cm before deploying the stent.

B.   Remove the delivery balloon while maintaining backward tension on the guide, to prevent it from advancing into the ostium and damaging the stent.

C.   Perform adjunctive PTCA with a high pressure balloon to ensure full stent expansion and apposition. Flaring the proximal end of the stent with a slightly larger balloon is useful.

D.   Final result.

References:
1.   Rechavia E, Litvack F, Macko G, Eigler N. Stent implantation of saphenous vein graft aorto-ostial lesions in patients with unstable ischemic syndromes: Immediate angiographic results and long-term clinical outcome. J Am Coll Cardiol 1995;25:866-870.
2.   Zampieri P, Colombo A, Almagor Y, Mairello L, Finci L. Results of coronary stenting of ostial lesions. Am J Cardiol 1994;73:901-903.
3.   Rocha-Singh K, Morris N, Wong C, Schatz R, Teirstein P. Coronary stenting for treatment of ostial stenoses of native coronary arteries or aortocoronary saphenous venous grafts. Am J Cardiol 1995;75:26-29.
4.   Maiello L, Hall P, Nakamura S, et al. Results of stent implantation for diffuse coronary disease assisted by intravascular ultrasound. J Am Coll Cardiol 1995;25:156A.
5.   Wong SC, Hong M, Popma J, et al. Stent placement for the treatment of aorto-ostial saphenous vein graft lesions. J Am Coll Cardiol 1994;23:118A.
6.   Fenton S, Fischman D, Savage M, et al. Does stent implantation in ostial saphenous vein graft lesions reduce restenosis? J Am Coll Cardiol 1994;23:118A.
7.   Wong SC, Popma J, Hong M, et al. Procedural results and long term clinical outcomes in aorto-ostial saphenous vein graft lesions after new device angioplasty. J Am Coll Cardiol 1995;25:394A.
8.   Eeckhout E, Stauffer J-C, Vogt P, Debbas N, Kappenberger L, Goy J-J. A comparison of intracoronary stenting with conventional balloon angioplasty for the treatment of new onset stenoses of the right coronary artery. J Am Coll Cardiol 1995;25:196A.

9. Colombo A, Itoh A, Maiello L, et al. Coronary stent implantation in aorto-ostial lesions: Immediate and follow-up results. J Am Coll Cardiology 1996;27:253A.
10. Schuhlen H, Hausleiter J, Elezi S, et al. Coronary stent placement in ostial lesions. Six-month clinical and angiographic follow-up. J Am Coll Cardiol 1997;29 (Suppl A):16A.
11. Jain SP, Liu MW, Dean LS, et al. Comparison of balloon angioplasty versus debulking devices versus stenting in right coronary ostial lesions. Am J Cardiol 1997;79:1334-1338.

275. Answer: b (false)

For aorto-ostial vein graft lesions, the results of stenting have been shown to be superior to those of DCA;[1] comparative studies of DCA and stents have not been performed on lesions at the LAD origin.

References:
1. Wong SC, Popma J, Hong M, et al. Procedural results and long term clinical outcomes in aorto-ostial saphenous vein graft lesions after new device angioplasty. J Am Coll Cardiol 1995;25:394A.

276. Answer: b (false)

There are several small observational studies of stents for chronic total occlusion and diffuse disease;[1-9,12,14-17] subacute thrombosis and restenosis occurred in 1.2-5% and 20-35%, respectively. A randomized study of stents versus PTCA for chronic total occlusions is in progress; preliminary data in 53 lesions suggest significantly better immediate angiographic results after stenting,[10] but angiographic restenosis (36% vs. 33%) and target lesion revascularization (32% vs. 29%) were similar at 3-6 months.[11] When optimally deployed, multiple stents may not be a strong predictor of late cardiac events according to one study,[13] but this issue remains controversial.[18-21]

Chronic Total Occlusions and Diffuse Lesions

Series	Stent	Morphology	N	Success (%)	SAT (%)	Comments
Sato[11] (1996)	-	CTO	30	-	0	ARS (36%); TLR (32%)[+]
Medina[1] (1995)	PSS	CTO	30	100	9	RS (22%)
Hsu[2] (1994)	PSS, Wiktor	CTO	36	-	5	RS (20%)*
Ooka[3] (1994)	PSS, GRS	CTO	33	-	5	RS (24%)**
Ooka[8] (1995)	PSS, GRS	CTO	47	-	10	RS (44%)***
Goldberg[9] (1995)	PSS	CTO	60	98	5	ARS (20%); 14-month EFS (77%)
Liu[12] (1997)	PSS, GRS	diffuse	48	100	-	

Series	Stent	Morphology	N	Success (%)	SAT (%)	Comments
Maiello[4] (1995)	PSS, GRS, Wiktor	diffuse	89	93	1.2	RS (35%)
Reimers[5] (1995)	PSS, GRS, Wall	diffuse	48	94	4	ARS (25%)
Shaknovich[6] (1995)	PSS	diffuse	54	98.2	3.7	

Abbreviations: ARS = angiographic restenosis; CRS = clinical restenosis; SAT - subacute thrombosis; DS = diameter stenosis; PSS = Palmaz-Schatz stent; GRS = Gianturco-Roubin stent; Wall; Wallstent; - = not reported; CTO = chronic total occlusion; TLR = target lesion revascularization; EFS = event-free survival; * Reocclusion 22% and restenosis 61% for PTCA; ** Reocclusion 35% and restenosis 68% for PTCA; *** Reocclusion 35% and restenosis 68% for PTCA; + Randomized study of stents vs. PTCA; for PTCA: ARS (33%), TLR (29%)

References:
1. Medina A, Melian F, deLezo J, et al. Effectiveness of coronary stenting for the treatment of chronic total occlusion in angina pectoris. Am J Cardiol 1994;73:1222-1224.
2. Hsu Y-S, Tamai H, Ueda K, et al. Clinical efficacy of coronary stenting in chronic total occlusions. Circulation 1994;90:I-613.
3. Ooka M, Suzuki T, Kosokawa H, Kukkutomi T, Yamashita K, Hayase M. Stenting vs. non-stenting after revascularization of chronic total occlusion. Circulation 1994;90:I-613.
4. Maiello, Luigi, Hall, Patrick, Nakamura, Shigeru Blengino, Simonetta, et al. Results of stent implantation for diffuse coronary disease assisted by ultravascular ultrasound. J Am Coll Cardiol 1995;25:156A.
5. Reimers B, Di Mario C, Nierop P, Pasquetto G, Camenzind E, Ruygrok P. Long-term restenosis after multiple stent implantation. A quantitative angiographic study. Circulation 1995;92:I-327.
6. Shaknovich A, Moses J, Undemir C, et al. Procedural and short-term clinical outcomes of multiple Palmaz-Schatz stents (PSS) in very long lesions/dissections. Circulation 1995;92:I-535.
7. Akira I, Hall P, Maielli L, et al. Coronary stenting of long lesions (greater than 20 mm)-A matched comparison of different stents. Circulation 1995;92:I-688.
8. Ooka M, Suzuki T, Yokoya K, et al. Stenting after revascularization of chronic total occlusion. Circulation 1995;92:I-94.
9. Goldberg SL, Colombo A, Maiello L, Borrione M, et al. Intracoronary stent insertion after balloon angioplasty of chronic total occlusion. J Am Coll Cardiol 1995;26:713-719.
10. Sato Y, Kimura T, Nosaka H, Nobuyoshi M. Randomized comparison of balloon angioplasty (BA) versus coronary stent implantation (CS) for total occlusion (TO): Preliminary result. Circulation 1995;92:I-475.
11. Sato Y, Nosaka H, Kimura AT, et al. Randomized comparison of balloon angioplasty versus coronary stent implantation for total occlusion. J Am Coll Cardiology 1996;27:152A.
12. Liu MW, Luo JF, Dean LS, et al. Coronary vessel reconstruction with multiple stents--a follow-up study. Circulation 1996;94:I-258.
13. Eccleston DS, Belli G, Penn IM, et al. Are multiple stents associated with multiplicative risk in the optimal stent era? Circulation 1996;94:I-454.
14. Nienaber CA, Fratz S, Lund GK, et al. Primary stent placement or balloon angioplasty for chronic coronary occlusions: A matched pair analysis in 100 patients. Circulation 1996;94:I-696.
15. Sievert H, Rohde S, Schulze R, et al. Stent implantation after successful balloon angioplasty of a chronic coronary occlusion-a randomized trial. J Am Coll Cardiol 1997;29 (Suppl A):15A.
16. Mathey DG, Seidensticker A, Rau T, et al. Chronic coronary artery occlusion: Reduction of restenosis - and reocclusion - rates by stent treatment. J Am Coll Cardiol 1997;29 (Suppl A):396A.
17. Elezi S, Schuhlen H, Hausleiter J, Pache J, et al. Six-month angiographic follow-up after stenting of chronic total coronary occlusions. J Am Coll Cardiol 1997;29 (Suppl A):16A.
18. Gaziola E, Vietstra RE, Browne KF, et al. Six-month follow-up of patients with multiple stents in a single coronary artery. J Am Coll Cardiol 1997;29 (Suppl A):276A.
19. Hamasaki N, Nosaka H, Kumura T, et al. Influence of lesion length on late angiographic outcome and restenotic process after successful stent implantation. J Am Coll Cardiol 1997;29 (Suppl A):238A.
20. Aliabadi D, Bowers TR, Tilli FV, et al. Multiple stents increase target vessel revascularization rates. J Am Coll Cardiol 1997;29 (Suppl A):276A.
21. Moussa I, DiMario C, Moses J, et al. Single versus multiple Palmaz-Schatz stent implantation: Immediate and follow-up results. J Am Coll Cardiol 1997;29 (Suppl A):276A.

277. Answer: c

Stenting may be reasonable if thrombus can be removed.[1] Potentially useful adjuncts include TEC atherectomy;[2-4] systemic or intracoronary infusion of thrombolytics;[5] or local delivery of heparin or lytics.[6] For patients who are clinically stable, a 3-7 day infusion of heparin or a 2-3 week course of warfarin may "clean-up" the vessel and permit stent implantation. Coronary angioscopy may be especially useful in saphenous vein grafts to help guide interventional strategy in clinical situations in which thrombus is likely to be present.[2,3] Stenting lesions with thrombus may be feasible,[7-9] despite conventional wisdom to suggest otherwise.

References:
1. Kaul U, Agarwal R, Mathur A, Wasir HS. Intracoronary stent placement in thrombus containing vein graft lesions. J Inv Cardiol 1995;7:248-250.
2. Kaplan BM, Safian RD, Grines CL, Goldstein JA, et al. Usefulness of adjunctive angioscopy and extraction atherectomy before stent implantation in high-risk aortocoronary saphenous vein grafts. Am J Cardiol 1995;76:822-824.
3. Annex BH, Ajluni SC, Larkin TJ, et al. Angioscopic guided interventions in a saphenous vein bypass graft. Cathet Cardiovasc Diagn 1994;31:330-333.
4. Hong MK, Pichard A, Kent KM, et al. Assessing a strategy of stand-alone extraction atherectomy followed by staged stent placement in degenerated saphenous vein graft lesions. J Am Coll Cardiol 1995;25:394A.
5. Denardo SJ, Morris NB, Rocha-Singh KJ, Curtis GP, et al. Safety and efficacy of extended urokinase infusion plus stent deployment for treatment of obstructed, older saphenous vein grafts. Am J Cardiol 1995;76:776-780.
6. Glazier J, Kiernan F, Bauer H, et al. Treatment of thrombotic saphenous vein graft stenoses/occlusions with local urokinase delivery with the dispatch catheter-initial results. Circulation 1995;92:I-671.
7. Kaul U, Agarwal R, Jain P, Wasir H. Safety and efficacy of intracoronary stenting for thrombus-containing lesions. Am J Cardiol 1996;77:425-7.
8. Alfonso F, Rodriguez P, Phillips P, et al. Clinical and angiographic implications of coronary stenting in thrombus-containing lesions. J Am Coll Cardiol 1997;29 (Suppl A):96A.
9. Alfonso F, Rodriguez P, Phillips P, et al. Clinical and angiographic implications of coronary stenting in thrombus-containing leisons. J Am Coll Cardiol 1997;29:725-733.

278. Answer: e

The primary concern about stenting in the setting of acute MI is stent thrombosis. Nevertheless, small observational studies have reported successful bailout stenting for failed PTCA in 80-94%; subacute thrombosis rates have varied between 1.8-30%.[1-15] In one report, major in-hospital complications were similar to those obtained after successful PTCA for acute MI.[4] Other studies using the heparin-bonded stent are now in progress. In reviewing 565 lesions treated by PTCA for acute MI, 63% were anatomically suitable for stent implantation based on vessel diameter ≥ 3 mm and other angiographic characteristics.[4] Taken together, these data suggest that stents should not be withheld from appropriate patients with acute MI.

References:
1. Walton AS, Oesterle SN, Yeung AC. Coronary artery stenting for acute closure complicating primary angioplasty for acute myocardial infarction. Cathet Cardiovasc Diagn. 1995;34:142-146.
2. Ahmad T, Webb JG, Carere RR, Dodek A. Coronary stenting for acute myocardial infarction. Am J Cardiol 1995;76:77-80.
3. Wong PH, Wong CM. Intracoronary stenting in acute myocardial infarction. Cathet Cardiovasc Diagn. 1994;33:39-45.
4. Benzuly KH, Goldstein JA, Almany SL, et al. Feasibility of stenting in acute myocardial infarction. Circulation 1995;92:I-616.
5. Iyer S, Bilodeau L, Cannon A, et al. Stenting the infarct related artery within 15 days of the acute event: Immediate and long term outcome using the Flexible Metallic Coil stent. J Am Coll Cardiol 1993;21:291A.
6. Capers Q, Thomas C, Weintraub W, King S, Douglas J, Scott N. Emergent stent placement: Worse out come in the patients with a recent myocardial infarction. J Am Coll Cardiol 1994;23:71A.
7. Levy G, De Boisgelin X, Volpiliere R, Gallay P, Bouvagnet P. Intracoronary stenting in direct angioplasty: Is it dangerous? Circulation 1995;92:I-139.
8. Saito S, Kim K, Hosokawa G, Hatano K, Tanaka S. Primary Palmaz-Schatz implantation without coumadine in acute myocardial infarction. Circulation 1995;92:I-796.
9. Monassier JP, Ellias J, Meyer P, et al. STENTIM I: The French Registry of stenting of acute myocardial infarction. J Am Coll Cardiology 1996;27:68A.
10. Garcia-Cantu E, Spaulding C, Corcos T, et al. Stent implantation in acute myocardial infation. Am J Cardiol 1996;77:451-4.
11. Turi ZG, McGinnity JG, Fischman D, et al. Retrospective comparative study of primary intracoronary stenting versus balloon angioplasty for acute myocardial infarction. Cathet Cardiovas Diagn 1997;40:235-239.
12. Stone GW, Brodie BR, Morice MC, et al. Primary stenting in acute myocardial infarction: Design and interim results of the PAMI stent pilot trial. J Invas Cardiol 1997;9 (Suppl B):24B-30B.
13. Moses J, Moussa I, Stone G. Clinical trials of coronary stenting in acute myocardial infarction. J Invas Cardiol 1997;10:3:225-229.
14. Garcia E. In-hospital results of the Wiktor stent in acute myocardial infarction. J Invas Cardiol 1997;10:3:231-235.
15. Schomig A, Neuman FJ, Walter H, et al. Coronary stent placement in patients with acute myocardial infarction: Comparison of clinical and angiographic outcome after randomization to antiplatelet or anticoagulant therapy. J Am Coll Cardiol 1997;29:28-34.

279. Answer: b (false)

The immediate and long-term results for stent implantation in patients with stable and unstable angina are similar.[1,2] In a study of 62 patients with unstable angina and post-MI angina, procedural success for Palmaz-Schatz stenting was 94%, with in-hospital death in 3%, Q-wave MI in 3%, and serious vascular complications in 5%. Stent thrombosis did not occur. Adjunctive lytic therapy was used in 38% and warfarin in 37% of patients.[3] Available data suggest that stenting is reasonable and safe in patients with unstable angina. The potential benefit of ReoPro is under investigation in the EPILOG-Stent trial.

References:
1. Malosky S, Hirshfeld J, Herrmann H. Comparison of results of intracoronary stenting in patients with unstable vs. stable angina. Cathet Cardiovasc Diagn 1994;31:95-101.
2. Marzocchi A, Piovaccari G, Marozzini C, et al. Results of coronary stenting for unstable versus stable angina pectoris. Am J Cardiol 1997;79:1314-1318.
3. Guameri EM, Schatz RA, Sklar MA, Norman SL, et al. Acute coronary syndromes: Is it safe to stent? Circulation 1995;92:I-616.

280. Answer: a, b

Stenting of a single patent coronary artery or bypass graft may be considered for patients who are not candidates for CABG, when the target lesion is anatomically suitable for stenting, and there is good distal runoff. Technical considerations include predilatation of the lesion (to ensure full balloon inflation and maximize the chance of rapid stent deployment); use of large lumen guides with sideholes (to permit passive perfusion during intervention); use of prophylactic IABP or CPS if necessary; and possible use of IVUS (to ensure optimal stenting). The target vessel and age of the patient are not important factors.

281. Answer: b (false)

There have been a few experimental[1] and clinical[2-4] reports of stents with vein allografts, which have been used to seal perforations and/or coronary pseudoaneurysms. This technique is technically challenging, and is not appropriate for inexperienced stent operators or for patients with profound hemodynamic collapse.

References:
1. Stefanadis C, Vlachopoulos C, Kallikazaros I, et al. Autologous vein graft coating applied to vascular stents: the ideal coated stent? J Am Coll Cardiol 1994;23:135A.
2. Dorros G, Jain A, Kumar K. Management of coronary artery rupture: Covered stent or microcoil embolization. Cathet Cardiovasc Diagn. 1995;36:148-154.
3. Kaplan BM, Stewart RE, Sakwa MP, et al. Repair of a coronary pseudoaneurysm with percutaneous placement of a saphenous vein allograft attached to a biliary stent. Cathet Cardiovasc Diagn 1996 (in-press).
4. Stefanadis C, Konstantinos T, Vlachopoulos C, et al. Autologous vein graft-coated stent for treatment of coronary artery disease. Cathet & Cardiovasc Diagn 1996;38:159.

282. Answer: a, c, e

A prospective randomized trial of aspirin, aspirin plus warfarin, and aspirin plus ticlopidine has been completed recently; preliminary data suggest superiority of aspirin plus ticlopidine after optimal stenting (STent Anti-Thrombotic Regimen Study, STARS) for patients treated successfully with elective Palmaz-Schatz stents.[1] The recent ISAR trial (Intracoronary Stenting and Antithrombotic Regimen) randomized 517 patients to ASA/ticlopidine or ASA/warfarin after high-risk stenting; antiplatelet therapy alone was associated with a 7-10 fold reduction in stent thrombosis, ischemic complications and bleeding.[2,3] Antiplatelet therapy without warfarin appears to be effective after stenting for suboptimal PTCA.[4,5] The value of soluble aspirin (compared to enteric coated aspirin) and subcutaneous heparin have not yet been demonstrated. The value of low-molecular weight heaprin is under evaluation in the ATLAST study.

References:
1. Schomig A, Schuhlen H, Blasini R, et al. Anticoagulation versus antiplatelet therapy after intracoronary Palmaz-Schatz placement-A prospective randomized trial. Circulation 1995;92:I-280.
2. Schomig A, Neumann FJ, Kastrati A, et al. A randomized comparison of antiplatelet and anticoagulant therapy after the placement of coronary artery stents. N Engl J Med 1996;334:1084-9.
3. Schuhlen H, Hadamitzky M, Walter H, et al. Major benefit from antiplatelet therapy for patients at high risk for adverse cardiac events after coronary Palmaz-Schatz stent placement. Analysis of a prospective risk stratification protocol in the intracoronary stenting and antithrombotic regiment (ISAR) trial. Circulation 1997;95:2015-2020.
4. Lablanche JM, Bonnet JL, Grollier G, et al. Combined antiplatelet therapy without anticoagulation after stent implantation: The Ticlopidine aspirin stent evaluation (TASTE) study. J Am Coll Cardiol 1997;29:95A.
5. Antoniucci D, Valenti R, Santoro GM, et al. Bailout coronary stenting without anticoagulation or intravascular ultrasound guidance: Acute and six-month angiographic results in a series of 120 consecutive patients. Cathet Cardiovasc Diagnos 1997;41:41:14-19.

283. Answer: b (false)

For all stent patients, adjunctive medical therapy is required to prevent stent thrombosis. Despite a multitude of studies testing a variety of different drug combinations, the medical regimen is largely empiric. However, no studies suggest that Dextran is useful.

284. Answer: b (false)

Available data suggest fewer bleeding and vascular complications, and a lower incidence of stent thrombus after therapy with aspirin/ticlopidine compared to aspirin/Warfarin.[1,2]

References:
1. Schomig A, Schuhlen H, Blasini R, et al. Anticoagulation versus antiplatetet therapy after intracoronary Palmaz-Schatz placement-A prospective randomized trial. Circulation 1995;92:I-280.
2. Schomig A, Neumann FJ, Kastrati A, et al. A randomized comparison of antiplatelet and anticoagulant therapy after the placement of coronary artery stents. N Engl J Med 1996;334:1084-9.

285. Answer: b (false)

In highly selected cases, heparin effect was reversed with protamine without complication;[1] however, the utility of this approach is uncertain, and it is not routinely recommended.

References:
1. Colombo A, Hall P, Nakamura S, et al. Preliminary experience using protamine to reverse heparin immediately following a successful coronary stent implantation. J Am Coll Cardiol 1995;25:182A.

286. Answer: a, b, d

General Patient Management After Stent Implantation

	Warfarin Regimen*	Antiplatelet Regimen**
Sheath removal	ACT < 140 sec	ACT < 140 sec
Groin compression	≥ 1 hour	Standard
Pressure dressing	Yes	No
Heparin bolus	No	No
Heparin infusion	10-13 ug/kg/hr	No
Bedrest	48 hrs	Standard
Ambulation	Gradual	Standard
PTT	60-80 sec	Not Applicable
Warfarin	INR 2.5-3.5	Not Applicable

*   Restart heparin after sheaths removed; oral anticoagulation with Warfarin
**   No additional heparin; no Warfarin

287. Answer: a, b, c, d

Potential uses of IVUS include accurate measurement of reference vessel dimensions, assessment of the degree and distribution of calcium (to guide the need for other adjunctive devices), identification of the adequacy of lesion coverage by the stent; and assessment of the parameters for optimal stent implantation.   Such parameters include stent *expansion* (minimum stent cross-sectional area/average reference cross-sectional area ≥ 0.8-0.9), *symmetry* (ratio of minimum/maximum stent diameter > 0.7), and *apposition* (flush axial and radial contact between the stent and vessel wall).   Current IVUS transducers are relatively insensitive for detection of thrombus.

288. Answer: b (false)

IVUS criteria have also been used to identify patients suitable for antiplatelet therapy with aspirin and ticlopidine after stenting.[1]   However, similar clinical results can be achieved without IVUS.[2-5]

References:
1.   Hong MK, Wong SC, Pichard AD, et al. Long-term results of patients enrolled in the anti-platelet treatment after intravascular ultrasound guided optimal stent expansion (APLAUSE) trial. Circulation 1996;94:I-686.
2.   Hall P, Nakamura S, Maiello L, et al. Clinical and angiographic outcome after Palmaz-Schatz stent implantation guided by intravascular ultrasound. J Inv Cardiol 1995;7:12A-22A.
3.   Blasini R, Mudra H, Schuhlen H, et al. Intravascular ultrasound guided optimized emergency coronary Palmaz-Schatz stent placement without post procedural systemic anticoagulation. J Am Coll Cardiol 1995;25:197A.
4.   Painter J, Mintz G, Wong C, et al. Intravascular ultrasound assessment of biliary stent implantation in saphenous vein graft. Am J Cardiol 1995;75:731-734.
5.   Nakamura S, Hall P, Gaglione A, et al. High pressure assisted coronary stent implantation accomplished without intravascular ultrasound guidance and subsequent anticoagulation. J Am Coll Cardiol 1997;29:21-27.

289. Answer: a, b, c, d

Although IVUS may add cost and time (21 minutes on average),[1] routine use of high-pressure PTCA does not ensure optimal stent implantation by IVUS criteria;[2-5] in a study of 96 stents implanted with "optimal technique," IVUS revealed improper stent expansion in 60%.[6] In another study, 80% of stents underwent further PTCA after IVUS because of inadequate results.[7] In addition, IVUS can improve stent apposition not discernible by angiography;[2,8-12] however, the discrepancy between IVUS and quantitative angiography decreases with progressively higher inflation pressures.[13] Despite data to suggest that IVUS can be used to optimize lumen enlargement and stent expansion, other data indicate that excellent results can be achieved using post-stent high-pressure (14-16 atm.) inflations without IVUS.[14] At the present time, the interventional community is divided over the routine use of IVUS-guided stenting. The prospective multicenter Angiography Versus Intravascular ultrasound-Directed stent placement (AVID) trial will help resolve this important issue; preliminary data in 280 patients indicated that even after high-pressure balloons, 30% of patients with angiographic optimal stenting failed to satisfy IVUS criteria, but IVUS had no impact on 30-day clinical event rates.[15]

References:
1. Mudra H, Klauss V, Blasini R, Kroetz M. Ultrasound guidance of Palmaz-Schatz intracoronary stenting with a combined intravascular ultrasound balloon catheter. Circulation 1994;90:1252-1261.
2. Caputo R, Lopez J, Ho K, et al. Intravascular ultrasound analysis of routine high pressure balloon post-dilatation after Palmaz-Schatz stent deployment. J Am Coll Cardiol 1995;25:49A.
3. Gorge G, Haude M, Ge J, et al. Intravascular ultrasound after low and high inflation pressure coronary artery stent implantation. J Am Coll Cardiol 1995;26:725-730.
4. Sato Y, Nosaka H, Kimura AT, et al. Randomized comparison of balloon angioplasty versus coronary stent implantation for total occlusion. J Am Coll Cardiology 1996;27:152A.
5. Golderberg SL, Hall P, Nakamura S, et al. Is there a benefit from intravascular ultrasound when high-pressure stent expansion is routinely performed prior to ultrasound imaging? J Am Coll Cardiology 1996;27:306A.
6. Gil R, Prati F, Ligthart J, von Birgelen C, van Camp G, Serruys P. Is quantitative angiography a substitute for intracoronary ultrasound in guidance of stent deployment? Circulation 1995;92:I-327.
7. Nakamura S, Colombo A, Gaglione A, et al. Intracoronary ultrasound observations during stent implantation. Circulation 1994;89:2026-2034.
8. Wong SC, Popma J, Mintz G, et al. Preliminary results from the Reduced Anticoagulation in Saphenous Vein Graft Stent (RAVES) Trial. Circulation 1994;90:I-125.
9. Popma J, Colombo A, Mintz G, Wong SC, Pichard A. The impact of intravascular (IVUS) on post-stent deployment balloon dilatation. J Am Coll Cardiol 1995;25:49A.
10. Jain S, Liu M, Iyer S, Parks M, Babu R, Yadav S. Do high-pressure balloon inflations improve acute gain within flexible metallic coil stents? An intravascular ultrasound assessment. J Am Coll Cardiol 1995;25:49A.
11. Mudra H, Klauss V, Blasini R, et al. Intracoronary ultrasound guidance of stent deployment leads to an increase of luminal gain not discernible by angiography. J Am Coll Cardiol 1994;23:71A.
12. Nunez B, Foster-Smith K, Berger P, Melby S, Garratt K, Higano S. Benefit of intravascular ultrasound guided high pressure inflations in patients with a "perfect" angiographic result: The Mayo Clinic Experience. Circulation 1995;92:I-545.
13. Blasini R, Schuhlen H, Mudra H, et al. Angiographic overestimation of lumen size after coronary stent placement impact of high pressure dilatation. Circulation 1995;92:I-223.
14. Caputo R, Ho K, Lopez J, Stoler R, Cohen D, Carrozza J. Quantitative angiographic comparison of Palmaz-Schatz stent implantation with and without intravascular ultrasound. Circulation 1995;92:I-545.
15. Russo RJ, Nicosia A, Teirstein PS. Angiography versus intravascular ultrasound-directed stent placement. J Am Coll Cardiol 1997;29 (Suppl A):60A.

290. Answer: c

IVUS may have an impact on complications: In one preliminary study, use of IVUS-guided stent deployment was associated with a lower incidence of subacute stent thrombosis (0% vs. 4.2%, p. < 0.01), but a higher incidence of emergency CABG (6.6% vs. 1.4%, p < 0.05) compared to angiography-guided stent deployment; there were no differences in overall success (98%) or major complications (8%).[1] Final balloon/artery ratio > 1.2 may be an independent predictor of ischemic complications; careful attention to balloon sizing (perhaps using IVUS guidance) may limit these complications.[2] Currently, the precise role of IVUS is uncertain and further study is needed.[3]

References:
1. Goldberg S, Colombo A, Almagor Y, et al. Has the introduction of intravascular ultrasound guidance led to different clinical results in the deployment of intracoronary stents? Circulation 1994;90:I-612.
2. Hall P, Nakamura S, Maiello L, Blengino S, Martini G, Colombo A. Factors associated with procedural complications during high pressure optimized Palmaz-Schatz intracoronary stent implantation. Circulation 1994;90:I-612.
3. Moussa I, DiMario C, Reimers B, et al. Subacute stent thrombosis in the era of intravascular ultrasound-guided coronary stenting without anticoagulation: Frequency, predictors, and clinical outcome. J Am Coll Cardiol 1997;29:6-12.

291. Answer: b

Although intracoronary urokinase was originally recommended for patients receiving the Wallstent, thrombolytic therapy is not routinely recommended for patients receiving stents.

292. Answer: a (true)

Intracoronary urokinase (250,000-500,000 U bolus over 5-15 min. or continuous infusion of 50,000-200,000 U/hr for 8-24 hr) has been used as an adjunct to recanalize vessels with stent thrombosis[1] or in degenerated vein grafts.[2] Urokinase is not recommended for intraluminal haziness unless thrombus in confirmed by angioscopy.

References:
1. Wong PH, Wong CM. Intracoronary stenting in acute myocardial infarction. Cathet Cardiovasc Diagn. 1994;33:39-45.
2. Denardo SJ, Morris NB, Rocha-Singh KJ, Curtis GP, et al. Safety and efficacy of extended urokinase infusion plus stent deployment for treatment of obstructed, older saphenous vein grafts. Am J Cardiol 1995;76:776-780.

293. Answer: b (false)

Most interventional cardiologists empirically treat stent patients with long-acting nitrates and calcium channel blockers, beginning 24 hrs prior to stent placement and continuing for 6 weeks after discharge. This regimen seems reasonable to prevent vasospasm in arterial segments adjacent to the stent, but its value has not been rigorously tested.

294. Answer: a (true)

There are no data to suggest the benefit of routine antibiotics in patients receiving intravascular stents. Although endovascular infections are rare in stent patients, it is reasonable to prescribe prophylactic antibiotics for patients who require dental procedures, endoscopy, or other invasive procedures within 3 months of stent placement (until intimal coverage is complete).

295. Answer: a, c, d

Stent thrombosis is the most feared complication of stenting, due to the high incidence of ischemic complications (death in 7-19%, MI in 57-85%, emergency CABG in 30-44%).[1] Acute stent thrombosis (i.e., before the patient leaves the cath lab) is rare (< 1%) and is virtually always associated with readily identifiable causes such as incomplete stent expansion and uncovered dissection. In general, the risk of stent thrombosis is highest at 3-5 days and is rare after 2 weeks, although the risk of Wiktor stent thrombosis is highest within the first 24 hours.[2] The strongest predictors of stent thrombosis include unstented distal disease or dissection (odds ratio 10.6), stent diameter < 3mm (odds ratio 14.7), residual filling defect inside the stent (odds ratio 14.7); and multiple stents (odds ratio 3.7);[3] the rate of stent thrombosis increased from 5.6% to 9.4% to 16.7%, when none, 1 or 2 of these factors were present, respectively.[4,5]

References:
1. Mak KH, Belli G, Ellis SG, Moliterno DJ. Subacute stent thrombosis: Evolving issues and current concepts. J Am Coll Cardiol 1996;27:494-503.
2. Holmes D, Garratt K, Schwartz R. Timing of stent occlusion/thrombosis after stent placement. J Am Coll Cardiol 1994;23:70A.
3. Agrawal S, Ho D, Liu M, et al. Predictors of thrombotic complications after placement of the flexible coil stent. Am J Cardiol 1994;73:1216-1219.
4. Haude M, Erbel R, Issa H, et al. Subacute thrombotic complication after intracoronary implantation of Palmaz-Schatz stents. Am Heart J 1993;126:15-22.
5. Liu MW, Voohees W, Agrawal S, Dean L, Roubin G. Stratification of the risk of thrombosis after intracoronary stenting for threatened or acute closure complicating coronary balloon angioplasty: A Cook registry study. Am Heart J 1995;130:8-13.

296. Answer: b (false)

The proper medical regimen for preventing stent thrombosis is a subject of intense investigation. Because of the tendency of intravascular metals to form blood clots, original guidelines for medical management focused on the use of aggressive anticoagulation regimens to prevent stent thrombosis. Aggressive anticoagulation regimens were associated with a high incidence of bleeding and vascular complications, prolonged hospital stay, and increased cost. Use of aspirin and ticlopidine, rather than aspirin and Warfarin, is associated with a lower incidence of stent thrombosis and bleeding complications. Largely due to the pioneering work of Colombo and colleagues, stent thrombosis is now viewed as a mechanical problem that can be prevented by optimal stent implantation technique without the need for aggressive anticoagulation.

297. Answer: a, c, d

"Optimal stenting" requires meticulous technique to ensure complete coverage of the lesion, complete apposition of the stent to the vessel wall, full stent expansion, and stent symmetry. Adjunctive angioplasty after stent implantation using high-pressure balloons inflated to at least 15 ATM is a key component of "optimal stenting," and IVUS may be valuable to confirm "optimal" technique. Although final diameter stenosis < 50% is the standard "definition" of successful PTCA, any residual stenosis > 10% would be considered "suboptimal" by stent standards.

298. Answer: b, c, d, e

In most cases, emergency catheterization and revascularization are recommended; potential remedial causes should be sought and corrected if possible, including inadequate stent apposition (IVUS may be useful), improper stent sizing, and failure to adequately cover distal disease or dissection. Rarely, stent occlusion may be secondary to intimal flaps protruding through stent struts or coils; this can be managed by overlapping stents. Most cases of stent thrombosis can be successfully managed by repeat PTCA. When crossing the stented segment with a guidewire, it is important to put a large J-curve on the wire tip; otherwise, the wire may pass between the stent and the vessel wall. If this occurs and goes unrecognized — excessive resistance to balloon advancement is an important clue — subsequent balloon inflations can separate the stent from the vessel wall and lead to stent compression, stent embolization, and further thrombus formation. Potentially useful adjuncts for treating stent thrombosis include an intracoronary bolus of thrombolytics (urokinase 250,000-500,000 over 2-5 min.); a prolonged (8-24 hr) intracoronary infusion of thrombolytics (urokinase 100,000-200,000 U/hr through an infusion wire); or local delivery of thrombolytic drugs directly into the stented segment. The use of new platelet glycoprotein receptor IIb/IIIa antagonists is theoretically attractive and reasonable, but of unproven value. For refractory stent thrombosis, CABG is usually advised. Stent thrombosis is associated with significant patient morbidity and mortality, including death in 7-19%, nonfatal myocardial infarction in 57-88%, and emergency CABG in 30-44%.

299. Answer: b (false)

In the recent multicenter randomized trials of PTCA vs. stents, significant bleeding or vascular repair occurred in 7.3-13.5% of stent patients due to the intensive anticoagulation regimen. In contrast, major bleeding occurred in 1% and major vascular complications in 2.5% of 1232 patients treated without warfarin after optimal stent technique.[1] Risk factors for vascular complications include age > 70 years, female gender, multiple procedures during the same hospitalization, and the use of warfarin.[2,3]

References:
1. Morice M-C. Advances in post stenting medication protocol. J Inv Cardiol 1995;7:32A-35A.
2. Mansour K, Moscucci M, Kent C, et al. Vascular complications following directional coronary atherectomy or Palmaz-Schatz stenting. J Am Coll Cardiol 1994;23:136A.
3. Dean L, Voorhees W, Sutor C, Roubin G. Female gender: A risk factor for complications following intracoronary stenting? A Cook multicenter registry report. Circulation 1994;90:I-620.

300. Answer: a (true)

Stent embolization occurs in < 1% of patients receiving coronary stents, may occur more often in those receiving biliary stents, and can be managed by stent deployment at the site of embolization.[1,2] Stent retrieval with a wire snare is feasible, but difficult.

References:
1. Cishek MB, Laslett L, Gershony G. Balloon catheter retrieval of dislodged coronary artery stents: A novel technique. Cathet Cardiovasc Diagn 1995;34:350-

Answers

352.
2. Rozenman Y, Burstein M, Hasin Y, Gotsman M. Retrieval of occluding unexpanded palamaz-Schatz stent from a saphenous aorto-coronary vein graft. Cathet Cardiovasc Diagn. 1995;34:159-161.

301. Answer: b, c, d, e

Coronary perforation occurs more often after percutaneous laser and atherectomy than after PTCA. In contrast, two contemporary studies of coronary perforation did not report perforation after coronary stenting, although coronary artery rupture was mentioned as a serious complication after high-pressure adjunctive PTCA.[1,2] In our own stent experience, we have observed several cases of coronary artery perforation, which were usually related to one of the following: Use of an oversized balloon (balloon-to-artery ratio > 1.2) during stent deployment or adjunctive PTCA; high-pressure balloon inflations outside the stent; stenting of vessels with significant tapering; stenting of contained perforations after other devices; recrossing lesions with antecedent severe dissections or abrupt closure; and stenting total occlusions when there has been unrecognized subintimal passage of the guidewire.

References:
1. Colombo A, Hall P, Nakamura S, et al. Intracoronary stenting without anticoagulation accomplished with intravascular ultrasound guidance. Circulation 1995;91:1676-1688.
2. Hall P, Nakamura S, Maiello L, Blengino S, Martini G, Colombo A. Factors associated with procedural complications during high pressure optimized Palmaz-Schatz intracoronary stent implantation. Circulation 1994;90:I-612.

302. Answer: a, c

Compared to PTCA, the elective use of Palmaz-Schatz stenting in the STRESS trial was associated with a 90% increase in length of hospital stay, a 37% increase in cath lab costs, and a 27% increase in initial hospital costs. However, stenting was associated with a 25% reduction in repeat revascularization at 1 year, and a 58% reduction in follow-up hospital costs — overall costs at 1 year were virtually identical.[1,2] It is anticipated that stent costs will be reduced by less intensive anticoagulation regimens, which will result in fewer bleeding and vascular complications, shorter hospital stay, and fewer repeat revascularizations.[2-6] In fact, preliminary data from the Reduced Anticoagulation VEin graft Stent trial (RAVES) suggest that IVUS-guided optimal stent implantation and reduced anticoagulation may reduce overall costs by 38% compared to conventional Warfarin-based regimens due to reductions in length of stay and complications.[7] In another study, IVUS-guided stent implantation and reduced anticoagulation resulted in a 13% increase in procedural cost, but an 18% reduction in total hospital cost compared to conventional treatment.[8] The cost-effectiveness of IVUS is under evaluation.

References:
1. Cohen D, Krumhotz H, Sukin C, et al. Economic outcomes in the randomized stent restenosis study (STRESS): In-hospital and one-year follow-up costs. Circulation 1994;90:I-620.
2. Cohen D, Breall J, Ho K, et al. Evaluating the potential cost-effectiveness of stenting as a treatment for symptomatic single-vessel coronary disease. Use of a decision-analytic model. Circulation 1994;89:1859-1874.
3. Cohen D, Baim D. Coronary stenting: Costly or cost-effective? J Inv Cardiol 1995;7:36A-42A.
4. Weintraub W, Bernard J, Hicks F, Canup D, Mauldin P, Becker E. How coronary stents impact costs in interventional cardiology. Circulation 1995;92:I-436.
5. Eccleston D, Eisenberg M. Ticlopidine without intravascular ultrasound or coumadin reduces high marginal costs of elective coronary stent deployment. Circulation 1995;92:I-796.

6. Goods C, Liu M, Iyer S. A cost analysis of coronary stenting without anticoagulation versus stenting with anticoagulation using warfarin. Circulation 1995;92:I-796.

7. Wong SC, Popma JJ, Chuang YC, et al. Economic impact of reduced anticoagulation after saphenous vein graft stent placement. J Am Coll Cardiol 1995;25:80A.

8. Blengino S, Nakamura S, Hall P, et al. A cost analysis of intravascular ultrasound guided coronary stenting without anticoagulation vs. the traditional method of stenting with anticoagulation. J Am Coll Cardiol 1995;25:197A.

303. Answer: a, d

When stenting a tortuous vessel, excellent guiding catheter support and coaxial alignment are essential. If the JL4 guide fails to adequately engage the left main stenosis while advancing it (failed "push test"), a larger curve (JL $\geq$ 4.5) or geometric guide may provide better support.

304. Answer: a, c, d

Predilation and postdilation of the target lesion is recommended for all stents. Unlike balloon-expandable stents, self-expanding stents cannot be expanded beyond their maximum (unconstrained) diameter, irrespective of the diameter of the final balloon.

305. Answer: c, d, e, f

Every effort should be made to post-dilate a stent with a high-pressure balloon, even if the angiographic result is excellent immediately after stent deployment, due to the high-incidence of angiographically-inapparent inadequate stent diameter, apposition and symmetry.

306. Answer: a, b, d

The stent delivery sheath is designed to protect the stent and decrease the risk of stent embolization, but increases the profile of this delivery system. In some cases, slight advancement of the delivery balloon relate to the delivery sheath can improve tracking and enhance delivery of the stent to the target lesion.

307. Answer: a (true)

The Palmaz-Schatz coronary stents are manufactured independently and then mounted on balloons of different size; the stents themselves are identical.

308. Answer: b (false)

For Gianturco-Roubin stents, manufacturing of the stent and delivery balloon is an integrated process; stents of different sizes are not structurally and geometrically identical.

309. Answer: b, c

A 3.0 mm Palmaz-Schatz stent can be easily post-dilated with a 4.0 mm balloon. In contrast, post-dilation of a 3.0 mm Gianturco-Roubin stent with a 4.0 mm balloon may result in separation and distortion of the stent coils; post-dilation of a Gianturco-Roubin stent is recommended with a balloon $\leq$ 0.5 mm larger than the nominal size of the stent itself.

310. Answer: b (false)

Eccentric lesions are readily treated by stents. Initial debulking of highly eccentric lesions by DCA or Rotablator is theoretically attractive but of unproven value.

311. Answer: c, d, e

Stent implantation is complicated by "no-reflow"; additional stents, perfusion balloons, and emergency CABG are ineffective, since microvascular flow is impaired. The patient should be stabilized, and if administration of intra-graft calcium antagonists does not improve flow and hemodynamic performance, a pacemaker and IABP should be inserted. Although nitroglycerin alone has not been effective in reversing most cases of no-flow, it can attenuate epicardial spasm and its use is not associated with adverse consequences or delays.

312. Answer: a, c

Marginal dissections should be treated by deployment of additional stents. As long as the initial stent is dilated at high pressure, it is usually feasible to deploy additional stents(s) distal or proximal to the original stent; extra-support guidewires are useful, if necessary. The procedure should not be terminated since aggressive anticoagulation regimens have not been shown to prevent stent thrombus and ischemic complications after "suboptimal" stenting. Verifying that the ACT > 300 seconds is reasonable, especially if additional stents are indicated.

313. Answer: a

314. Answer: a, b, d

Heparin coating is available on a newer design of the Palmaz-Schatz coronary stent, which is utilized in the BENESTENT-II and stent-PAMI trials.

315. Answer: b (false)

Intravenous ReoPro is under investigation as an alternative or adjunct to Palmaz-Schatz intracoronary stenting, in the EPILOG-Stent trial. Although theoretically attractive, the value of ReoPro as an adjunct to stenting has not been established.

316. Answer: c

The GR stent is useful when stenting across a significant bifurcation. Because of its flexibility and coil design, sidebranches are readily accessible to most balloons and guidewires; the coils will usually separate sufficiently to allow passage of balloons, and return to their normal position after removal of the balloon. In selected bifurcation lesions, "kissing" stents may be considered if the parent vessel and sidebranch are > 2.5-3.0 mm.

317. Answer: b (false)

Severe focal dissection is a clear indication for the Gianturco-Roubin Flex-Stent®; dissections < 10 mm in length can be treated with a single stent. It is essential that multiple orthogonal views be used to identify the distal extent of dissection, and confirm that the stent completely covers the entire length of dissection. Stenting should not be performed if the distal extent of dissection cannot be identified. Although some operators have expressed concern that the use of adjunctive PTCA may cause further vessel injury, there are no data to support this impression and post-stent high-pressure balloon inflations are strongly recommended to ensure optimal stent deployment.

ROTABLATOR

318. Answer: b

The Rotablator system consists of a reusable console that controls the rotational speed of an olive-shaped, nickel-plated, brass burr, which is coated on its leading edge with 20-30 micron diamond chips and is bonded to a flexible drive shaft. The drive shaft is enclosed in a 4.3 F flexible Teflon sheath, which protects the arterial wall from the rotating drive shaft and serves as a conduit for saline flush solution, which cools and irrigates the system. The speed of burr rotation is regulated by a compressed-air or nitrogen-driven turbine, which is controlled by the console and activated by a foot pedal; rotational speed is monitored by a fiberoptic tachometer. The Rotablator requires a specialized 0.009-inch stainless steel guidewire.

Answers

319. Answer: a (true)

Differential cutting is defined as the ability of a device to selectively cut one material while maintaining the integrity of another, based on differences in substrate composition. In the case of high-speed rotational atherectomy, this results in pulverization of inelastic material such as fibrotic atheromatous plaque and lipid-rich tissue; in contrast, nondiseased vessel segments, which retain their viscoelastic properties, are deflected away from the advancing burr and spared from ablation.

320. Answer: a (true)

Orthogonal displacement of friction explains the easy passage of the burr through tortuous and diseased segments of the coronary vasculature. At a rotational speed of 60,000 RPM, the longitudinal friction vector is virtually eliminated, resulting in reduced surface drag and unimpeded advancement and withdrawal of the burr.

321. Answer: b (false)

Histological[1] and IVUS[2,3] studies have demonstrated that fibrotic, calcified, and soft plaque are removed after Rotablator, leaving a smooth internal surface devoid of endothelium without medial injury. The segments proximal and distal to the treatment site show no change in diameter at follow-up angiography 3 and 6 months after atherectomy, suggesting that Rotablator does not accelerate atherosclerosis.[4]

References:
1. Fourrier JL, Stankowiak C, Lablanche JM, et al. Histopathology after rotational angioplasty of peripheral arteries in human beings. J Am Coll Cardiol 1988;11:109A.
2. Kovach J, Mintz G, Pichard A, Kent K, et al. Sequential intravascular ultrasound characterization of the mechanisms of rotational atherectomy and adjunct balloon angioplasty. J Am Coll Cardiol 1993;22:1024-32.
3. Mintz G, Potkin B, Keren G, Satler L, et al. Intravascular ultrasound evaluation of the effect of rotational atherectomy in obstructive atherosclerotic coronary artery disease. Circulation 1992; 86:1383-1393.
4. Cowley M, Buchbinder M, Warth D, Dorros G, et al. Effect of coronary rotational atherectomy abrasion on vessel segments adjacent to treated lesions . J Am Coll Cardiol 1992;19:333A.

322. Answer: a, b, c

The size of microparticulate debris generated during Rotablator is determined by the size of the diamond chips and by the speed and pressure of the advancing burr. Larger particles are generated at slow (< 75,000 RPM)[1] burr speeds and heat is generated by forceful advancement of the burr characterized by a fall in RPM > 5000.[2] Conversely, smaller particles and a lower particulate burden are generated at speeds > 140,000 RPM and during gentle advancement of the burr. Experimental studies have found that 77% of the particles generated by the Rotablator were < 5 microns and 88% were < 12 microns,[1] and that particulate concentrations 10-30 times greater than those observed in human Rotablator studies were needed to reduce coronary blood flow.[3]

References:

1. Prevosti LG, Cook JA, Unger EF, Sheffield CD, et al. Particulate debris from rotational atherectomy: size distribution and physiologic effect. Circulation 1988;78:II-83.
2. Reisman M, DeVore LJ, ferguson M, et al. Analysis of heat generation during high-speed rotational ablation: Technical implications. J Am Coll Cardiol 1996;27:292A.
3. Friedman HZ, Elliott MA, Gottlieb GJ, O'Neill WW. Mechanical rotary atherectomy: The effects of microparticle embolization on myocardial blood flow and function. J Interv Cardiol 1989;2:77-83.

323. Answer: a, c

Most particles pass harmlessly through the circulation and are cleared by the liver, lungs, and spleen;[1] studies using positron emission tomography (PET)[2] and simultaneous transesophageal echocardiography[3] found no effect on hemodynamic performance, global LV function, or regional wall motion. In contrast, another study[4] demonstrated a transient (30-40 minutes) decrease in regional wall motion of 28% due primarily to myocardial stunning[5] The need for pharmacologic or mechanical support is unusual in the absence of complications or severe baseline LV impairment.

References:

1. Hansen DD, Auth DC, Hall M, Ritchie JL. Rotational endarterectomy in normal canine coronary arteries: preliminary report. J Am Coll Cardiol 1988; 11:1073-77.
2. Sherman C, Brunken R, Chan A, et al. Myocardial perfusion and segmental wall motion after coronary rotational atherectomy. Circulation 1992;86:I-652.
3. Pavlides G, Hauser A, Grines C, et al. Clinical, hemodynamic, electrocardiographic, and mechanical events during nonocclusive coronary atherectomy and comparison to balloon angioplasty. Am J Cardiol 1992;70:841-845.
4. Williams MJA, Dow CJ, Newell JB, et al. Prevalence and timing of regional myocardial dysfunction after rotational coronary atherectomy: J Am Coll Cardiol 1996;28:861-9.
5. Huggins GS, Williams MJA, Yang J, et al. Transient wall motion abnormalities following rotational atherectomy are reflective of myocardial stunning more than myocardial infarction. J Am Coll Cardiol 1995;25:96A.

324. Answer: a, b, d

Quantitative angiographic analyses suggest that Rotablator atherectomy achieves a lumen that is 90% of the selected burr size;[1] lumen dimensions may increase even further over the following 24 hours,[2] possibly due to release of elastic recoil and/or vasospasm. Intravascular ultrasound (IVUS) studies show that the primary mechanism of lumen enlargement after the Rotablator is plaque ablation; Kovach et al[3] demonstrated a decrease in plaque plus media area (plaque removal), an increase in lumen diameter, no change in external elastic membrane area (no arterial expansion), and a significant decrease in the arc of target lesion calcium. In contrast, adjunctive PTCA was shown to enlarge the lumen primarily through arterial expansion (an increase in external elastic membrane in 80% of lesions) and not by plaque removal (no change in plaque plus media). Typical IVUS findings after Rotablator atherectomy included an intimal-luminal interface that was distinct and circular, and lumen dimensions that were frequently in excess of final burr diameter. Deviations from cylindrical geometry were noted only in areas of calcified plaque manifesting superficial tissue disruption, and in areas of soft plaque.[4]

References:

1. Safian R, Freed M, Lichtenberg A, et al. Are residual stenoses after excimer laser angioplasty and coronary atherectomy due to inefficient or small devices? Comparison with balloon angioplasty. J Am Coll Cardiol 1993;22:628-1634.
2. Reisman M, Buchbinder M, Bass T, et al. Improvement in coronary dimensions at early 24-hour follow-up after coronary rotational ablation: Implications for restenosis. Circulation 1992;86:I-332.
3. Kovach JA, Mintz GS, et al. Sequential intravascular ultrasound characterization of the mechanisms of rotational atherectomy and adjunct balloon angioplasty. J Am Coll Cardiol 1993;22:1024-32.
4. Mintz GS, Douek P, et al. Target lesion calcification in coronary artery disease: An intravascular ultrasound study. J Am Coll Cardiol 1992;20:1149-55.

325. Answer: b

In an environment of cost containment, any incremental cost of a procedure must be weighed against its ability to improve acute and long-term outcome. In the case of the Rotablator, limited data are available concerning cost-effectiveness.[1,2] In a randomized trial of PTCA, Rotablator atherectomy and excimer laser angioplasty, the incremental cost of Rotablator over PTCA was 23%; however, this was accompanied by an increase in procedural success (93% vs. 83% for PTCA) and a decrease in length of stay (3.5 days vs. 4.2 days for PTCA). To date, no studies have been reported which suggest any benefit in reducing restenosis.

References:
1. Nino C, Freed M, Blankenship L, et al. Procedural cost and benefits of new interventional devices. Am J Cardiol 1994;74:1165-1166.
2. Vandormael M, Reifart N, Preusler W, et al. In-hospital costs comparison of excimer laser angioplasty, rotational atherectomy (Rotablator) and balloon angioplasty for complex coronary lesions: A randomized trial (ERBAC). J Am Coll Cardiol 1994;89:223A.

326. Answer: a, b

The approach to Rotablator is similar to PTCA; however, several factors are worth special emphasis. For target lesions in a dominant RCA, dominant circumflex or ostial LAD, or when using a 2.5 mm burr, the high incidence of bradyarrhythmias and heart block warrants prophylactic atropine or insertion of a temporary pacemaker. Bradycardia usually occurs immediately upon burr activation and typically reverses within 5-60 seconds after ablation is terminated. The mechanism of bradycardia is unknown, but may be due to microcavitation, microparticulate embolization, vasospasm, guidewire vibration or an unknown reflex. Continuous monitoring of pulmonary artery pressure and prophylactic placement of an intra-aortic balloon pump are strongly recommended when Rotablator atherectomy is used in patients with significant baseline LV dysfunction,[1] or when the target vessel supplies a large myocardial territory, to prevent hemodynamic instability should transient myocardial dysfunction occur.

References:
1. O'Murchu B, Foreman RD, Shaw RE, et al. Role of intraaortic balloon pump counterpulsation in high risk coronary rotational atherectomy. J Am Coll Cardiol 1995;26:1270-5.

327. Answer: c, e

As for all interventions, aspirin (325 mg/d beginning at least 1 day prior to atherectomy) is mandatory. Adequate hydration and calcium channel blockers are also recommended prior to the case and may reduce the frequency of vasospasm, which may occur in up to 15% of patients. During the procedure, heparin (10,000 units IV bolus with supplements as needed) is used to maintain the ACT > 350 seconds throughout the case. Although severe vasospasm is uncommon, generous doses of intracoronary nitroglycerin are recommended; a common technique is to administer a 100-150 mcg bolus after each ablation run. Intracoronary verapamil or Diltiazem (injected through a balloon or transport catheter into the distal vessel) may be helpful in reversing cases of slow-flow or no-reflow. Finally, some operators prepare a "cocktail" of nitroglycerin, verapamil and heparin in the flush solution, to provide continuous delivery of coronary vasodilators during Rotablation, which may reduce the incidence of no-reflow.[1-3]

References:
1. Cohen B, et al. Intracoronary cocktail infusion during rotational ablation: Safety and Efficacy. Cathet Cardiovasc Diagn (in press).
2. Coletti RH, Haik BJ, Wiedermann JG, et al. Marked reduction in slow-reflow after rotational atherectomy through the use of a novel flushing solution. TCT Meeting 1996;Washington DC
3. Stertzer SH, Pomerantsev EV, Fitzgerald PJ, et al. Effects of technique modification on immediate results of high speed rotational atherectomy in 710 procedures on 656 patients. Cathet Cardiovasc Diagn 1995;304-310.

328. Answer: a

A critical step during Rotablator atherectomy is selection of the guide catheter: Coaxial alignment will ensure that the guidewire is oriented in the center of the lumen. Since ablation occurs along the path of the guidewire, tangential orientation of the guidewire (guidewire bias) may result in directing the burr into the arterial wall, thereby increasing the risk of dissection or perforation.[1] The internal diameter of the guiding catheter must be 0.004-inch larger than the burr: The 1.25 mm, 1.50 mm, 1.75 mm and 2.0 mm burrs can be advanced through a giant-lumen 8F guide (ID ≥ 0.086-inch); 2.25 mm burrs through a 9F guide (ID > 0.092-inch); 2.38 mm burrs through a giant-lumen 9F guide (ID ≥ 0.098-inch); and 2.50 mm burrs through a 10F guiding catheter.

References:
1. Reisman M, Harms V. Guidewire bias: A potential source of complications with rotational atherectomy. Cathet Cardiovasc Diagn (in press).

329. Answer: b, c, d

A multiple burr approach, beginning with a burr-to-artery ratio of 0.5-0.6 and ending with a burr-to-artery ratio of 0.75-0.8, is often recommended to minimize the microparticulate burden and allow the operator to assess the progress of the procedure. After the burr is tested outside the body, it is advanced to a position just proximal to the target lesion (i.e., the "platform segment"). The burr must have free unimpeded rotation in the platform segment; if the burr is activated while in contact with the arterial wall, the risk of vessel injury is greatly increased. Free flow of contrast dye around the burr will confirm adequate positioning. Prior to activating the burr, all forward tension accumulated by advancing the device should be neutralized by gentle pulling back on the drive shaft itself; no resistance should be felt when the advancer knob is loosened and "jiggled." If tension remains in the drive shaft, activation of the device will cause the burr to lurch forward, possibly resulting in dissection. Once tension is released, the burr is activated in the platform segment and platform speed (RPM proximal to lesion) is adjusted according to the burr size; burrs > 2 mm should have a platform speed of 160,000 RPM while burrs ≤ 2 mm should have a platform speed of 180,000 RPM.

330. Answer: e

The most recent modification of Rotablator technique is the use of RPM surveillance to guide slow and careful advancement of the burr through the lesion. Aggressive burr advancement, indicated by excessive deceleration (rotational speed falls > 5,000 RPM below the platform speed), increases the risk of vessel trauma and ischemic complications caused by frictional heat and the formation of large particles. In general, the technician should never adjust the rotational speed while the burr is activated during ablation. If the burr decelerates, the operator should withdraw the burr slightly; excessive forward pressure on the burr (to "pop it" through the lesion) or abrupt discontinuation of the run while the burr is in the lesion, can increase the risk of vessel injury.

331. Answer: b, c, d

Contrast injections are intermittently performed to provide visual assessment of burr advancement; these injections identify the borders of the lesion, the orientation of the device in tortuous segments, the burr-to-artery relationship, and may also provide secondary benefit by inducing reactive hyperemia. If egress of contrast is not observed, the burr should be withdrawn slightly to re-establish antegrade flow and allow clearance of particles.

332. Answer: a, b, d

The optimal duration of ablation is based on lesion morphology, distal runoff, and hemodynamic and clinical parameters. In general, each run lasts 15-30 seconds, with time between runs (30 seconds to 2 minutes depending on patient's response) sufficient to allow particle clearance and the administration of vasodilators. When ECG changes, significant chest discomfort, or hemodynamic compromise occurs, the interval between ablation runs should be increased until the patient is clinically stable. Several (average 2-4) ablation runs are usually required to completely treat the lesion (i.e., minimal tactile resistance and no drop in RPM during burr advancement). Meticulous attention to technical details can produce excellent results with few complications even in very complex lesions.[1]

References:
1. Stertzer SH, Pomerantsev EV, Fitzgerald PJ, et al. Effects of technique modification on immediate results of high speed rotational atherectomy in 710 procedures on 656 patients. Cathet Cardiovasc Diagn 1995;304-310.

333. Answer: c, d

Since most burrs are small in relation to the target vessel, adjunctive PTCA (or other devices) is required to achieve definitive lumen enlargement in about 90% of lesions; the technique of adjunctive PTCA (low-pressure inflations with slightly oversized balloons vs. standard inflation pressures using balloons matched to the reference vessel diameter) is under evaluation. Rotablator atherectomy followed by directional atherectomy has been applied synergistically to calcified lesions in large diameter vessels. In one report,[1] diameter stenosis decreased from 79% pretreatment to 50% after the Rotablator to 17% after directional atherectomy; the arc of calcium decreased with each procedure and the Rotablator appeared to render calcified plaque more susceptible to directional atherectomy. In another study using IVUS, adjunctive DCA after

Rotablator achieved lumen enlargement which was superior to adjunctive PTCA.[2] There is growing interest in the use of Rotablator followed by stenting (RotaStent) for calcified stenoses. Compared to adjunctive PTCA, adjunctive stenting resulted in a larger lumen and smaller final stenosis.[3] An IVUS study of Rotablator followed by PTCA, DCA, or stent for calcified lesions in vessels > 3 mm found that Rotablator/stent resulted in the largest lumen and lowest residual stenosis.[4] Finally, IVUS has been used to assess the extent and distribution of lesion calcium and guide interventional strategy: The preferred treatment of superficial calcium is the Rotablator, whereas lesions with deep calcium (without superficial calcium) can be treated by many types of devices.

References:
1. Mintz GS, Pichard AD, et al. Transcatheter device synergy: preliminary experience with adjunct directional coronary atherectomy following high-speed rotational atherectomy or excimer laser angioplasty in the treatment of coronary artery disease. Cathet Cardiovasc Diagn 1993;28:37-44.
2. Dusaillant GR, Mintz GS, Pichard AD, et al. Mechanisms and immediate and long-term results of adjunct directional coronary atherectomy after rotational atherectomy. J Am Coll Cardiol 1996;27:1390-1397.
3. Mintz GS, Dussaillsnt GR, Wong SC, et al. Rotational atherectomy followed by adjunct stents: The preferred therapy for calcified large vessels? Circulation 1995;92:I-329.
4. Dussaillant GR, Mintz GS, Pichard AD, et al. The optimal strategy for treating calcified lesions in large vessels: Comparison of intravascular ultrasound results of rotational atherectomy + adjunctive PTCA, DCA, or stents. J Am Coll Cardiol 1996;27:153A.

334. Answer: b (false)

In uncomplicated cases, the pacemaker may be removed at the end of the procedure. Bradycardia and heart block are usually transient and occur at the time of burr activation (if at all); recurrent or sustained bradyarrhythmia is unusual.

335. Answer: a, b, c, d

Available Rotablator data are based on earlier techniques; important modifications in technique (adjustment of platform speed, RPM surveillance, awareness of guidewire bias) may have significant beneficial impact on immediate and long-term results. In a multicenter registry of 2976 patients (3717 lesions), procedural success was achieved in 94.5%.[1] In the majority of cases (~ 90%), adjunctive angioplasty was needed to obtain a residual stenosis < 30%. Procedural success was greater in restenotic lesions than de novo lesions, but was not predicted by patient age, gender, multivessel disease or unstable angina, or baseline lesion morphology. An angiographic study revealed further lumen enlargement 24 hours post-Rotablator, suggesting release of elastic recoil and/or vasospasm.[2]

Rotablator Atherectomy: Procedural Success and Restenosis

Series	N	Success[†]	PTCA	Final Stenosis	Restenosis
Reisman[15] (1997)	200 (1994) 2953 (1988-94)	96 95	-	-	-
Stertzer[4] (1995)	656	96	65	-	-

Series	N	Results (%)			
		Success[†]	PTCA	Final Stenosis	Restenosis
MacIsaac[5] (1995)	2161	94.5	74	22	-
Safian[6] (1994)	116	95.2	77	30	51
Vandormael[7] (1994)	215	91	-	31	62
Ellis[8] (1994)	400	89.9	-	27	-
Warth[9] (1994)	874	94.7	42	-	38
Barrione[10] (1993)	166	95	100	24	-
Guerin[11] (1993)	67	93.4	100	-	-
Gilmore[12] (1993)	143	91.7	-	-	-
Stertzer[13] (1993)	346	94	77	-	37
Dietz[14] (1991)	106	73	67	32	42

Abbreviation: - = not reported

†   Residual stenosis < 50% without death, Q-wave MI, or emergency bypass surgery

††   PTCA = adjunctive PTCA

*   Subsets of the multicenter Registry

References:
1. MacIsaac A, Whitlow P, Cowley M, Buchbinder M. Angiographic predictors of outcome of coronary rotational atherectomy from the completed multicenter registry. J Am Coll Cardiol 1994;23:353A.
2. Reisman M, Buchbinder M, Bass T, et al. Improvement in coronary dimensions at early 24-hour follow-up after coronary rotational ablation: Implications for restenosis. Circulation 1992;86:I-332.
3. Reisman M, Harms V, et al. Comparison of early and recent results with rotational atherectomy. J Am Coll Cardiol 1997;29:353-7.
4. Stertzer SH, Pomerantsev EV, Fitzgerald PJ, et al. Effects of technique modification on immediate results of high speed rotational atherectomy in 710 procedures on 656 patients. Cathet Cardiovasc Diagn 1995;304-310.
5. MacIsaac AI, Bass TA, Buchbinder M, et al. High speed rotational atherectomy: Outcome in calcified and noncalcified coronary artery lesions. J Am Coll Cardiol 1995;26:531-6.
6. Safian RD, Niazi KA, et al. Detailed angiographic analysis of high-speed mechanical rotational atherectomy in human coronary arteries. Circulation 1993;88:961-8.
7. Vandormael M, Reifart N, Preusler W, et al. Comparison of excimer laser, rotablator and balloon angioplasty for the treatment of complex lesions: ERBAC study final results. J Am Coll Cardiol, 1994;23:57A.
8. Ellis SG, Popma JJ, et al. Relation of clinical presentation, stenosis morphology, and operator technique to the procedural results of rotational atherectomy and rotational atherectomy facilitated angioplasty. Circulation 1994;89:882-92.
9. Warth DC, Leon MB, et al. Rotational atherectomy multicenter registry: Acute results, complications and 6-month angiographic follow-up in 709 patients. J Am Coll Cardiol 1994;24:641-8.
10. Borrions M, Hall P, et al. Treatment of simple and complex coronary stenosis using rotational ablation followed by low pressure balloon angioplasty. Cath Cardiovasc Diagn 1993;30:131-7.
11. Guerin Y, Rahal S, et al. Coronary angioplasty combining rotational atherectomy and balloon dilatation. Results in 67 complex stenoses. Arch Mal du Coeur 1993;86:1535-41.
12. Gilmore PS, Bass TA, et al. Single site experience with high-speed coronary rotational atherectomy. Clin Cardiol 1993;16:311-6.

13. Stertzer SH, Rosenblum J, et al. Coronary rotational ablation: initial experience in 302 procedures. J Am Coll Cardiol 1993;21:287-95.
14. Dietz UR, Erbel R, et al. Angiographic and histologic findings in high frequency rotational ablation in coronary arteries in vitro. Zeitschrift fur Kardiologie 1991;80:222-9.
15. Reisman M, Harms V, Whitlow P, et al. Comparison of early and recent results with rotational atherectomy. J Am Coll Cardiol 1997;29:353-7.

336. Answer: c, e

Restenosis rates appear comparable to balloon angioplasty and have ranged from 39% in the multicenter registry to 57% in the randomized Excimer Laser Rotablator Balloon Angioplasty Comparison (ERBAC) trial.[1] A study of restenosis by lesion length and calcium showed that restenosis was 1.86 times more likely in long lesions and 2.54 times more likely in noncalcified lesions;[2] restenosis rates were lowest (6.3%) for short calcified lesions and highest (37.2%) for noncalcified lesions greater than 20 mm in length.[2-4]

References:
1. Reifart N, Vandormael M, Krajear M, et al. Randomized comparison of angioplasty of complex coronary lesions at a single center. Excimer laser, rotational atherectomy, and balloon angioplasty comparison (ERBAC) study. Circulation 1997;96:91-98.
2. Leguizamon JH, Chambre DF, Torresani EM, et al. High speed coronary rotational atherectomy: Are angiographic factors predictive of failure, major complications or restenosis? J Am Coll Cardiol 1995;25:95A.
3. MacIsaac AI, Bass TA, Buchbinder M, et al. High speed rotational atherectomy: Outcome in calcified and noncalcified coronary artery lesions. J Am Coll Cardiol 1995;26:531-6.
4. Altmann D, Popma J, Kent K, et al. Rotational atherectomy effectively treats calcified lesions. J Am Coll Cardiol 1993;21:443A.

337. Answer: e

Although Rotablator may be used successfully in a wide variety of lesions, there are relatively little data suggesting its superiority to other devices. Nevertheless, Rotablator is the treatment of choice for undilatable lesions, which are not readily managed by other devices.

Procedural Success by Lesion Morphology

Series	Lesion Type	N	Success (%)
MacIsaac[1]	Calcified	1078	94
(1995)	Non calcified	1083	95
Altmann[2]	No/mild Calcified	-*	96
(1993)	Moderate Calcified	-	96
	Heavy Calcified	-	92
Vandormael[3]	Complex**	215	91
(1994)			
Reisman[4]	< 10 mm	953	95
(1993)	11-15 mm	180	97
	15-25 mm	143	92
Favereau[5]	10-20 mm	215	95
	20 mm	73	84
Koller[6]	Ostial	29	93
(1994)			

Answers

Series	Lesion Type	N	Success (%)
Zimarino[7] (1994)	Ostial	69	92
Popma[8] (1993)	Ostial	105	97
Omoigui[9] (1995)	Chronic TO	145	91
Reisman[10] (1993)	Undilatable	34	97
Brogan[11] (1993)	Undilatable	41	90
Sievert[12] (1993)	Undilatable	32	97
Rosenblum[13] (1992)	Undilatable	40	97
Bass[14] (1992)	Restenotic	428	97
Chevalier[15] (1994)	Angulated	123	86

Abbreviation: TO = total occlusion
*   Total number of lesion = 675; subgroup data not available
**   Type B$_2$ (72%), Type C (13%)

References:
1. MacIsaac AI, Bass TA, Buchbinder M, et al. High speed rotational atherectomy: Outcome in calcified and noncalcified coronary artery lesions. J Am Coll Cardiol 1995;26:531-6.
2. Altmann D, Popma J, Kent K, et al. Rotational atherectomy effectively treats calcified lesions. J Am Coll Cardiol 1993;21:443A.
3. Vandormael M, Reifart N, Preusler W, et al. Comparison of excimer laser, rotablator and balloon angioplasty for the treatment of complex lesions: ERBAC study final results. J Am Coll Cardiol, 1994;23:57A.
4. Reisman M, Cohen B, Warth D, Fenner J, et al. Outcome of long lesions treated with high speed rotational ablation. J Am Coll Cardiol 1993;21:443A.
5. Favereaux X, Chevalier B, Commeau P, et al. Is rotational atherectomy more effective than balloon angioplasty for the treatment of long coronary lesions? SCA & I Meeting Abstracts, 92.
6. Koller PT, Freed M, Grines CL, O'Neill WW. Success, complications, and restenosis following rotational and transluminal extraction atherectomy of ostial stenoses. Cathet and Cardiovas Diagn 1994;31:255-260.
7. Zimarino M, Corcos T, Favereau X, et al. Rotational coronary atherectomy with adjunctive balloon angioplasty for the treatment of ostial lesions. Cathet Cardiovas Diagn 1994;33:22-27.
8. Popma J, Brogan W, Pichard A, et al. Rotational coronary atherectomy of ostial stenoses. Am J Cardiol 1993;71:436-438.
9. Omoigui N, Booth J, Reisman M, et al. Rotational atherectomy in chronic total occlusions. J Am Coll Cardiol 1995;25:97A.
10. Reisman M, Devlin P, Melikian J, et al. Undilatable noncompliant lesions treated with the Rotablator: outcome and angiographic follow-up. Circulation 1993;88: I-547.
11. Brogan W, Popma J, Pichard A, Satler L, et al. Rotational coronary atherectomy after unsuccessful coronary balloon angioplasty. Am J Cardiol 1993;71:794-798.
12. Sievert H, Tonndorf S, Utech A, Schulze R. [High frequency rotational angioplasty (rotablation) after unsuccessful balloon dilatation] Z Cardiol 1993;82:411-414.
13. Rosenblum J, Stertzer S, Shaw R, et al. Rotational ablation of balloon angioplasty failures. J Inva Cardiol 1992;4:312-317.
14. Bass T, Gilmore P, Buchbinder M, et al. Coronary rotational atherectomy (PTCA) in patients with prior coronary revascularization: a registry report. Circulation 1992;86:I-653.
15. Chevalier B, Commeau P, Favereau X, et al. Limitations of rotational atherectomy in angulated coronary lesions. J Am Coll Cardiol 1994;23:285A.

338. Answer: a, b, d

The Rotablator is not recommended in thrombus-containing lesions or saphenous vein grafts due to the risk of distal embolization and no-reflow. Fibrous plaque at graft anastomoses, however, has been successfully treated. The incidence of sidebranch occlusion after Rotablator was 7.5% in one study; persistent sidebranch occlusion >24 hours was unusual.[1] Rigid, undilatable lesions in nondegenerated vein grafts can be treated with Rotablator.

References:
1. Walton AS, Pomerantsev EV, Oesterle SN, et al. Outcome of narrowing related sidebranches after high-speed rotational atherectomy. Am J Cardiol 1996;77:370-3.

339. Answer: a, b, c

The "DYNAGLIDE" light is located adjacent to the "STALL" light, and is visible only when illuminated. Dynaglide™ provides controlled low-speed rotation (50,000-90,000 RPM) when the burr is removed from the patient. The Dynaglide™ foot pedal button activates Dynaglide™, and the word "DYNAGLIDE" is illuminated in green; the foot pedal must be depressed again to deactivate Dynaglide™ If the "DYNAGLIDE" light cannot be extinguished, there may be insufficient pressure in the gas tank. Check the pressure gauge, and replace the tank if necessary.

340. Answer: b (false)

Guiding catheters must be selected to ensure coaxial alignment; sidehole guides are recommended to allow passive perfusion. Amplatz curves are beneficial for treating lesions in the circumflex artery because of ideal coaxial alignment. The following guiding catheter internal diameters (ID) are recommended:

Burr size (mm)	Guide ID (inches)
≤ 2.0	0.086
≤ 2.25	0.092
≤ 2.38	0.098
≤ 2.5	1.102

341. Answer: a, b, c, d

"Guidewire bias", defined as an eccentrically-oriented guidewire (secondary to non-coaxial guiding catheter alignment, a tortuous vessel, or an angulated target lesion), requires modification in burr sizing and technique. Failure to recognize guidewire bias can lead to complications.

342. Answer: a (true)

Answers

343. Answer: a, b, c, d, e

Severely angulated lesions (> 60°) should not be routinely considered for the Rotablator. For angulated lesions that are highly calcified, initial debulking may be considered, using a burr/artery ratio of 0.05-0.6. All angulated lesions need to be assessed for guidewire bias, which may result in tangential ablation. Lesions on the outer curve may be better suited for the Rotablator than lesions on the inner curve.

344. Answer: c, d

Protection of a sidebranch is not feasible during Rotablator of bifurcation lesions. If both limbs of the bifurcation exceed 2.5mm in diameter, first treat the vessel that is more difficult to wire. Some operators recommend gentle predilation of the sidebranch before Rotablator of the parent vessel, to minimize sidebranch occlusion. Kissing balloons are commonly employed after Rotablator. If the branch origin is angulated, a conservative burr strategy is recommended using final burr/artery ratio ≤ 0.6.

345. Answer: a, b, e

Calcified lesions are the most frequent indication for Rotablator; no other devices are as effective. In heavily calcified lesions, ablation may liberate large amounts of microparticles. Techniques to minimize complications include initial use of a 1.5mm burr, further incremental steps in burr size of 0.25-0.5mm, ablation runs not to exceed 30 seconds, and extended (occasionally several minutes) intervals between runs until hemodynamics and ECG normalize, and symptoms resolve.

346. Answer: b (false)

Focal lesions should be treated with slow ablation runs to ensure engagement of the plaque, particularly in the aorto-ostial location.

347. Answer: b, d, f

Long lesions (> 15mm) require a different approach due to the risk of distal embolization. Rather than attempt to completely ablate the entire lesion in one pass, a segmental ablation technique is recommended: Advance the burr into the lesion (pecking motion; RPM surveillance; ablation time not to exceed 1530 seconds); discontinue run, administer intracoronary nitroglycerin (100-200 mcg), and allow time for particle clearance; and repeat as many times as needed to treat the entire lesion.

348. Answer: a (true)

A stepped-burr approach is recommended for most lesions; based on the response to the initial burr, further increments in burr size may be considered. Long lesions do not necessarily indicate overall longer ablation times: A heavily calcified 10 mm lesion may require more ablation time than a noncalcified 30 mm lesion.

349. Answer: b, c, d

Eccentric lesions can be effectively and safely treated with the Rotablator. Since guidewire bias may occur, a lesion modification strategy should be considered. Careful repositioning of the guiding catheter and/or guidewire may direct the burr towards the lesion, resulting in "favorable" guidewire bias. This strategy ("active guidewire technique" or "directional rotational atherectomy") may improve angiographic outcome for eccentric lesions.

350. Answer: c, d

Unsuccessful PTCA can be secondary to failure to cross or dilate the lesion with the balloon; both are readily amenable to Rotablator. However, if antecedent PTCA results in dissection, Rotablator should be deferred for 2-4 weeks, to allow the dissection to heal. Rotablator should not be performed if there is angiographic dissection.

351. Answer: c

Treatment of aorto-ostial disease requires coaxial guiding catheter alignment. A guide catheter that "kicks out" into the aorta during atherectomy is acceptable as long as the guidewire remains coaxial. Initial burr activation should occur in the guide catheter, while the guide is engaged with the ostium. The platform speed should be adjusted proximal to the primary curve in the guiding catheter; RPM surveillance is mandatory. Under no circumstances should the burr be activated while in direct contact with the target lesion.

352. Answer: a (true)

Restenotic lesions are readily treated; the initial burr may be 0.25 mm greater than that used for de novo lesions.

353. Answer: b, c

For ostial lesions, which may be rigid and fibrotic, Rotablator and adjunctive PTCA or stenting are reasonable strategies. For lesions in the body of vein grafts (often associated with soft grumous and thrombus), a device other than the Rotablator should be used. In contrast, lesions at the distal anastomosis are favorable for the Rotablator. Ostial and distal anastomotic lesions evident within 6 weeks of surgery should not be treated with Rotablator because of the risk of disruption of the suture line; the exact time at which Rotablator is safe is not known.

354. Answer: a, b, c, d

Severe proximal tortuosity can significantly impact the results of Rotablator since the guidewire may deform the vessel and preclude advancement of the nonactivated burr. Activation of the burr in segments where the guidewire deforms the vessel may result in dissection; low speeds to pass these segments (100,000 RPM) and small burrs should be used, or Rotablator should be avoided. Distal tortuosity may result in pseudolesions, which resolve after guidewire removal.

355. Answer: b (false)

If the occluded segment can be crossed with a guidewire, Rotablator can be performed. A 1.25 mm burr is initially recommended when there is no distal flow, as long as the operator is certain that the guidewire is not extra-luminal. A conventional stepped-burr approach can be used for maximal debulking once distal flow is present. Rotablator is contraindicated if the total occlusion cannot be crossed with a guidewire.

356. Answer: c

Slow-flow (TIMI flow = 2) and no-reflow (TIMI flow ≤ 1) represent a spectrum of flow disturbances caused by rotational atherectomy (and other devices). The etiology is multifactorial, but most likely results from severe microvascular spasm and distal microembolization. If no-reflow occurs, further ablation should not be performed. If slow-flow occurs, but resolves after treatment , further ablation may be considered after resumption of normal antegrade flow. Severe chest pain (with or without ECG changes, hemodynamic compromise, or angiographic flow impairment) may be a harbinger of no-reflow; further ablation should be deferred until chest pain resolves. Intracoronary (not intravenous) calcium antagonists are effective for reversing no-reflow.

357. Answer: a, b, c, e

If no-reflow (TIMI flow ≤ 1) occurs, further Rotablator should be avoided. Intracoronary nitrates, calcium channel blockers, and/or adenosine are useful to reverse no-reflow, and must be delivered through a balloon or transport catheter to the distal microvascular bed; delivery through the guiding catheter is usually unsuccessful, since the agent will not reach the distal vessel.

358. Answer: b

When no-reflow occurs, intracoronary calcium antagonists must be delivered to the distal microvascular bed. Urokinase is usually ineffective in reversing no-reflow, but will be useful if there is distal embolization of thrombus. If no-reflow persists, microvascular dysfunction obviates the value of emergency CABG, which is not recommended.

359. Answer: b, c

The cause of dissection or perforation is usually relative "oversizing" of the treated segment. The following strategies may avoid these complications: Use frequent, small contrast injections to assess the cutting vector of the burr in the vessel; use burr-to-artery ratio < 0.6 in severely angulated segments; assess the presence of guidewire bias leading to preferential cutting ("directional" rotational atherectomy); burr-to-artery ratio < 0.6 is recommended in eccentric lesions and tortuous vessels; ensure proper platform speed in the platform segment before burr advancement; and do not allow burr speed to fall by more than 5000 RPM when engaging the lesion.

360. Answer: a (true)

Burr detachment is very rare. Since the platinum spring tip is larger than the central orifice of the burr, it prevents the burr from coming off the guidewire. Should burr detachment occur, the burr can be retrieved by removing the guidewire.

361. Answer: a, b, c, d

The following situations may be associated with burr stall:
- A kink in the airhose at the connection to the advancer.
- Over-tightening the Y-connector, which crimps the drive shaft.
- The 1.25mm burr is trapped by the sheath during advancement into the vessel (sheath telescopes over the burr); this is solved by retracting the burr into the guide catheter and advancing the burr beyond the sheath.
- The gas tank is empty.
- Improper connections to the console.
- Aggressive burr advancement, which is addition to burr stall, can result in dissection and perforation; these can be avoided by proper technique. A kink in the fiberoptic cable has no impact on burr speed unless the cable is fractured).

362. Answer: a, c

The following steps should be employed to prevent guidewire fracture:
- Always use the wireClip™, especially when depressing the brake defeat button when the

Rotablator is activated (e.g., "burping" the burr forward, or removing the burr by Dynaglide).
- Never place the guidewire into small branches.
- Avoid prolapsing the platinum spring.
- Avoid prolonged ablation runs at a single point on the guidewire (excessive guidewire wear); if unavoidable, advance or withdraw the guidewire a short distance to "expose" a new area.
- If a loop develops in the guidewire outside the vessel ostium due to inadvertent displacement of the guide catheter, pulling the wire may result in fracture; it is best to rotate the burr and reduce the loop (must depress the brake defeat button on the Advancer).

DIRECTIONAL CORONARY ATHERECTOMY

363. Answer: b (false)

Contemporary designs of the Simpson AtheroCath require 9.5F and 10F guiding catheters.

364. Answer: a (true)

365. Answer: b, c

A "stepped" approach is commonly employed for Rotablator atherectomy, but is not necessary for directional atherectomy.

Selection of AtheroCath Based on Vessel Diameters

Size (F)	Vessel diameter (mm)*	Vessel diameter (mm) Practical **
5F	2.5-2.9	2.5
6F	3.0-3.4	2.5-3.0
7F	3.5-3.9	3.0-3.5
7FG	4.0	3.5-4.0

Abbreviations: F = French size; G = graft cutter
* These guidelines are based on the product label
** These guidelines are not approved by the FDA, but may allow for more "optimal atherectomy"

366. Answer: c, d, e

Use only dilute (50:50 mix) contrast; higher concentrations will prolong balloon inflation/deflation times, and prolonged interruption of blood flow. Any 0.014-inch guidewire is compatible with the AtheroCath. If the guidewire is already across the lesion, the AtheroCath can be tracked over an exchange length (300 cm) or extendable wire. Many operators prefer the bare-wire technique to cross the lesions, followed by back-loading the wire into the AtheroCath; this approach may be easier technically and allows better contrast opacification of the target vessel. After attaching the MDU, the cutter should be "locked" before advancing the AtheroCath into the guiding catheter. A pressure bag with heparinized thresh is required for TEC and Rotablator, but not directional atherectomy.

367. Answer: a (1); b (2); c (3); d (4); e (5); f (6)

Left Coronary Artery	DVI Guide Catheter
• Normal	JL 4.0
• Narrow aortic root or superior origin	JL 3.5
• Wide aortic root or posterior origin	JL 4.5, JL 5.0
Right Coronary Artery	
• Normal	JR 4.0 ST, JR 4.0
• Anterior origin	Hockey stick
• Horizontal origin	Hockey stick
• Superior origin or Shepherd Crook	Hockey stick, JRG
• Inferior origin	JR 4.0 IF, JR 4.0 ST
Vein Grafts to Left Coronary Artery	
• Normal	JR 4.0, JR 4.0 ST, Hockey stick
• Superior origin	Hockey stick, JRG, JLG
Vein Grafts to Right Coronary Artery	
• Normal	Multipurpose, JR 4.0 IF
• Horizontal origin	JR 4.0, Hockey stick

Abbreviations: LCA = left coronary artery; RCA = right coronary artery; JL = Judkins left; JR = Judkins right; ST = short tip; JRG = modified right graft; IF = inferior; JLG = modified left graft

368. Answer: b (false)

Over-rotation and deep-seating of the guide greatly increase the risk of vessel injury and should be avoided. Avoid aggressive manipulation of an engaged guiding catheter because of extreme torque-responsiveness, which increases the risk of ostial dissection.

369. Answer: b (false)

Predilatation of the lesion with a 2.0 or 2.5 mm balloon is occasionally needed to allow smooth passage of the AtheroCath into calcified or ostial lesions, but is rarely needed for other lesions.

370. Answer: d

Under fluoroscopy, the AtheroCath is advanced by applying gentle forward pressure; gentle torquing (screwing motion) of the proximal rotator is recommended. Over torquing the AtheroCath can result in catheter damage and loss of torsional reponse. Unidirectional rotation is recommended; bidirectional rotation increases the risk of damage to the shaft. Forced advancement of the AtheroCath against resistance increases the risk of vessel trauma; "jack-hammering" the device is never indicated and should be avoided. Advancement of the AtheroCath when the guiding catheter is not coaxially aligned may damage the device and cause vessel injury.

371. Answer: a, c, d

With the AtheroCath positioned in the target lesion, ensure the guidewire tip is in a straight portion f a major artery and extends ~ 3-5 cm beyond the tip of the AtheroCath. Monitor the location and freedom of the guidewire tip during cutting. If the guidewire does not move freely, reposition it before initiating the cutting sequence. Guidewire entrapment in a branch vessel increases the risk of tip fracture during activation of the MDU. Before and during each cut, make sure the guidewire moves freely. During each cut, hold the guidewire to prevent its proximal migration.

372. Answer: a, c, d

Initial cuts should be directed towards angiographically-apparent plaque. Brief cutter activation is recommended to advance and retract the advancement control level. Inflate the balloon to 5-15 psi (0.3 to 1.0 atm) using the low-pressure inflation device; the balloon is not designed to dilate the stenosis, but rather to hold the housing securely within the vessel. Do not inflate the balloon over 60 psi (4 atm) due to the risk of balloon rupture, arterial injury, and air embolization. Fully advance the cutter through the lesion over 5-7 seconds until it reaches the mechanical cutter stop; excised atheroma will be packed into the collection chamber nosecone.

373. Answer: a, b, c, d, e

Failure to fully advance and lock the cutter increases the risk of tissue embolization and may produce an incomplete cut, leaving an intimal flap and the potential for abrupt closure. It is reasonable to perform additional cuts at higher balloon inflation pressures (15-40 psi). Immobility of the guidewire is an indication that the collection chamber is full. If a cut cannot be completed, partially deflate the balloon and attempt to achieve full cutter advancement. The collection chamber may be full after 5-7 cuts, necessitating removal of the catheter and emptying of the collection chamber.

374. Answer: d

If a residual stenosis > 15% is still evident, the decision to perform directional coronary atherectomy (with a larger cutter or higher pressure), PTCA or stenting depends on the cutter-to-artery ratio: If upsizing to the next largest cutter complies with the sizing guidelines, Directional coronary atherectomy is performed; if the next size cutter is too large for the target vessel, PTCA or stenting is performed. PTCA should be performed using a balloon-to-artery ratio of 1.0-1.2 and inflation pressures of 4-6 ATM.

Selection of AtheroCath Based on Vessel Diameters

Size (F)	Vessel diameter (mm)*	Vessel diameter (mm) Practical **
5F	2.5-2.9	≤ 2.5
6F	3.0-3.4	2.5-3.0
7F	3.5-3.9	3.0-3.5
7FG	≥ 4.0	3.5-4.0

Abbreviations: F = French size; G = graft cutter
* These guidelines are based on the product label; recommended by the FDA
** These guidelines are not approved by the FDA, but may allow for more "optimal atherectomy"

375. Answer: c, d

376. Answer: a, b, c, d

For residual stenosis > 20%, reasonable options include using the same AtheroCath at higher inflations pressures (30-40 psi), a larger AtheroCath at low inflation pressures (15-20 psi), adjunctive PTCA, or stenting.

377. Answer: b (false)

In the EPIC and EPILOG trials, ReoPro improved outcome in patients undergoing PTCA and directional atherectomy.[1-3]

Answers

References:
1. The EPIC Investigators. Use of a monoclonal antibody directed against the platelet glycoprotein IIb/IIIa receptor in high-risk coronary angioplasty. N Engl J Med 1994;330:956-61.
2. Simoons M. The CAPTURE study, as presented at the 45th Annual Session of the American College of Cardiology in Orlando, Florida, USA, 1996.
3. Lefkovits J, Blankenship JC, Anderson K, et al. Increased risk of non-Q-wave MI after directional atherectomy is platelet dependent: Evidence from the EPIC trial. J Am Coll Cardiol 1996;28:849.

378. Answer: a, b, c

Directional coronary atherectomy should be used cautiously in the setting of acute myocardial infarction; culprit lesions are frequently totally occluded, which may preclude accurate assessment of extent of disease, length of occlusion, thrombus burden, and normal vessel diameter distal to the occlusion. For some focal occlusions in vessels $\geq$ 3mm in diameter without a large clot burden, directional coronary atherectomy may be considered; bolus and infusion of ReoPro improve outcome (EPIC trial).

379. Answer: b, d

Lesions with moderate or extreme angulation should be treated cautiously if at all with directional coronary atherectomy. Techniques that may enhance success include coaxial alignment of the guiding catheter, use of extra-support or Platinum-Plus guidewires to facilitate tracking, and use of slightly undersized short-cut devices at low-pressure (15-20 psi). Atherectomy cuts should be limited to angiographically-evident disease; adjunctive PTCA with a balloon-to-artery ratio of 1.0 should be employed at low inflation pressures (2 ATM) to achieve optimal results. Oversized devices or balloons should be avoided. Long (40 mm) balloons may be especially useful to conform to vessel angulation and minimize straightening forces.

380. Answer: a, b, d

Directional coronary artery is well-suited for many bifurcation lesions because of the potential for minimizing "snow-plow injury"due to shifting plaque. The simplest approach involves using a single-wire and directional coronary atherectomy of the parent-vessel; if possible, it is best to avoid cutting across the origin of a diseased sidebranch. For sidebranches $\geq$ 2.5mm with ostial disease, PTCA or directional coronary atherectomy may be performed by repositioning the first wire in the diseased sidebranch. If necessary, adjunctive PTCA may be performed after directional coronary atherectomy using a kissing balloon technique at low-pressure; excellent angiographic results should be anticipated. Directional coronary atherectomy should not be performed in vessels < 2.5mm. Some experienced operators prefer a double-wire technique for bifurcation lesions: A nitinol guidewire is positioned in the sidebranch for protection, while directional coronary atherectomy is performed on the parent vessel. After successful revascularization of the parent vessel, the guidewire is removed, and directional coronary atherectomy or PTCA is performed on the sidebranch.

381. Answer: a, b, c, d

In vessels with fluoroscopic calcification, it is virtually impossible to identify the extent and depth of calcification without IVUS. Extensive superficial calcification is predictive of directional coronary atherectomy failure; such lesions should be pretreated with Rotablator before considering directional coronary atherectomy. Rotablator can be easily performed through all directional coronary atherectomy guiding catheters, and directional coronary atherectomy can be performed over Rotablator guidewire. For lesions with deep calcification or in vessels with calcification proximal to the target lesion, directional coronary atherectomy may be considered; coaxial guiding catheter alignment, extra-support or Platinum-Plus guidewires, and short-cut devices may enhance the likelihood of success in difficult anatomic situations.

382. Answer: a, d, e

Directional coronary atherectomy may be considered in selected lesions complicated by focal dissection; spiral dissections, contrast staining beyond the lumen margins, target vessels < 3mm, and inability to visualize the distal extent of dissection are absolute contraindications to directional coronary atherectomy.

383. Answer: a (true)

In suitable focal dissections, directional coronary atherectomy may be performed with undersized cutters at low inflations pressures (15-20 psi); aggressive tissue resection is not recommended. If further lumen enlargement is necessary after resection of obstructive flaps, adjunctive PTCA (4-6 atm.) or stenting should be performed.

384. Answer: a, b, c, d, e

Directional coronary atherectomy may be performed in aorto-ostial lesions; predilation with a 2.0 mm balloon may be necessary to facilitate passage of the AtheroCath. It is important to ensure ideal coaxial alignment of the guiding catheter; extra-support guidewires and initial use of undersize cutters may facilitate directional coronary atherectomy. For lesions < 5 mm in length, short-cutter devices are preferred. If necessary, further lumen enlargement may be achieved with adjunctive angioplasty or stenting.

385. Answer: a (true)

Isolated focal lesions involving the origin of sidebranches ≥ 2.5 mm are well suited for directional coronary atherectomy; short-cutter devices are particularly useful to facilitate cornering and limit resection of nondiseased vessel wall components.

Answers

386. Answer: b (false)

Directional coronary atherectomy should not be performed in degenerated vein grafts because of the risk of no-reflow and myocardial infarction. Focal lesions proximal to severely degenerated segments may be considered.

387. Answer: a, b, c, d, e

Mild degrees of proximal vessel tortuosity pose no particular problems for directional atherectomy. For moderate degrees of tortuosity, atherectomy technique may be facilitated by ideal co-axial alignment of the guiding catheter, use of an extra-support or Platinum-Plus guidewire to straighten tortuous segments, and use of a short-cutter device to facilitate cornering, and predilation of the target lesion to ease passage of the device. Continuous device rotation during advancement is important to reduce friction. Severe proximal tortuosity, especially when calcified, is a relative contraindication.

388. Answer: a, b, c, d, e

389. Answer: a (true)

The GTO is a third generation AtheroCath which is available in all sizes except the 7F Graft. The GTO has a redesigned shaft with better support and torque control than the EX. Within the next year, further additions to the line of available AtheroCaths will include a GTO-short housing device; better cutters for treating large vessels (3.75-5.0 mm); a Power Blade device with a tungsten carbide-coated cutter for enhanced excision of heavily calcified lesions; and an ultrasound-guided atherectomy device.

390. Answer: a, d

Adjunctive medical therapy for directional coronary atherectomy is similar to PTCA, including preprocedural aspirin (325 mg/d starting at least 1 day prior) and intraprocedural heparin (to maintain the ACT >300 seconds). Long acting nitrates and/or calcium antagonists are administered at the discretion of the operator to minimize vasospasm. If a satisfactory angiographic result is obtained, heparin is discontinued at the end of the case and the vascular sheaths are removed 4-6 hours later. Other platelet antagonists such as dipyridamole, Dextran, and sulfinpyrazone are not routinely prescribed. In high-risk patients (e.g, unstable ischemic syndromes, high-risk lesion morphology), bolus and infusion of ReoPro has been shown to decrease the incidence of major complications and possibly restenosis.[1]

References:
1. Topol E, Califf R, Weisman H, et al. Randomized trial of coronary intervention with antibody against platelet IIb/IIIa integrine for reduction of clinical

restenosis: results at six months. Lancet 1994;343:881-886.

391. Answer: a, d

Although preliminary data suggest that intravascular ultrasound can be used to achieve larger lumen diameters,[1-4] other data suggest that comparable lumen enlargement can be achieved using angiography alone.[5,6] The "ideal" residual stenosis is unknown; one study suggested a reduction in late cardiac events when the final diameter stenosis was 10-20%, with no incremental benefit for residual stenoses < 10%.[7] Most operators attempt to achieve a residual stenosis < 15-20%.

References:
1. Leon M, Kuntz R, Popma J, et al. Acute angiographic, intravascular ultrasound and clinical results of directional atherectomy in the optimal atherectomy restenosis study. J Am Coll Cardiol 1995;25:137A.
2. Simonton CA, Leon MB, Kuntz RE, et al. Acute and late clinical and angiographic results of directional atherectomy in the optimal atherectomy restenosis study (OARS). Circulation 1995;92:I-545.
3. Doi T, Tamai H, Ueda K, Hsu YS, Ono S, et al. Impact of intracoronary ultrasound-guided directional atherectomy on restenosis. Circulation 1995;92:I-545.
4. Bauman RP, Yock PG, Fitzgerald PJ, Annex BH, et al. "Reference Cut" method of intracoronary ultrasound guided directional coronary atherectomy: Initial and six month results. Circulation 1995;92:I-546.
5. Baim D, Kuntz R, Popma J, Leon M. Results of directional atherectomy in the "Pilot" phase of BOAT. Circulation 1994;90:I-214.
6. Baim DS, Kuntz RE, Sharma SK, Fortuna R, Feldman R, et al. Acute results of the randomized phase of the balloon versus optimal atherectomy trial (BOAT). Circulation 1995;92:I-544.
7. Waksman R, Weintraub WS, Ghazzal ZMB, Douglas JS, et al. Directional coronary atherectomy (Directional coronary atherectomy): Is much bigger much better? Circulation 1995;92:I-329.

392. Answer: a (true)

Although directional coronary atherectomy can excise tissue and plaque, the amount of tissue removal (usually 6-45 mg) may not fully account for the magnitude of luminal enlargement. IVUS studies suggest that tissue removal accounts for about 75% of the luminal improvement after directional coronary atherectomy, [1-4] the rest being due to a combination of Dotter and balloon dilating effects.

References:
1. Matar F, Mintz G, Farb A, Douek P. The contribution of tissue removal to lumen improvement after directional coronary atherectomy. Am J Cardiol 1994;74:647-650.
2. Tenaglia AN, Buller CE, Kisslo KB, Stack RS. Mechanisms of balloon angioplasty and directional coronary atherectomy as assessed by intracoronary ultrasound. J Am Coll Cardiol 1992;20:685-691.
3. Braden G, Herrington D, Downes T, et al. Qualitative and quantitative contrasts in the mechanisms of lumen enlargement by coronary balloon angioplasty and directional coronary atherectomy. J Am Coll Cardiol 1994;23:40-48.
4. Umans V, Baptisla J, di Mario C, et al. Angiographic, ultrasound, and angioscopic assessment of the coronary artery wall and lumen area configuration after directional atherectomy: The mechanism revisited. Am Heart J 1995;130.217-227.

393. Answer: a, d

The results of directional coronary atherectomy have been reported in numerous single and multicenter observational studies, and in three large multicenter prospective randomized trials. Further studies of optimal atherectomy (with and without ultrasound guidance) are also in progress. In the three largest randomized studies comparing directional coronary atherectomy and PTCA in native vessels (CAVEAT-I, CCAT)[1,2] and vein grafts (CAVEAT-II) , directional coronary atherectomy resulted in better immediate lumen enlargement, higher procedural success, and similar major complications rates. Although adjunctive PTCA after directional coronary atherectomy was initially discouraged, PTCA may actually improve directional coronary atherectomy outcome and can often result in residual stenoses <10%.[4-7]

Results of Randomized Trials of PTCA Vs. Directional Coronary Atherectomy

In-hospital (%)	CAVEAT-I[1]		CCAT[2]		CAVEAT-II[3]	
	PTCA (n=500)	DCA (n=512)	PTCA (n=136)	DCA (n=138)	PTCA (n=156)	DCA (n=149)
Final DS	36	29	33	25**	38	32**
Success	76	82*	88	94+	79	89*
Abrupt closure	3	7	5.1	4.3	2.6	4.7
Death, QMI, CABG	4.4	5	4.4	2.1	5.7	4.7
Any MI	8	19**	3.7	4.3	11.5	17.4
Distal embolization	-	-	-	-	5.1	13.4*
Follow-up (6 months) (%)						
Final DS ≥ 50%	57	50	4.3	46	46	51
TLR	37.2	36.5	26.4	28.3	26	19
EFS	63	60	71	71	56	60

Abbreviations: CAVEAT = Coronary Angioplasty Versus Excisional Atherectomy Trial (I = native vessels; II = saphenous vein grafts); CCAT = Canadian Coronary Atherectomy Trial (LAD only); DS = diameter stenosis; QMI = Q-wave myocardial infarction; CABG = emergency coronary artery bypass surgery; TLR = target lesion revascularization; EFS = event-free survival; N = number of patients; - = not reported
* p < 0.05
+ p = 0.06
** p < 0.01

References:
1. Topol E, Leya F, Pinkerton C, et al. A comparison of directional atherectomy with coronary angioplasty in patients with coronary artery disease. N Engl J Med 1993;329:221-227.
2. Adelman A, Cohen E, Kimball B, et al. A comparison of directional atherectomy with balloon angioplasty for lesions of the left anterior descending coronary artery. N Engl J Med 1993;329:228-233.
3. Holmes D, Topol E, Califf R, et al. A multicenter, randomized trial of coronary angioplasty versus directional atherectomy for patients with saphenous vein bypass graft lesions. Circulation 1995;91:1966-1974.
4. Leon M, Kuntz R, Popma J, et al. Acute angiographic, intravascular ultrasound and clinical results of directional atherectomy in the optimal atherectomy restenosis study. J Am Coll Cardiol 1995;25:137A.
5. Simonton CA, Leon MB, Kuntz RE, et al. Acute and late clinical and angiographic results of directional atherectomy in the optimal atherectomy restenosis study (OARS). Circulation 1995;92:I-545.
6. Baim D, Kuntz R, Popma J, Leon M. Results of directional atherectomy in the "Pilot" phase of BOAT. Circulation 1994;90:I-214.
7. Baim DS, Kuntz RE, Sharma SK, Fortuna R, Feldman R, et al. Acute results of the randomized phase of the balloon versus optimal atherectomy trial (BOAT). Circulation 1995;92:I-544.

394. Answer: a (true)

Although angiography is often insensitive for detecting thrombus, local thrombosis is felt to complicate approximately 2% of directional atherectomy procedures, and may account for ≥ 50% of acute vessel closures after atherectomy.[1,2] Treatment includes PTCA and thrombolytic agents (local drug delivery, intracoronary, or intravenous), or CABG for refractory cases.

References:
1. Popma J, Topol E, Hinohara T, et al. Abrupt vessel closure after directional coronary atherectomy. J Am Coll Cardiol 1992;19:1372-1379.
2. Carrozza J, Baim J. Complications of directional coronary atherectomy: Incidence, causes, and management. Am J Cardiol 1993;72:47E-54E.

395. Answer: a (true)

In CAVEAT-I, abrupt closure was more common after directional coronary atherectomy (8% vs. 3.8%, p = 0.005) and occurred at a site *other* than the target lesion in 42% (from guide catheter or nosecone trauma).[1]

References:
1. Holmes DR, Simpson JB, Berdan LG, et al. Abrupt closure: The CAVEAT I Experience. J Am Coll Cardiol 1995;26:1494-500.

396. Answer: a, b, c

Coronary artery perforation is an important complication because of its associated morbidity and mortality. The incidence of perforation after directional coronary atherectomy is < 1%, which is probably lower than other devices that ablate or remove plaque (TEC, Rotablator, ELCA), but higher than the 0.2% incidence after PTCA. Some perforations occur when directional coronary atherectomy is used to reverse abrupt closure by excising flow-limiting dissection; vessel perforation can be minimized in this situation by use of an undersized device and low-pressure (10 psi) atherectomy.[1] Treatment is identical to perforation of any cause including prolonged balloon inflations and pericardiocentesis. Contained perforations treated without surgery may lead to focal ectasia, pseudoaneursym, and restenosis.[2]

References:
1. Van Suylen RJ, Serruys PW, Simpson JB, et al. Delayed rupture of right coronary artery after directional coronary atherectomy for bail-out. Am Heart J 1991;121:914-917.
2. Selmon MR, Robertson GC, Simpson JB, et al. Retrieval of media and adventitia by directional coronary atherectomy and angiographic correlation. Circulation 1990;82:III-624.

397. Answer: a, b, c, d

In most observational studies of directional atherectomy, the reported incidence of non-Q-wave MI is 3-12.5%. In CAVEAT-I, but not in CCAT or CAVEAT-II, there was a higher incidence of non-Q-wave MI after directional coronary atherectomy compared to PTCA. Risk factors for CK-MB elevation include high-risk patients, de novo lesions, and complex lesion morphology.[1] The clinical significance of non-Q-wave MI in the absence of other signs of ischemia is uncertain; while some

Answers

studies suggest an adverse prognosis,[2] others do not. [3] Patients with high CK-MB levels (i.e., > 50 IU/L) appear to be at risk for adverse clinical outcome at 2 years.[3] Results from the EPIC trial suggest that the risk of non-Q-MI can be reduced by ReoPro, invoking a platelet-dependent mechanism.[4] The CK-MB ratio may be useful for identifying significant enzyme elevations.[5]

Immediate Results and Clinical Complications after Directional Coronary Atherectomy

Series	N (pts)	Final DS (%)	Success (%)	MC (%)	Comments
Fortuna[6] (1995)	310	16	95%	5	VSR (1.3%), TLR (28%)
Safian[7] (1990)	67	5	88	1.5	VSR (3%); nQMI (4.5%)
Umans[8] (1994)	150	29	90	10	Worse 2 year EFS with unstable angina
Popma[9] (1993)	306	14	95	2.6	nQMI (5.6%); CRS (28% at 1 year)
Cowley[10] (1993)	300	-	95%	4.6	
Baim[11] (1993)	873	-	92%	4.9	US Directional coronary atherectomy Registry: ARS (42%); nQMI (5%); VSR (1.1%)
Feld[12] (1993)	116	8	99	4%	Matched comparison with PTCA;* nQMI (6%)
Fishmann[13] (1992)	190	7	97	3	nQMI (7.4%); ARS (32%); 1 yr. EFS (74%); nQMI (7.4%)
Popma[14] (1992)	1020	-	83	-	Death (0.2%), MI (1.7%); CABG (2.5%)
Garratt[15] (1992)	158	-	91	7	ARS (58%)
Ellis[16] (1991)	378	-	88	6.3	
Hinohara[17] (1991)	339	15	94	3.4	Success: 78% (noncalcified), 52% (calcified)
Rowe[18] (1990)	83	14	95	2.2	
Kaufmann[19] (1989)	50	15	89	4%	nQMI (4.2%), VSR (1.4%)

Abbreviations: MC = major in-hospital complication (death, Q-wave myocardial infarction, emergency coronary artery bypass surgery); nQMI = non-Q-wave myocardial infarction; VSR = vascular surgical repair; TLR = target lesion revascularization; EFS = event-free survival; - = not reported; ARS = angiographic restenosis, CRS = clinical restenosis
* After PTCA: Success 98%; fewer dissections with Directional coronary atherectomy (13% vs. 22%); major complications 1.6%

References:
1. Hinohara T, Vetter JW, Robertson GC, Selmon MR, et al. CK MB elevation following directional coronary atherectomy. Circulation 1995;92:I-544.
2. Tauke JT, Kong TW, Meyers SN, et al. Prognostic value of reatinine kinase elevation following elective coronary artery interventions. J Am Coll Cardiol 1995;25:269A.
3. Kugelmass AD, Cohen DJ, Moscucci M, et al. Elevation of the creatine kinase myocardial isoform following otherwise successful directional coroanry atherectomy and stenting. Am J cardiol 1994;74:748-754.
4. Lelkovits J, Blankenship JC, Anderson K, et al. Increased risk of non-Q MI after directional atherectomy is platelet dependent: Evidence from the EPIC trial. J Am Coll Cardiol 1996;28:849.
5. Cutlip DE, Ho KKI, Senerchia C, Baim DS, et al. Classification of myocardial infarction after directional coronary atherectomy and relation to clinical outcome. Results of the OARS trial. Circulation 1995;92:I-616.
6. Fortuna R, Walston D, Hansell H, Schulz G. Directional coronary atherectomy: Experience in 310 patients. J Invas Cardiol 1995;7:57-64.
7. Safian R, Gelbfish J, Erny R, Schnitt S, Schmidt D, Baim D. Coronary atherectomy. Clinical, angiographic, and histological findings and observations regarding potential mechanisms. Circulation 1990;82:69-79.
8. Umans V, de Feyter P, Deckers J, et al. Acute and long-term outcome of directional coronary atherectomy for stable and unstable angina. Am J Cardiol 1993;74:641-646.
9. Popma J, Mintz G, Satler L, et al. Clinical and angiographic outcome after directional coronary atherectomy: A qualitative and quantitative analysis using coronary arteriography and intravascular ultrasound. Am J Cardiol 1993;72:55E-64E.
10. Cowley M, DiSciascio G. Experience with directional coronary atherectomy since pre-market approval. Am J Cardiol 1993;72:12E-20E.
11. Baim D, Tomoaki H, Holmes D, et al. Results of directional coronary atherectomy during multicenter preapproval testing. Am J Cardiol 1993;72:6E-11E.
12. Feld H, Schulhoff N, Lichstein E, et al. Coronary atherectomy versus angioplasty: The CAVA study. Am Heart J 1993;126:31-38.
13. Fishman R, Kuntz R, Carrozza J, et al. Long-term results of directional coronary atherectomy: Predictors of restenosis. J Am Coll Cardiol 1992;20:1101-1110.
14. Popma J, Topol E, Hinohara T, et al. Abrupt vessel closure after directional coronary atherectomy. J Am Coll Cardiol 1992;19:1372-1379.
15. Garratt K, Holmes D, Bell M, et al. Results of directional atherectomy of primary atheromatous and restenosis lesions in coronary arteries and saphenous vein grafts. Am J Cardiol 1992;70:449-454.
16 Ellis S, DeCesare N, Pinkerton C, Whitlow P. Relation of stenosis morphology and clinical presentation to the procedural results of directional coronary atherectomy. Circulation 1991;84:644-653.
17. Hinohara T, Rowe MH, Robertson GC, et al. Effect of lesion characteristics on outcome of directional coronary atherectomy. J Am Coll Cardiol 1991;17:1112-20.
18. Rowe MH, Hinohara T, White NW, Robertson GC. Comparison of dissection rates and angiographic results following directional coronary atherectomy and coronary angioplasty. Am J Cardiol 1990;66:49-53.
19. Kaufmann UP, Garratt KN, Vlietstra RE, Menke KK. Coronary atherectomy: First 50 patients at the Mayo Clinic. Mayo Clin Proc 1989;64:747-752.

398. Answer: a, b, c, d

Multicenter Trials of Directional Coronary Atherectomy in Native Coronary Arteries

	CAVEAT-I[1]	CCAT[2]	OARS[3]	BOAT[4]
N (pts)	1012	548	200	1000
Year[a]	1993	1993	1995	1995
# Cases/Operator[b]	50	-	> 200	> 200
Qualify[c]	No	No	Yes	Yes
AtheroCath[d]	Surlyn, EX	Surlyn, EX	EX, GTO	EX, GTO
PTCA[e]	No	No	Yes	Yes
IVUS[f]	No	No	Yes	No
Goal (final DS %)[g]	< 50	< 50	< 15	< 15

Abbreviations: CAVEAT-I = Coronary Angioplasty Versus Excisional Atherectomy Trial (native vessels); CCAT = Canadian Coronary Atherectomy Trial (LAD); OARS = Optimal Atherectomy Restenosis Study; BOAT = Balloon vs. Optimal Atherectomy Trial; - not reported
a. Year of primary publication
b. Co-investigators had to perform a minimum number of Directional coronary atherectomy cases
c. Co-investigators had to submit angiograms to Core Lab to document their ability to achieve good results
d. Type of AtheroCaths used during study period
e. Use of adjunctive PTCA: No = not permitted; Yes = permitted
f. Routine use of IVUS
g. Co-investigators attempted to achieve a predefined target diameter stenosis

References:
1. Topol E, Leya F, Pinkerton C, et al. A comparison of directional atherectomy with coronary angioplasty in patients with coronary artery disease. N Engl J Med 1993;329:221-227.
2. Adelman A, Cohen E, Kimball B, et al. A comparison of directional atherectomy with balloon angioplasty for lesions of the left anterior descending coronary artery. N Engl J Med 1993;329:228-233.
3. Leon M, Kuntz R, Popma J, et al. Acute angiographic, intravascular ultrasound and clinical results of directional atherectomy in the optimal atherectomy restenosis study. J Am Coll Cardiol 1995;25:137A.
4. Baim D, Kuntz R, Popma J, Leon M. Results of directional atherectomy in the "Pilot" phase of BOAT. Circulation 1994;90:I-214.

399. Answer: b (false)

Deep wall components (media and adventitia) can be identified in up to 2/3 of directional coronary atherectomy cases.[1,2] Although immediate post-procedure lumen diameter is an important determinant of restenosis and is the central theme of the "bigger-is-better" hypothesis,[3] there is concern among some interventionalists that achieving large lumen diameters by partial excision of plaque and deep vessel wall components may increase the risk of perforation, restenosis, and aneurysm formation.[4] Although perforation is slightly more frequent after directional coronary atherectomy than PTCA, there does not appear to be any relationship between retrieval of deep wall components and perforation. The controversy surrounding restenosis[4,5] appears to have been recently resolved by a report from the CAVEAT I and II investigators, who found that deep wall resection does not increase the risk of restenosis.[6]

References:
1. Safian R, Gelbfish J, Erny R, Schnitt S, Schmidt D, Baim D. Coronary atherectomy. Clinical, angiographic, and histological findings and observations regarding potential mechanisms. Circulation 1990;82:69-79.
2. Garratt KN, Kaufmann UP, Edwards WD, Vlietsra RE. Safety of percutaneous coronary atherectomy with deep arterial resection. Am J Cardiol 1989;64:538-542.
3. Kuntz RE, Gibson MC, Nobuyoshi M, Baim DS. Generalized Model of Restenosis After Conventional Balloon Angioplasty, Stenting and Directional Atherectomy. J Am Coll Cardiol 1993;21:15-25.
4. Garratt K, Holmes D, Bell M, et al. Restenosis after directional coronary atherectomy: Differences between primary atheromatous and restenosis lesions and the influence of subintimal resection. J Am Coll Cardiol 1990;16:1665-1671.
5. Kuntz R, Hinohara T, Safian R, Selmon M, Simpson J, Baim D. Restenosis after directional coronary atherectomy. Effects of luminal diameter and deep wall excision. Circulation 1992;86:1394-1399.
6. Holmes DR, Garratt KN, Isner JM, et al. Effect of subintimal resection on initial outcome and restenosis for native coronary lesions and saphenous vein graft disease treated by directional coronary atherectomy: A report from the CAVEAT I and II investigators. J Am Coll Cardiol 1996;28:645-651.

400. Answer: a (true)

In the CAVEAT-II study, directional coronary atherectomy resulted in better lumen enlargement and higher procedural success, but no difference in angiographic restenosis, target lesion revascularization, or event-free survival compared to PTCA.[1]

References:
1. Holmes D, Topol E, Califf R, et al. A multicenter, randomized trial of coronary angioplasty versus directional atherectomy for patients with saphenous vein bypass graft lesions. Circulation 1995;91:1966-1974.

401. Answer: b (false)

The application of directional atherectomy to patients with peripheral vascular and coronary artery disease has provided the first opportunity for sampling of atherosclerotic vascular tissue from living patients. The availability of such tissue has led to several interesting observations, which may have important implications for further understanding and treatment of atherosclerosis. De novo lesions frequently consist of fibrosis, necrotic debris, foam cells, cholesterol, and calcium, typical findings of atherosclerosis. In 20% of de novo lesions, intimal proliferation is evident and is indistinguishable from similar cellular proliferation in restenotic lesions.[1] Thus, intimal proliferation is not specific for restenosis, but is a nonspecific response to injury. Such injury may be due to spontaneous events (plaque rupture), to interventional devices, or to other causes. Intimal hyperplasia is observed in 93% of restenotic lesions and in 44% of de novo lesions.[2] Intimal hyperplasia in de novo lesions was associated with younger age and lesions in the LAD, and was not associated with higher rates of restenosis than de novo lesions without intimal hyperplasia.

References:
1. Escaned J, van Suylen R, MacLeod D, et al. Histologic characteristics of tissue excised during directional coronary atherectomy in stable and unstable angina pectoris. Am J Cardiol 1993;71:1442-1447.
2. Miller M, Kuntz R, Friedrich S, et al. Frequency and consequences of intimal hyperplasia in specimens retrieved by directional atherectomy of native primary coronary artery stenoses and subsequent restenoses. Am J Cardiol 1993;71:652-657.

TRANSLUMINAL EXTRACTION ATHERECTOMY

402. Answer: a, b

TEC cutters for coronary application are available in sizes from 5.5-7.5 F (1.8-2.5 mm). The conical cutter head — fabricated from a cylindrical base of proprietary stainless steel — is bonded to the distal end of the catheter and contains microtome-sharp cutting edges that rotate at 750 rpm when the motor-drive is activated. The shaft of the cutter consists of a hollow inner-core through which excised material is aspirated and evacuated. Special 10F tungsten-braided, soft-tip guiding catheters are available in the following sizes and tip configurations: JR 4.0; JL 3.5, 4.0, 5.0; modified Amplatz; hockey stick; multipurpose; and right bypass graft. A special rotating hemostatic valve (RHV), connects the TEC motor-drive handle to the guiding catheter. To minimize the risk of air embolism, it is extremely important to aspirate blood from the guiding catheter (once attached to the RHV), and to thoroughly flush all air from the RHV. A special 0.014-inch stainless steel guide wire allows coaxial passage of the catheter and has a radiopaque floppy tip with a terminal 0.021" ball to prevent wire tip entrapment or advancement of the cutting blades beyond the guidewire.

Cutters for TEC Atherectomy

Cutter Size (F)	Cutter Diameter (mm)	Vessel Diameter* (mm)	Guide ID** (inch)
5.5	1.8	2.5	0.086
6.0	2.0	2.75	0.092
6.5	2.17	3.0	0.092

Cutter Size (F)	Cutter Diameter (mm)	Vessel Diameter* (mm)	Guide ID** (inch)
7.0	2.33	3.25	0.104
7.5	2.5	3.5	0.104

* Minimum vessel diameter to be used with TEC cutters
** Minimum guide catheter internal diameter

Guiding Catheters for TEC Atherectomy

Target Vessel	Configuration	Guiding Catheter
RCA	Normal	JR 4
	Anterior origin	Mod.-Amplatz, Hockey Stick
	Horizontal origin	Hockey Stick
	Superior origin; Shepherd Cook	Hockey Stick, RBG
	Inferior origin	JR 4, Multipurpose
LCA	Normal	JL 4.0
	Narrow root or superior origin	JL 3.5
	Wide root or posterior origin	JL 5.0
SVG to LCA	Normal	JR 4
	Superior origin	Mod.-Amplatz, Hockey Stick
		Mod.-Amplatz, RBG
SVG to RCA	Normal	Mod.-Amplatz, Multipurpose, RBG
	Horizontal origin	JR 4, Hockey Stick, Mod.-Amplatz

Abbreviations: JR = right Judkins; JL = left Judkins; Mod.-Amplatz = modified Amplatz; RBG = right bypass graft; RCA = right coronary artery; LCA = left coronary artery; SVG = saphenous vein graft

403. Answer: a (true)

For TEC cutters ≤ 6.5F (2.2mm), 9F guiding catheters may be used; the 8F giant lumen (ID = 0.086 inches) guide can only accommodate the 5.5F cutter. Pressure damping and poor contrast opacification are common when using guiding catheters < 10F. 10F guides from other manufacturers can be used, if necessary.

404. Answer: b (false)

The TEC guiding catheters are stiffer than conventional angioplasty guides; over-rotation and deep-seating greatly increase the risk of vessel injury and should be avoided. During advancement of the TEC guide to the aortic root, blood loss can be minimized by tracking the guide over a 0.063-inch guidewire, or alternatively, over a 0.035-inch guidewire through a 6F multipurpose catheter.

405. Answer: a, c, d

TEC atherectomy must be performed with the special TEC guidewire. Because the stiff 300-cm stainless-steel TEC guidewire is less steerable than conventional PTCA guidewires, a conventional guidewire should be used to cross tortuous vessels or complex lesions. Once in position, the PTCA guidewire can be exchanged for the TEC guidewire using any suitable transport catheter that will accommodate the 0.021-inch ball. For simple anatomy, the TEC guidewire can be used as the primary wire, but a bare-wire tecnique must be employed (i.e., TEC wire advanced beyond the lesion without the TEC cutter). It is important to advance the floppy, radiopaque portion of the wire well beyond the lesion to ensure that atherectomy is performed along the stiff, radiolucent segment. Due to the stiffness of the TEC guidewire, pseudolesions are common but generally resolve after removal of the guidewire.

406. Answer: a, d

Ideal cutter selection criteria have not been identified; a common recommendation is to undersize the cutter by at least 1mm in relation to the distal reference segment (i.e., cutter/artery ratio of 0.5-0.7). In diffusely diseased vessels, subtotal stenoses, angulated lesions, or vessels < 3 mm, many operators recommend a 5.5F cutter followed by definitive lumen enlargement with adjunctive PTCA or stenting. The TEC cutter must be activated proximal to the lesion; activation within the lesion increases the risk of distal embolization and dissection, and should be avoided. The cutter should be advanced slowly (10 mm/30 seconds) through the lesion to achieve a continuous stream of blood entering the vacuum bottle. The cutter should not be activated in the guiding catheter or in nondiseased segments, particularly when traversing a bend. After completing 2-5 slow passes through the lesion, the TEC cutter should be retracted and the lesion reassessed. If a filling defect persists and there is no evidence for dissection, a larger TEC cutter may be used. If there is significant residual stenosis but no residual filling defect, adjunctive PTCA, DCA, or stenting should be performed.

407. Answer: a, b, c

Medications are the same as those prescribed for PTCA: All patients should receive aspirin ($\geq$ 325 mg/d at least 1 day prior to the procedure), heparin (to achieve and maintain an ACT $\geq$ 300 seconds during the case), and intracoronary nitroglycerin (100-200 mcg just prior to cutting to attenuate spasm). Intracoronary verapamil (100 mcg/min up to 1-1.5 mg), intracoronary urokinase (250,000-500,000 units over 5-30 min), and IV ReoPro may be of value for no-reflow, intraluminal thrombus, and high-risk angioplasty intervention, respectively, but are not recommended for routine TEC.

408. Answer: a

Angioscopy studies demonstrate partial or complete thrombus removal in 75-100% of thrombotic lesions after TEC;[1,2] dissection, however, has been noted in virtually all cases by angioscopy[1,2] (including occlusive dissections in 75% in one report)[3] and in 36% of cases by IVUS.[4] Although gross examination of aspirated material sometimes demonstrates yellowish debris, histologic studies have failed to reveal evidence for tissue removal. It is likely that a "Dotter" effect contributes to angiographic improvement after TEC.[5]

References:
1. Annex BH, Larkin TJ, O'Neill WW, Safian RD. Evaluation of thrombus removal by transluminal extraction coronary atherectomy by percutaneous coronary angioscopy. Amer J Cardiol 1994;74:606-9.
2. Kaplan BM, Safian RD, Grines CL, Goldstein JA, et al. Usefulness of adjunctive angioscopy and extraction atherectomy before stent implantation in high risk narrowings in aorto-coronary artery saphenous vein grafts. Amer J Cardiol 1995;76:822-824.
3. Moses JW, Lieberman SM, Knopf WD, et al. Mechanism of transluminal extraction catheter (TEC) atherectomy in degenerative saphenous vein grafts (SVG): An Angioscopic Observational Study. J Am Coll Cardiol 1993;21:442A.
4. Popma JJ, Leon MB, Mintz GS, et al. Results of coronary angioplasty using the transluminal extraction catheter. Am J Cardiol 1992;70:1526-1532.
5. Pizzulli L, Kohler U, Manz M, Luderitz B. Mechanical dilatation rather than plaque removal as major mechanism of transluminal extraction atherectomy. J Intervent Cardiol 1993;6:31-39.

409. Answer: a, b, c, d

Procedural success in native coronary arteries was achieved in 84-94%,[1,2] although adjunctive PTCA was required in 79-84% of lesions to enlarge lumen dimensions (72%), salvage technical failures (1%), or manage TEC-induced vessel occlusion (11%).[2] In one study, quantitative angiography revealed a residual diameter stenosis of 61% after TEC and 36% after adjunctive PTCA.[2]

In-hospital Results of TEC Atherectomy in Native Coronary Arteries[1,2]

	IVT (1995)	Safian (1994)
No. lesions	783	181
Adjunctive PTCA (%)	79	84
Success (%)	94	84
Complications (%)		
MI	0.6	3.4
Death	1.4	2.3
Acute closure	8.0	11.0
Distal embolization	1.6	0.5
No-reflow	0	0

References:
1. IVT Coronary TEC Atherectomy Clinical Database. 1995.
2. Safian RS, May MA, Lichtenberg A, et al. Detailed clinical and angiographic analysis of complex lesions in native coronary arteries. J Am Coll Cardiol 1995;25:848-854.

410. Answer: a (true)

The extent of elastic recoil after TEC was approximately 30%, similar to conventional PTCA.[1]

References:
1. Safian RD, Freed M, Reddy V, et al. Do excimer laser and rotational atherectomy facilitate balloon angioplasty? Implications for lesion-specific coronary intervention. J Am Coll Cardiol (in-press)

411. Answer: b (false)

The ideal treatment of degenerated vein grafts is unknown; serious angiographic complications after vein graft TEC include distal embolization in 2-17%, no-reflow in 8.8%, and abrupt closure in 2-5%. No-reflow occasionally responds to intragraft verapamil (100-300 mcg),[1-3] and the value of prophylactic intragraft verapamil prior to intervention is currently under investigation. In one report, distal embolization was more likely to occur in grafts with one or more intraluminal filling defects, and in older grafts.[4] In a recent NACI Registry report, distal embolization was associated with a higher incidence of in-hospital mortality and myocardial infarction; multivariate predictors of distal embolization included noncardiac disease, stand-alone TEC, thrombus, and large vessel size.[5] To minimize the risk of distal embolization and no-reflow, some operators recommend TEC followed by staged (1-2 months later) rather than immediate stent implantation; in one report, this approach resulted in less distal embolization,[6,7] although 15% of grafts occluded before stenting.[6] A multicenter randomized trial comparing TEC vs. PTCA followed by stent (TEC-BEST) has been initiated.

References:
1. Kaplan BM, Benzuly KH, Bowers TR, et al. Prospective study of intracoronary verapamil and nitroglycerin for the treatment of no-reflow after interventions on degenerated saphenous vein grafts. Circ 1995; 92:I-330.
2. Piana RN, Paik GY, Moscucci M, Cohen DJ, et al. Incidence and treatment of "no-reflow" after percutaneous coronary intervention. Circulation 1994; 89(6): 2514-2518.
3. Pomerantz RM, Kuntz RE, Diver DJ, Safian RD, Baim DS. Intracoronary verapamil for the treatment of distal microvascular coronary artery spasm following PTCA. Cathet Cardio Diagn 1991; 24: 283-285.
4. Hong MK, Popma JJ, Pichard AD, Kent KM, et al. Clinical significance of distal embolization after transluminal extraction atherectomy in diffusely diseased saphenous vein grafts. Am Heart J 1994; 127(6): 1496-1503.
5. Moses JW, Yeh W, Popma JJ, Sketch Jr. MH, NACI Investigators. Predictors of distal embolization with the TEC catheter: A NACI Registry Report. Circ 1995; 92:I-329.
6. Hong MH, Pichard AD, Kent KM, et al. Assessing a strategy of stand-alone extraction atherectomy followed by staged stent placement in degenerated saphenous vein graft lesions. J Amer Coll Cardiol 1995;27:394A.
7. Al-Shaibi KF, Goods CM, Jain SP, et al. Does transluminal extraction atherectomy reduce distal embolization in saphenous vein grafts? Circ 1995; 92:I-329.

412. Answer: b (false)

Angiographic restenosis has been reported in 64-69% of vein graft lesions treated with TEC,[1,2] with a 29% incidence of late total occlusion in one report.[2] There are no data to suggest that TEC decreases restenosis.

References:
1. IVT Coronary TEC Atherectomy Clinical Database. 1995.
2. Safian RS, Grines CL, May MA, et al. Clinical and angiographic results of transluminal extraction coronary atherectomy in saphenous vein bypass grafts. Circulation 1994; 89(1): 302-312.

Answers

413. Answer: a (true)

TEC may have a role in primary revascularization for acute MI, rescue after failed thrombolysis, post-infarct MI angina, and unstable angina associated with a thrombotic lesion. In a study of 110 patients with acute ischemic syndromes, overall procedural success was 94%; in-hospital complications included death in 4.3% (only 1.4% of patients not presenting in cardiogenic shock), CABG in 2.9%, repeat PTCA in 5.7%, and blood transfusion in 20%.[1] At 6 months, vessel patency was 90% and angiographic restenosis was 68%. A multicenter randomized trial comparing TEC vs. PTCA (TOPIT) in acute ischemic syndromes has been completed; preliminary data suggest a lower incidence of CK elevation after TEC.[2]

References:
1. Kaplan BM, Larkin TJ, Safian RS, O'Neill WW, et al. A Prospective pilot trial of direct and rescue extraction atherectomy for acute myocardial infarction. 1995 (to be submitted for publication).
2. Kaplan BM, Gregory M, Schreiber TL, et al. Transluminal extraction atherectomy versus balloon angioplasty in acute ischemic syndromes: An interim analysis of the TOPIT trial. 1996;October issue:AHA abstract book.

414. Answer: a (true)

Angiographic thrombus increases the risk of an adverse outcome in virtually all studies of percutaneous interventional devices. However, in the initial TEC registry, procedural success was equally high with and without thrombus, offering hope that TEC's ability to excise and aspirate thrombus would fill an important void in the interventional arena. More recent studies of TEC in thrombotic vein grafts reported lower procedural success, and more angiographic and clinical complications.[1,2] Nevertheless, TEC is currently under investigation as a bailout technique after failed PTCA in the setting of acute MI,[3] and to pretreat thrombotic lesions prior to stenting.[4]

References:
1. Popma JJ, Leon MB, Mintz GS, et al. Results of coronary angioplasty using the transluminal extraction catheter. Am J Cardiol 1992;70:1526-1532.
2. Dooris M, Hoffman M, Glazier S, et al. Comparative results of transluminal extraction coronary atherectomy in saphenous vein graft lesions with and without thrombus. J Am Coll Cardiol 1995; 25: 1700-1705.
3. Kaplan BM, O'Neill WW, Grines CL, et al. Rescue extraction atherectomy after failed primary angioplasty in right coronary artery infarction. Am J Cardiol (in-press).
4. Kaplan BM, Safian RS, Grines CL, Goldstein JA, et al. Usefulness of adjunctive angioscopy and extraction atherectomy before stent implantation in high risk narrowings in aorto-coronary artery saphenous vein grafts. Amer J Cardiol 1995;76:822-824.

415. Answer: a, b, c, d, e

Certain lesions are unsuitable for TEC, including moderate-to-heavily calcified lesions, severely angled stenoses, highly eccentric lesions, bifurcation lesions, and lesions in vessels < 2.5 mm. TEC is absolutely contraindicated in the setting of dissection caused by another device due to the risk of extending the dissection and perforating the vessel. Since it is often difficult to distinguish dissection from thrombus by angiography alone, adjunctive imaging techniques such as angioscopy and intravascular ultrasound can be used to guide subsequent use of TEC (for thrombus) or stents (for dissection).

416. Answer: a (true)

DOPPLER FLOW MEASUREMENTS

417. Answer: a, b, c, d

Myocardial blood flow is regulated by changes in vascular resistance at the level of the coronary arteriole. As myocardial O_2 demand increases (e.g., exercise), there is a decrease in resistance (coronary vasodilatation) and an increase in blood flow. Coronary flow reserve (CFR), defined as the ratio of hyperemic-to-resting blood flow velocity,[1] is typically > 2. In the presence of a flow-limiting epicardial stenosis, the distal microvasculature dilates to preserve resting basal blood flow;[2] however, maximal hyperemic flow is impaired and CFR is < 2. CFR and other blood flow measurements can be safely, easily, and reliably obtained in the cath lab with the use of the Cardiometrics FloWire, a flexible, steerable 0.014" or 0.018" guidewire with a tip-mounted piezoelectric Doppler crystal.[3-5] The Doppler wire measures coronary blood flow velocity, not absolute blood flow.

References:
1. Gould KL, Lipscomb K, Hamilton GW. Physiologic basis for assessing critical coronary stenosis. Am J Cardiol 1974;33:87-94.
2. Wilson RF, Laxson DD. Caveat Emptor: A clinician's guide to assessing the physiologic significance of arterial stenoses. Cathet Cardiovasc Diagn 1993;29:93-98.
3. Doucette JW, Corl PD, Payne HM, et al. Validation of a Doppler guidewire for intravascular measurement of coronary artery flow velocity. Circulation 1992;85:1899-1911.
4. Segal J, Kern MJ, Scott NA, King III SB, et al. Alterations of phasic coronary artery flow velocity in humans during percutaneous coronary angioplasty. J Am Coll Cardiol 1992;20:276-286.
5. Ofili EO, Kern MJ, Labovitz AJ, St. Vrain JA, et al. Analysis of coronary blood flow velocity dynamics in angiographically normal and stenosed arteries before and after endoluminal enlargement by angioplasty. J Am Coll Cardiol 1993;21:308-316.

418. Answer: a, b, c, d

Spectral flow velocity data, along with ECG and arterial blood pressure recording, are displayed in real time on the FlowMap monitor. In addition to coronary flow reserve — the parameter used to assess the functional significance of a lesion before and after intervention — other blood flow measurements can be obtained including the beat-to-beat phasic average peak velocity (APV), diastolic-to-systolic velocity ratio (DSVR), APV trend over 1.5-90 minutes, and the proximal-to-distal translesional velocity ratio. The "normal" range of Doppler-derived flow velocity variables has been defined,[1-9] but interpretation of each variable must be considered in the context of other Doppler variables, angiographic features, and clinical characteristics of the patient.[1,10] One possible limitation to the use of Doppler is that it measures changes in coronary blood flow velocity rather than volumetric flow. However, if the cross-sectional area of the artery remains constant between basal and hyperemic conditions, changes in flow velocity parallel changes in volumetric flow. Administration of intracoronary nitroglycerin can be used to minimize differences in vessel dimensions between basal and hyperemic conditions, and improve the reliability of CFR measurements.[11]

Answers

Doppler-Derived Flow Velocity Parameters

Variable	Normal Reference Range	Reference
Average Peak Velocity (APV)		1-3
Basal	≥ 20 cm/sec	
Hyperemic	≥ 30 cm/sec	
Diastolic/Systolic Mean Velocity Ratio (DSVR)		1-4
LAD	> 1.7	
LCX	> 1.5	
RCA	> 1.2*	
Proximal/Distal Mean Velocity Ratio (PDR)†	< 1.7	1-5
Distal Coronary Flow Reserve (CFR)	≥ 2.0	6-9

*   Normal DSVR > 1.4 in distal RCA or PDA
†   Also called Translesional Velocity Gradient (TVG)

References:
1. Segal J, Kern MJ, Scott NA, King III SB, et al. Alterations of phasic coronary artery flow velocity in humans during percutaneous coronary angioplasty. J Am Coll Cardiol 1992;20:276-286.
2. Ofili EO, Kern MJ, Labovitz AJ, St. Vrain JA, et al. Analysis of coronary blood flow velocity dynamics in angiographically normal and stenosed arteries before and after endoluminal enlargement by angioplasty. J Am Coll Cardiol 1993;21:308-316.
3. Ofili EO, Lasovitz AJ, Kern MJ. Coronary flow velocity dynamics in normal and diseased arteries. Am J Cardiol 1993;71:3D-9D.
4. Kajiya F, Ogasawara Y, Tsujioka K, et al. Analysis of flow characteristics in post-stenotic regions of the human coronary artery during bypass graft surgery. Circulation 1987;76:1092-1100.
5. Donohue TJ, Kern MJ, Aguirre FV, Bach RG, et al. Assessing the hemodynamic significance of coronary artery stenosis. Analysis of translesional pressure-flow velocity relations in patients. J Am Coll Cardiol 1993;22:449-458.
6. Kern MJ, Aguirre FV, Bach RG, Caracole EA, Donohue TJ. Translesional pressure-flow velocity assessment in patients: Part I. Cathet Cardiovasc Diagn 1994;313:49-60.
7. Kern MJ, Deligonul, Tatineni S, Serota H, et al. IV adenosine continuous infusion and low dose bolus administration for determination of coronary vascular reserve in patients with and without coronary artery disease. J Am Coll Cardiol 1991;18:718-729.
8. Miller DD, Donohue TJ, Younis LT, Bach RG, et al. Correlation of pharmacologic Technesium 99m-Sestamibi myocardial perfusion imaging with post-stenotic coronary flow reserve in patients with angiographically intermediate coronary artery stenoses. Circulation 1994;89:2150-2160.
9. Joye JD, Schulman DS, Lesorde D, Farah T, et al. Intracoronary Doppler guide wire versus stress single-photon emission computer tomographic thallium 201 imaging in assessment of intermediate coronary stenoses. J Am Coll Cardiol 1994;24:940-947.
10. Doucette JW, Corl PD, Payne HM, et al. Validation of a Doppler guidewire for intravascular measurement of coronary artery flow velocity. Circulation 1992;85:1899-1911.
11. Shammas NW, Thondapu V, Gerasimou EM, Antonio J, et al. Effect of pretreatment with nitroglycerin on coronary flow reserve measured using bolus intracoronary adenosine. Circulation 1995;92:I-264.

419. Answer: a, c, d

Coronary flow reserve (CFR) is defined as the ratio of hyperemic-to-baseline coronary blood flow velocity. Values > 2 are normal, while values < 2 suggest the presence of a functionally-significant epicardial obstruction. Several pharmacologic agents can be used to induce maximum (hyperemic) flow velocity and/or microvascular disease. In our cath lab, intracoronary adenosine is the preferred vasodilator because of its short duration of action, ease of use, and proven safety, but papaverine is also effective. CFR is the most useful of all the Doppler measurements; it is used primarily to assess the physiologic significance of a stenosis and the functional status of the distal microvascular bed before and after coronary intervention.

Drugs for Maximal Vasodilations

Drug	Dose	Duration	Reference
Adenosine			1-3
IC	RCA 6-10 mcg (bolus) LAD/LCX 12-20 mcg (bolus)	20-45 seconds	
IV	100-150 mcg/kg/min	45 seconds after drip discontinued	
Papaverine			4
IC	5-10 mg	45-150 seconds	
IV	*	*	
Dipyridamole			5
IV	0.56 mg/kg over 4 minutes	Peak 4-minutes Duration 20-40 minutes	

*	Intravenous infusion is not recommended because of a slow systemic excretion; drug accumulation may lead to systemic hypotension.

References:
1. Kern MJ, Deligonul, Tatineni S, Serota H, et al. IV adenosine continuous infusion and low dose bolus administration for determination of coronary vascular reserve in patients with and without coronary artery disease. J Am Coll Cardiol 1991;18:718-729.
2. Zijlstra F, Juilliere Y, Serruys PW, Roelandt JRTC. Value and limitations of intracoronary adenosine for the assessment of coronary flow reserve. Cathet Cardiovasc Diagn 1988;15:76-80.
3. Wilson RF, Wych K, Christensen BV, Zimmer S, Laxson DD. Effects of adenosine on human coronary arterial circulation. Circulation 1990;82:1595-1606.
4. Wilson RF, White CW. Intracoronary papaverine: An ideal vasodilator for studies of the coronary circulation in conscious humans. Circulation 1986;73:444-452.
5. Ranhosty A, Kempthorne-Rawson J. Intravenous Dipyridamole Thallium Imaging Study Group. The safety of intravenous dipyridamole thallium myocardial perfusion imaging. Circulation 1990;81:1205-1209.

420. Answer: a, b, c

The application of intracoronary Doppler velocimetry demands an in-depth understanding of the limitations of the technique.[1-3] Importantly, abnormalities of the microcirculation may decrease CFR and confound its interpretation. CFR may also be sensitive to changes in hemodynamic conditions, such as tachycardia (increases CFR), hypertension (decreases CFR), and increased contractility (increases CFR); fractional flow reserve (FFR), defined as the ratio of distal hyperemic APV-to-mean aortic pressure, may be independent of hemodynamic changes and particularly useful in the presence of hemodynamic changes.[4] CFR may be less useful for assessing the functional significance of a residual stenosis in acute MI patients treated with PTCA because of the known impairment of CFR in this setting.[5] Since conditions associated with impaired microcirculation have little regional variability, normal CFR in a vessel without an epicardial stenosis reliably excludes small vessel disease as a cause of decreased CFR in a vessel with a significant epicardial stenosis.

Answers

Technical and Anatomic Factors: Impact on Doppler Data

Factor	Potential Effect
Doppler Wire Technical Considerations	
1. Inappropriate on-line IPV tracking	APV and DSVR may be falsely low; CFR and TVG calculated from APV may be erroneous.
2. Inappropriate ECG gating from QRS	False diastolic and systolic time intervals; Erroneous DSVR.
3. Unstable phasic Doppler signal	APV may be falsely low.
4. Doppler probe not positioned to assess peak flow velocity	APV may be falsely low.
Translesional Velocity Gradient (TVG, PDR) may be influenced by:	
1. Ostial lesions	No proximal value to assess lesion.
2. Single unbranched conduits	TVG may be falsely low.
3. Tortuous vessels	Unable to obtain reliable distal peak velocity.
4. Diffuse distal disease	Falsely low TVG secondary to falsely elevated distal velocity.
5. Tandem/sequential lesions	Falsely low TVG secondary to falsely elevated distal velocity (distal lesional flow acceleration).
6. Eccentric lesions	Falsely high TVG secondary to falsely elevated proximal velocity (acceleration at lesional flow convergence).
Coronary Flow Reserve (CFR) may be influenced by:	
1. Abnormal microcirculation (hypertrophy, diabetes, connective tissue disease, prior myocardial infarction, Syndrome X)	May falsely lower CFR.
2. Sequential lesions	Distal CFR is the result of the combined physiologic effect of all lesions.
3. Changes in vasomotor tone	May falsely lower CFR.
4. Submaximal vasodilator dose	May falsely lower CFR.
5. Transient increase in distal flow	May falsely lower CFR.
6. Varying Doppler wire position between baseline and hyperemic assessment	May falsely lower CFR.
7. Varying hemodynamic conditions	May falsely lower CFR

References:
1. Doucette JW, Corl PD, Payne HM, et al. Validation of a Doppler guidewire for intravascular measurement of coronary artery flow velocity. Circulation 1992;85:1899-1911.
2. White CW, Wilson RF, Intracoronary Doppler Ultrasound in Nanda P (ed): Doppler Ultrasound. Philadelphia, Lea & Febiger, 1994, pp 403-412.
3. McGinn AL, White CW, Wilson RF. Interstudy variability of coronary flow reserve. Influence of heart rate, arterial pressure and ventricular preload. Circulation 1990;81:1319-1330.
4. De Bruyne B, Bartunek J, Stanislas US, et al. Feasibility and hemodynamic dependency of invasive indexes of coronary stenosis. Circulation 1995;92:I-324.
5. Claeys MJ, Vrints CJ, Bosmans JM, Cools F, et al. Coronary flow reserve measurement during coronary angioplasty in the infarct related vessel. Circulation 1995;92:I-326.

421. Answer: a (true)

422. Answer: b, c, d

Comparison of Imaging and Doppler Techniques

	Digital Angiography	Angioscopy	IVUS	Doppler Flowire
Vessel lumen detail	+	++++	++	-
Vessel wall detail	-	-	++++	-
Vessel dimensions	++	-	++++	-
Coronary flow	++	-	+	++++
Borderline lesions	+	++	+++	++++
Ostial lesions	+	-	+++	++
Detect diffuse disease	+	+++	++++	-
Suboptimal results	+	+++	+++	+++
Clot vs dissection	±	++++	+++	-
Continuous record	-	-	-	+++
Predict complications	+	Possible	Possible	+++
Predict restenosis	±	-	Possible	Possible
Microvascular disease	-	-	-	+++
Cause ischemia	-	+++	++	-

Abbreviation: IVUS = intravascular ultrasound
- = no value
± = limited value
+ - ++++ = increasing value

423. Answer: a, b, d

CFR is a reliable means of assessing the physiologic significance of intermediate or borderline lesions.[1-12] CFR can often identify the "culprit" lesion in patients with multivessel coronary disease who present with "unstable" angina without ECG changes, and can be used to identify borderline lesions requiring intervention. Normal translesional velocity gradient and/or CFR suggest the presence of non-flow-limiting obstruction(s); intervention may be safely deferred in such lesions.[13,14]

Answers

References:
1. Gould KL, Lipscomb K, Hamilton GW. Physiologic basis for assessing critical coronary stenosis. Am J Cardiol 1974;33:87-94.
2. Gould KL, Lipscomb K, Calvert J. Compensatory changes of the distal coronary vascular bed during progressive coronary constriction. Circulation 1975;51:1085-1094.
3. Kirkeeide R, Gould KL, Parsel L. Assessment of coronary stenoses by myocardial imaging during coronary vasodilation. VII. Validation of coronary flow reserve as a single integrated measure to stenosis severity accounting for all its geometric dimensions. J Am Coll Cardiol 1986;7:103-113.
4. Gould KL, Kirkeeide R, Buchi M. Coronary flow reserve as a physiologic measure of stenosis severity. Part I. Relative and absolute coronary flow reserve during changing aortic pressure. Part II. Determination from arterographic stenosis dimensions under standardized conditions. J Am Coll Cardiol 1990;15:459-474.
5. Demer L, Gould KL, Kirkeide RL. Assessing stenosis severity: Coronary flow reserve, collateral function, quantitative coronary arteriography, position imaging, and digital subtraction angiography: a review and analysis. Prog Cardiovasc Dis 1988;30:307-322.
6. Gould KL. Identifying and measuring severity of coronary artery stenosis: quantitative coronary arteriography and position emission tomography. Circulation 1988;78:237-245.
7. Wilson RF, Marcus ML, White CW. Prediction of the physiologic significance of coronary arterial lesions by quantitative lesion geometry in patients with limited coronary artery disease. Circulation 1987;75:723-732.
8. Donohue TJ, Kern MJ, Aguirre FV, Bach RG, et al. Assessing the hemodynamic significance of coronary artery stenosis. Analysis of translesional pressure-flow velocity relations in patients. J Am Coll Cardiol 1993;22:449-458.
9. Kern MJ, Aguirre FV, Bach RG, Caracole EA, Donohue TJ. Translesional pressure-flow velocity assessment in patients: Part I. Cathet Cardiovasc Diagn 1994;313:49-60.
10. Kern MJ, Deligonul, Tatineni S, Serota H, et al. IV adenosine continuous infusion and low dose bolus administration for determination of coronary vascular reserve in patients with and without coronary artery disease. J Am Coll Cardiol 1991;18:718-729.
11. Miller DD, Donohue TJ, Younis LT, Bach RG, et al. Correlation of pharmacologic Technesium 99m-Sestamibi myocardial perfusion imaging with post-stenotic coronary flow reserve in patients with angiographically intermediate coronary artery stenoses. Circulation 1994;89:2150-2160.
12. Joye JD, Schulman DS, Lesorde D, Farah T, et al. Intracoronary Doppler guide wire versus stress single-photon emission computer tomographic thallium 201 imaging in assessment of intermediate coronary stenoses. J Am Coll Cardiol 1994;24:940-947.
13. Kern MJ, Donohue TJ, Aguirre FV, Bach RG, et al. Clinical outcome of deferring angioplasty in patients with normal translesional pressure-flow velocity measurements. J Am Coll Cardiol 1995;25:178-187.
14. Lesser JT, Wilson RF, White CW. Physiologic assessment of coronary stenosis of intermediate severity can facilitate patient selection for coronary angioplasty. Coronary Art Dis 1990;1:697-705.

424. Answer: a, b, c

425. Answer: a (true)

Since conditions associated with impaired microcirculation have little regional variability, normal CFR in a vessel without an epicardial stenosis reliably excludes small vessel disease as a cause of decreased CFR in a vessel with a significant epicardial stenosis.

426. Answer: a (2); b (1); c (4); d (3)

EXCIMER LASER CORONARY ANGIOPLASTY

427. Answer: a, b, c

The name "excimer" is an acronym for e*x*cited di*mer*. Laser energy is produced when the active medium (e.g. HCl gas) is excited by electrical energy and emits monochromatic, coherent light. Laser energy can be emitted as a continuous or pulsed wave. The excimer laser emits pulsed ultraviolet laser light at 308 mm. Excimer laser energy ablates inorganic material by photochemical mechanisms that involve the breaking of molecular bonds without generation of heat.[1] In vivo, the precise mechanism of tissue ablation is unknown, but it probably consists of photochemical, localized thermal, and mechanical effects. Some ultrasound studies in humans have demonstrated lumen enlargement due to atheroablation and vessel expansion,[2] while others demonstrate little or no plaque ablation.[3] In blood or radiographic contrast, ultraviolet laser energy is avidly absorbed, inducing significant acoustic effects, tissue disruption, and dissection.[4] Accordingly, ELCA should be performed only after blood and contrast are displaced from the coronary artery.

References:
1. Grundfest WS, Segalowitz J, Laudenslager J, et al. The physical and biological basis for laser angioplasty: In coronary laser angioplasty. Litvack F (ed), Blackwell Scientific Publications, 1992.
2. Mintz GS, Kovach JA, Javier SP, et al. Mechanisms of lumen enlargement after excimer laser coronary angioplasty: An intravascular ultrasound study. Circulation. 1995;92:3408-3414.
3. Honye J, Mahon DJ, Nakamura S, Wallis J, et al. Intravascular ultrasound imaging after excimer laser angioplasty. Cathet Cardiovasc Diagn 1994;32:213-222.
4. van Leeuwen TG, Meertens JH, Velema E, et al. Intraluminal vapor bubble induced by excimer laser pulse causes microsecond arterial dilation and invagination leading to extensive wall damage in the rabbit. Circulation 1993;87:1258-1263.

428. Answer: a, b, c

Conventional excimer laser catheters are front-firing, concentric, and track over conventional coronary angioplasty guidewires. The current concentric designs use greater than 200 individual, small fibers concentrically arranged around the guidewire lumen. Limitations of concentric catheters include the inability to treat highly eccentric lesions on an inner curve of a severe bend; the catheter may deflect off the plaque and into the normal wall, resulting in dissection and/or perforation. Other limitations include the need for definitive lumen enlargement by PTCA or stenting. To overcome some of these limitations, the directional excimer laser catheter has been developed. The catheter shaft has an eccentric fiberoptic bundle opposite the guidewire lumen, which runs through a tapered tip. During the procedure, the catheter is rotated so the fiberoptic bundle is in contact with the plaque; the guidewire and protective tip are positioned along the normal wall. Directional ELCA allows selective ablation of eccentric plaque, minimizing injury to the normal wall.

Excimer Laser Catheters

Catheter Type	Diameter mm	Diameter French	Guidewire* (inch)	Guide ID * (inch)	Vessel Diameter* (mm)
Over-the-Wire					
Extreme	1.4	4.3	0.014	0.084	2.4
Extreme	1.7	4.7	0.018	0.084	2.7
Extreme	2.0	5.9	0.018	0.092	3.0
Monorail					
Vitesse	1.4	4.3	0.014	0.072	2.4
Vitesse	1.7	4.7	0.018	0.080	2.7
Vitesse	2.0	5.9	0.018	0.092	3.0

Abbreviations: F = French; ID = internal diameter; * = maximum guidewire, minimum guide ID, maximum vessel diameter

Answers

429. Answer: b (False)

Currently available excimer laser catheters cannot be used to revascularize target lesions which cannot be crossed with a guidewire. However, a laser guidewire (Prima™) has been developed for crossing chronic total occlusions. This wire has a shapeable tip and 12 individual front firing, small diameter (45 micron) laser fibers running through it. The device is currently in clinical trial in the U.S. and Europe.[1]

References:
1. Serruys PW, Leon MB, Hamburger JN, et al. Recanalization of chronic total coronary occlusions using a laser guide wire: The European and US total experience. J Am Coll Cardiol 1996;March Special Issue.

430. Answer: b, c, d

Early randomized clinical trials showed similar angiographic results for conventional PTCA and ELCA, but restenosis rates were higher after ELCA. In the Dutch AMRO study,[1-3] there were no differences in angiographic success, dissection, or perforation; however, there was a 10-fold higher incidence of transient vessel occlusion and a trend toward higher restenosis after ELCA. However, lesions >20 mm were excluded. The German ERBAC study[4] randomized complex lesions to conventional PTCA, ELCA and Rotablator; higher rates of acute complications and restenosis were observed after ELCA compared to PTCA. However, chronic total occlusions and long lesions were excluded (these were unsuitable for Rotablator). These studies may have been biased against ELCA because of failure to use the saline-infusion technique.

Dutch AMRO Study: Comparison of ELCA and Conventional PTCA[1-3]

	PTCA (n = 157)	ELCA (n = 151)
Angiographic Success (%)	79	80
Angiographic Complications (%)		
Dissection	55	47
Spasm	1	4
Perforation	1	3
Transient Occlusion	0.7	7*
Clinical Events at 6 months (%)		
Death	0	0
Myocardial Infarction	5.7	4.6
Coronary artery bypass surgery	10.8	10.6
Repeat PTCA	18.5	21.2
Overall clinical events	29.9	33
Restenosis stenosis > 50%	41.3	51.6

* p = 0.005

References:
1. Foley DP, Appelman YE, Piek JJ on behalf of the AMRO group. Comparison of angiographic restenosis propensity of excimer laser coronary angioplasty (ELCA) and balloon angioplasty (BA) in the Amsterdam Rotterdam (AMRO) Trial. Circulation 1995;92: I-477.
2. Koolen J, Appelman Y, Strikwerda S, et al. Initial and long-term results of excimer laser coronary angioplasty versus balloon angioplasty in functional and total coronary occlusions. Eur Heart Journal 1994:832.
3. Appelman YEA, Piek JJ, Strikwerda S, et al. Randomized trial of excimer laser angioplasty versus balloon angioplasty for treatment of obstructive coronary artery disease. Lancet 1996;347:79-84.
4. Reifart N, Vandormael M, Krajear M, Gohring S, Preusler W, Schwart F, Storger H, Hofmann M, Klopper J, Muller S, Haase J. Randomized comparison of angioplasty of complex coronary lesions at a single center. Excimer laser, rotational atherectomy, and balloon angioplasty comparison (ERBAC) study. Circulation 1997;96:91-98.

431. Answer: a, b, c

The saline infusion technique eliminates blood and contrast from the laser field, resulting in a significant decrease in dissection.[1,2] In addition, many operators are now using smaller laser probes and slightly larger balloons to achieve better angiographic results, as well as the directional laser for lesions unfavorable for the conventional laser.[3]

ELCA Results: Influence of Saline Infusion Technique[1]

	Saline	No Saline
Baseline Stenosis (%)	79	71
ELCA Success (%)	97	96
Dissection (%)	7	24

References:
1. Deckelbaum LI, Natarajan MK, Bittl JA, et al. For the percutaneous excimer laser coronary angioplasty (PELCA) investigators: Effect of intracoronary saline infusion on dissection during excimer laser coronary angioplasty: A randomized trial. J Am Coll Cardiol 1995;26:1264-9.
2. Tcheng JE, Wells LD, Phillips HR, et al. Development of a new technique for reducing pressure pulse generation during 308-nm excimer laser coronary angioplasty. Cathet Cardiovasc Diagn 1995;34:15-22.
3. Rechavia E, Federman J, Shefer A, et al. Usefulness of a prototype directional catheter for excimer laser coronary angioplasty in narrowings unfavorable for conventional excimer or balloon angioplasty. Am J Cardiol 1995;76:1144-1146.

432. Answer: a

The new Prima™ laser wire was designed to treat total occlusions refractory to conventional PTCA guidewires.[1]

References:
1. Hamburger JN, Gomes R, et al. Recanalization of chronic total coronary occlusions using a laser guidewire: The European TOTAL multicenter surveillance study. J Am Coll Cardiol 1997;29(Suppl A):69A.

433. Answer: a, b, c, d

It is reasonable to exchange for a more flexible, smaller catheter. Never apply additional laser energy if dissection has occurred. If the 1.4 mm catheter cannot cross a rigid lesion on a straight segment of the artery, the energy density may be increased to 60 mJ/mm^2, or the frequency increased to 30 Hz, to facilitate crossing. If the catheter will not cross, ELCA should be abandoned, and another revascularization technique should be employed.

434. Answer: c

The saline infusion technique has been shown to decrease the incidence of dissection, but has little influence on procedural success and restenosis. A special pressurized flush solution is recommended for Rotablator and TEC, but not ELCA; saline infusion is performed by hand-injection.

435. Answer: a, b

Administer heparin (10,000-15,000 units as IV bolus) to obtain (and maintain) an ACT > 300 sec. Aspirin is recommended in all patients; there are no data to suggest utility of intracoronary verapamil or ReoPro.

436. Answer: a, c

Coaxial alignment of the guiding catheter with the vessel ostium is crucial, especially when treating ostial lesions. When the guiding catheter is not coaxial with the vessel, the laser catheter may be difficult to advance and control. Improper guide catheter alignment may also lead to misalignment of the laser catheter tip when addressing lesions in the proximal vessel. Short-tipped guiding catheters are generally more easily aligned than long-tipped guiding catheters. In most cases, conventional large lumen, soft-tip, non-aggressive guiding catheters are recommended (unless anatomic variations require more aggressive designs); special guiding catheters are not manufactured by Spectranetics.

Guiding Catheter Sizing Recommendations

Laser Catheter	Guide Catheter (minimum ID)*
1.4mm	7F (≥ .072") or 8F (ID .076")
1.7mm	8F large lumen (≥ .080")
2.0mm	9F large lumen (≥ .092")

437. Answer: a (true)

In the majority of cases, .014"-.018" guidewires have been used in conjunction with ELCA. For the Extreme® family of over-the-wire laser catheters, a 300cm exchange-length guidewire is recommended to facilitate transfer to adjunctive devices. The use of guidewire dimensions < .014" decreases the ability to approach and align the laser catheter; larger diameter guidewires with stiffer characteristics may enhance trackability and laser alignment, depending on the lesion geometry.

Guidewire Recommendations

Laser Catheter	Guidewire Compatibility
1.4mm	≤ .014" guidewire
1.7mm	≤ .018" guidewire
2.0mm	≤ .018" guidewire
1.7 mm Vitesse E II	≤ 0.14" guidewire

438. Answer: a, b, c, d

Excimer laser energy levels depend on plaque composition (hard vs. soft) and vessel type (native coronary vs. saphenous vein graft). The two energy settings are the fluence (40-60 mJ/mm^2) and repetition rate (20-40 Hz). When fluence is increased, the potential for ablating tissue at higher densities is increased. When the pulse repetition rate is increased, the cutting rate is increased. In general, if there is resistance due to ancillary equipment (guiding catheter or guidewire) these issues should be resolved first. If resistance is due to lesion density, increase the fluence prior to the next lasing train, then increase the repetition rate, if necessary. The Spectranetics CVX-300 excimer laser system is equipped with computer software which enables custom (push-button) adjustment of energy parameters during the laser procedure without the need for recalibration. This allows the physician to quickly adjust and control the energy to treat a variety of lesions (utilized in the same manner that a physician adjusts pressure and duration for balloon inflations).

Energy Parameters for Excimer Laser Ablation

Lesion/Vessel characteristics:	Fluence (mJ/mm)	Rate (H$_z$)
De Novo (Restenotic) Lesions in Native Vessels	50 (45)	25
If lesion resistance is encountered increase fluence	60	25
Continued lesion resistance, increase repetition rate	60	40
When area of resistance is passed, reduce settings	50	25
Bypass Graft Lesions	40	25
If resistant to ablation, increase fluence	50	25
Continued resistance, increase fluence further	60	25
If still resistant, increase repetition rate	60	40
Reduce energy when resistance is passed	50	25

Lesion/Vessel characteristics:	Fluence (mJ/mm)	Rate (H$_z$)
Ostial Lesions	50	25
If calcified and resistant to ablation increase repetition rate	60	40
If non-calcified and resistant to ablation increase fluence	60	25
Reduce energy when resistance is passed	50	25

439. Answer: a (true)

The laser catheter must be *in contact* with the target lesion at the time of lasing. For the Vitesse-E II eccentric catheter, align the fiber face to the bulk of the lesion by slowly rotating the torque knob until the slot in the radiopaque tip is visible. If necessary, inject contrast to help position the tip of the laser catheter. If contrast is trapped between the catheter tip and the lesion, retract the catheter 1-2 mm, and flush with saline to allow antegrade flow and egress of contrast. However, before lasing, ensure the laser catheter tip is in contact with the lesion.

440. Answer: b (false)

Prior to activating the CVX-300 Excimer Laser System, it is imperative to flush and rinse all residual contrast from the lasing site and all ancillary equipment (extension tubes, manifold, injection syringe, Y adapter, guiding catheter). Introducing excimer laser energy into a field of contrast media (with a concentration as low as 0.3%) can result in acoustic shockwaves and dissection. Since 10% contrast is not detectable by fluoroscopy, an aggressive, conscientious approach to flushing contrast away from the lasing site is mandatory.

441. Answer: a

The lasing sequence (train) should last for 2-5 seconds (maximum 5 seconds) and the laser catheter advanced at 1 mm/sec. For longer lesions, the catheter tip is often embedded in the lesion at the end of a lasing train. Several trains may be required to treat the entire lesions; each train should be proceeded by a bolus of saline and performed with continuous saline infusion; terminate the saline injection at the end of the lasing train, and refill the control syringe with 20cc of saline in preparation for the next lasing sequence. Any electrocardiographic changes induced by saline infusion should be permitted to resolve before repeating the sequence.

442. Answer: a (true)

443. Answer: a (true)

Lesions involving a significant sidebranch (> 2.0mm) should not be treated with ELCA; the presence of a bifurcation lesion is an important predictor of complications.

444. Answer: a, b

It is difficult to assess the degree of vessel calcification by fluoroscopy. Mild calcification (confirmed by IVUS) is amenable to ELCA, using short laser trains (~ 3 seconds) and high energy densities (50-60 mJ/mm^2). In contrast, severe calcification is not amenable to ELCA using currently recommended energy densities; Rotablator is preferred.

445. Answer: a, b, c

Eccentric lesions are best treated with the eccentric laser catheter, to maximize the efficiency of laser ablation and minimize vessel injury. In general, the laser fiber should not exceed 70% of the normal reference vessel diameter. Laser trains of 3-4 seconds at energy densities of 50 mJ/mm^2 are recommended. Adjunctive PTCA or other devices are routinely necessary for definitive lumen enlargement.

446. Answer: b (false)

Focal lesions are readily treated by ELCA, although there may not be any advantage compared with PTCA or other techniques.

447. Answer: a, c

Long lesions are amenable to ELCA. The laser fiber should not exceed 70% of the normal reference vessel diameter. Laser trains of 3-5 seconds at energy densities of 45-50 mJ/mm^2 are recommended. When the laser fiber is near the end of the lesions, laser trains should be decreased to < 3 seconds to minimize the chance of lasing the normal vessel segment. There is no known restenosis advantage for ELCA.

448. Answer: c

Aorto-ostial lesions are readily treated by ELCA. Coaxial guiding catheter alignment is extremely important. Energy densities usually start at 50 mJ/mm^2 for noncalcified lesions (native vessels or saphenous vein grafts), and 60 mJ/mm^2 for calcified lesions. The saline infusion technique is mandatory for all lesions.

449. Answer: b (false)

Branch-ostial lesions are amenable to ELCA, as long as the branch originates at a mild angle from the parent vessel. Angulated branches, particularly at the origin of the left circumflex, should be treated with caution, if at all, with ELCA.

450. Answer: b (false)

Nondegenerated vein graft (particularly aorto-ostial) lesions are amenable to ELCA. A 2.0 mm laser fiber is recommended in most grafts to achieve maximal debulking, at energy densities of 40-50 mJ/mm^2. There is relatively little experience with ELCA in degenerated vein grafts. However, some operators have found that a 2.0 mm laser catheter at a fluence of 40-50 mJ/mm^2 may be useful for debulking prior to more definitive lumen enlargement. Thrombolytic therapy should be considered prior to ELCA when thrombus is suspected.

451. Answer: b (false)

Total occlusions are amenable to ELCA if they can be crossed by a guidewire. However, ELCA should not be performed if there is any question of subintimal wire passage or guidewire-induced dissection. In most cases, the initial laser fiber should not exceed 1.4 mm. Selected chronic total occlusions that cannot be crossed with a guidewire may be considered for the excimer laser guidewire (investigational device in the United States).

CORONARY INTRAVASCULAR ULTRASOUND

452. Answer: a, b

Unlike angiography, which displays the coronary artery as a silhouette of the contrast-filled lumen, IVUS generates a cross-sectional tomographic image of the lumen and vessel wall. IVUS equipment consists of two principal components: A catheter with a miniaturized transducer, and a console to reconstruct the image. IVUS catheters range in size from 2.9-3.5F (0.96-1.17 mm). Excellent image quality is a result of high operating frequency (20-30 MHZ) and close proximity of the transducer to the target; nominal axial and lateral resolution are approximately 0.08 mm and 0.20 mm, respectively. Special software can be installed to reconstruct 3-dimensional images.

Intravascular Ultrasound Systems

Manufacturer	Type	Diameter (F)	Frequency (MHZ)	Catheter Configuration	Ultrasound Scanner
Boston Scientific	Mechanical	3.5	30	Short Monorail; No Sheath	HP Sonos 100™
	Mechanical	3.0	30	Shared Lumen; Moveable Imaging Core in Sheath	HP Sonos 100™
	Mechanical	2.9	30	Shared Lumen; Moveable Imaging Core in Sheath	CVIS Clearview™ or HP Sonos 100™
	Mechanical	3.2	30	Short Monorail; Moveable Imaging Core in Sheath	CVIS Clearview™ or HP Sonos 100™
Endosonics Corporation	Synthetic Phased Array	3.5	20	Monorail or over-the-wire	Endosonics Cathscanner™

Boston Scientific products are marketed by Scimed Life Systems

453. Answer: a, b, c, d

Mechanical devices employ an external motor and drive shaft to rotate a single piezoelectric transducer mounted near the distal end of the catheter. Mechanical transducers typically operate at 1800 rpm, which yields 30 frames per second. Excellent image quality is associated with a high operating frequency (30 MHz).

454. Answer: a, b, c, d

Synthetic phased array devices employ an annular array of 32-64 elements mounted near the distal tip of the catheter. Advantages of this design include excellent flexibility, absence of rotational artifacts, and excellent guidewire tracking; however, many experts feel that the image quality of synthetic phased array devices is inferior to mechanical devices. A unique version of an electronic IVUS catheter employs an imaging transducer mounted proximal to a standard angioplasty balloon; this device was recently approved by the FDA (Oracle-Micro ™ Endosonics Corp) and allows examination of the vessel before and after PTCA, without a catheter exchange. Despite their current limitations, synthetic phased array devices have tremendous potential; once perfected, the small size, lack of moving parts, and freedom from rotational artifacts may allow these transducers to be readily coupled to a variety of interventional devices.

Answers

455. Answer: a (true)

The normal coronary artery has been characterized by IVUS.[1-3] With low frequency transducers (20 MHz), the vessel lumen is sonolucent; at higher frequencies (≥ 30 MHz), blood appears as faint, finely textured specular echoes that move and swirl during active blood flow. Blood echogenicity assists image interpretation by identifying the communication between tissue planes and the lumen, thereby confirming the presence of a dissection channel; lumen echogenicity can identify the lumen-wall interface.

References:
1. Nissen SE, Gurley JC, Grines CL, Booth DC, et al. Intravascular ultrasound assessment of lumen size and wall morphology in normal subjects and coronary artery disease patients Circulation 1991;84:1087-1099.
2. St. Goar FG, Pinto FJ, Alderman EL, Fitzgerald PJ, et al. Detection of coronary atherosclerosis in young adult hearts using intravascular ultrasound, Circulation 1992;86:756-763.
3. Fitzgerald PJ, St. Goar FG, Connolly AJ, Pinto JF, et al. Intravascular ultrasound imaging of coronary arteries. Is three layers the norm? Circulation 1992;86:154-158.

456. Answer: a, b, c, d

Normal coronary artery morphology consists of a circular lumen surrounded by distinct layers exhibiting variable echogenicity.[1-3] Some normal vessels demonstrate three discrete vessel wall layers: 1) an inner layer, which represents the internal elastic lamina; 2) a middle sonolucent layer, which represents the media; and 3) an outer layer, which has a characteristic "onionskin" appearance and represents the adventitia and peri-adventitial tissues. About 50% of normal coronary arteries have a monolayered appearance. At frequencies ≥ 30 MHZ, blood echogenicity can be used to identify the path of blood flow.

References:
1. Nissen SE, Gurley JC, Grines CL, Booth DC, et al. Intravascular ultrasound assessment of lumen size and wall morphology in normal subjects and coronary artery disease patients Circulation 1991;84:1087-1099.
2. St. Goar FG, Pinto FJ, Alderman EL, Fitzgerald PJ, et al. Detection of coronary atherosclerosis in young adult hearts using intravascular ultrasound, Circulation 1992;86:756-763.
3. Fitzgerald PJ, St. Goar FG, Connolly AJ, Pinto JF, et al. Intravascular ultrasound imaging of coronary arteries. Is three layers the norm? Circulation 1992;86:154-158.

457. Answer: d

Advantages of IVUS

Precise quantitative measurements

    Lumen diameter

    Reference vessel diameter

    Cross-sectional area (CSA)

Characterization of plaque

    Distribution

        Eccentric

        Concentric

    Composition

        Soft plaque

        Fibrous plaque

        Calcified plaque

        Mixed plaque

        Depth of calcium (deep vs. superficial)

    Dissection

        Severity of lumen compromise

        Length of dissection

458. Answer: a (true)

Patients with coronary disease have a wide spectrum of abnormal features reflecting the distribution, severity, and composition of the atheroma.[1-4] Mild lesions are characterized by intimal thickening ≤ 0.30 mm; often missed by angiography, these lesions are readily identified by IVUS. Advanced lesions appear as large echogenic masses that encroach upon the lumen.

References:
1. Nissen SE, Gurley JC, Grines CL, Booth DC, et al. Intravascular ultrasound assessment of lumen size and wall morphology in normal subjects and coronary artery disease patients Circulation 1991;84:1087-1099.
2. Fitzgerald PJ, St. Goar FG, Connolly AJ, Pinto JF, et al. Intravascular ultrasound imaging of coronary arteries. Is three layers the norm? Circulation 1992;86:154-158.
3. Tobis JM, Mallery J, Mahon D, Lehmann K, et al. Intravascular ultrasound imaging of human coronary arteries in vivo. Analysis of tissue characterizations with comparison to in vitro histological specimens. Circulation 1991;83:913-926.
4. Nissen SE, Tuzcu EM, De Franco AC. Coronary intravascular ultrasound: Diagnostic and interventional applications. In: Topol EJ ed. Update to Textbook of Interventional Cardiology, W B Saunders, Philadelphia, PA, pages 207-222, 1994.

459. Answer: a, c

"Soft" plaques are less echogenic than surrounding adventitia due to their high lipid content; "fibrous" plaques have echodensity similar to adventitia *(in vitro* studies demonstrate that increasing echogenicity correlates with fibrous tissue content); and "calcified" lesions are more echogenic than surrounding adventitia. Calcified plaques attenuate transmission of the ultrasound signal and obscure architectural detail of deeper layers ("acoustic shadowing"), ultrasound is more sensitive than fluoroscopy in detecting and localizing calcium.

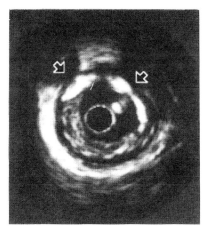 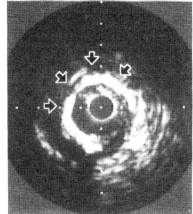

Hard Calcified Atheroma with Acoustic Shadowing

460. Answer: b (false)

All available ultrasound devices generate artifacts that can adversely affect image quality. The external motor drive and transducer must rotate in a precise one-to-one relationship to generate accurate images; mechanical transducers exhibit cyclical oscillations in rotational speed, or *non-uniform rotational distortion* (NURD) due to mechanical drag on the catheter drive-shaft. NURD is most evident when the drive-shaft bends in a small radius of curvature (such as tortuous vessel), and is recognized as "stretching" and compression of the image. In contrast, geometric distortion arises when the ultrasound beam is not perpendicular to the vessel wall, making the circular lumen appear elliptical.

461. Answer: a (true)

Transducer ring-down arises from acoustic oscillations that obscure the near-field imaging; inability to image structures immediately adjacent to the transducer yields a device with an "acoustic" size larger than its physical size.

462. Answer: a (true)

Visual interpretation of IVUS images is dependent upon differences in acoustic impedance of adjacent tissues. Although currently available devices produce remarkably detailed views of the vessel wall, image reconstruction is based upon acoustic reflections, not actual histology. The acoustic properties (echogenicity) of different histologic entities may appear similar.

463. Answer: c

Calcified plaques attenuate transmission of the ultrasound signal and obscure architectural detail of deeper layers ("acoustic shadowing").

464. Answer: c

Although angioscopy requires blood-free field, IVUS does not.

465. Answer: b

A sonolucent lesion may represent intracoronary thrombus or soft atherosclerotic plaque with a high lipid content. The identification of thrombus by IVUS is often unreliable and inferior to angioscopy.

466. Answer: a, b, c

Serious untoward effects are uncommon.[1] Transient coronary spasm occurs in 5% of patients, but responds rapidly to intracoronary nitroglycerin. The imaging transducer may cause transient ischemia when imaging severe stenoses or small vessels, but usually resolves after catheter withdrawal. Despite the safety of IVUS, any intracoronary instrumentation carries the risk of vessel injury; the necessary personnel and equipment should be immediately available to restore vessel patency. Intravenous heparin is recommended prior to IVUS, but the ideal ACT level is unknown.

References:
1. Nissen SE, Gurley JC, Grines CL, Booth DC, et al. Intravascular ultrasound assessment of lumen size and wall morphology in normal subjects and coronary artery disease patients Circulation 1991;84:1087-1099.

467. Answer: b, c

IVUS can detect atherosclerosis at sites that appear angiographically normal;[1] this angiographic appearance may be due to compensatory remodeling of the vessel wall.[2] IVUS provides precise quantitation of stenoses independent of the radiographic projection,[3] and can clarify the severity of angiographically borderline lesions. Angiography is still the "gold standard" for assessment of left main stenoses, despite greater accuracy of IVUS. IVUS can readily characterize ostial and bifurcation lesions, which may be particularly difficult to image by angiography. Identification of cardiac allograft atherosclerosis is important and clinically challenging since most patients do not experience angina. Many centers now routinely perform IVUS at the time of annual catheterization.[4]

References:
1. Nissen SE, De Franco AC, Raymond RE, Franco I, et al. Angiographically unrecognized disease at "normal" reference sites: a risk factor for sub-optimal results after coronary interventions. Circulation 1993;88:I-412A.
2. Glagov S, Weisenberg E, Zarins CK et al. Compensatory enlargement of human coronary arteries. N Engl J of Med 1987;316:1371-1375.
3. White CJ, Ramee SR, Collin TJ, Jain A, Mesa JE. Ambiguous coronary angiography: clinical utility of intravascular ultrasound. Cathet Cardiovasc Diagn 1992;26:200-203.
4. Tuzcu EM, Hobbs H, Rincon G, Bott-Silverman C, et al. Occult and frequent transmission of atherosclerosis coronary disease with cardia transplantation. Circulation 1995; 91:1706-1713.

468. Answer: d

Uses of IVUS: Interventional Applications

Definite uses

- Precise vessel sizing for device sizing

- Precise characterization of plaque for device selection

- Assess severity of borderline lesions

- Understanding mechanisms of lumen enlargement

Possible uses

- Predict complications

- Predict restenosis

- Guide "optimal" stenting or atherectomy

Not useful

- Unreliable identification of thrombus

---

469. Answer: a

IVUS facilitates greater lumen enlargement than angiography alone because of its precision in estimating vessel dimensions. However, a clear need for IVUS has not yet been demonstrated;

further studies are needed to determine if IVUS-guided intervention will improve immediate and long-term outcome compared to angiography-guided therapy.

470. Answer: b, c, d

IVUS is very useful for identifying the mechanisms of lumen enlargement after all devices. IVUS has shown that dissection represents the most common mechanism of luminal enlargement after PTCA, but stretching of the vessel wall constitutes the principal or exclusive mechanism in some patients;[1,2] lumen enlargement from plaque "compression" or redistribution is an unusual mechanism of PTCA. In contrast to balloon angioplasty, plaque removal is the primary mechanism of luminal enlargement after directional coronary atherectomy; however, tissue removal is incomplete since 40-60% of the cross-sectional area of the target lesion is still occupied by plaque.[3,4] IVUS has also shown that Rotablator works by plaque ablation, ELCA results in dissection and minimal vessel expansion without plaque ablation, and stenting results in the greatest lumen enlargement and virtually eliminates elastic recoil.

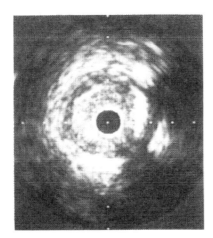 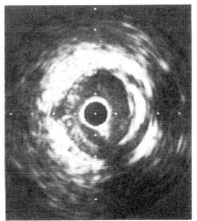

IVUS Before and After DCA

Although the angiogram shows an eccentric lesion, IVUS demonstrates a concentric plaque (left). There is little residual plaque after DCA (right).

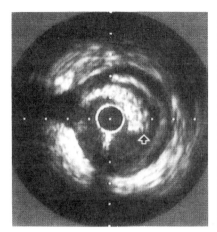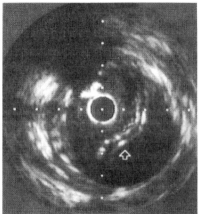

Complex Dissection After PTCA

A deep dissection (black arrow, left) is associated with a large intimal flap (black arrow, right)

References:
1. Waller BF: "Crackers, breakers, stretchers, drillers, scrapers, shavers, burners, welders, and melters": The future treatment of atherosclerotic coronary artery disease? A clinical-morphologic assessment. J Am Coll Cardiol 1989;13:969-87.
2. DeFranco AC, Tuzcu E, Abdelmeguid A, Lincoff AM, et al. Intravascular ultrasound assessment of PTCA results: Insights into the mechanisms of balloon angioplasty. J Am Coll Cardiol 1993,21:485A.
3. Popma JJ, Mintz GS et al. Clinical and angiographic outcome after directional coronary atherectomy. A qualitative and quantitative analysis using angiography and intravascular ultrasound. Am J Cardiol 1994;72:55E-64E.
4. DeFranco AC, Tuzcu EM, Moliterno DJ, et al. "Directional" coronary atherectomy removes atheroma more effectively from concentric than eccentric lesions: intravascular ultrasound predictors of lesional success. J Am Coll of Cardiol 1995;25:137A.
5. Kovach JA, Mintz GS, Pichard AD, Kent KM, et al. Sequential intravascular ultrasound characterization of the mechanism of rotational atherectomy and adjunct balloon angioplasty. J Am Coll Cardiol 1993;22:1024-1032.

471. Answer: a, c

Therapeutic decisions often hinge upon assessment of lumen dimensions, stenosis severity, diameter of the "normal" reference diameter, and the gain in lumen diameter after intervention. Precise quantitation of vascular dimensions represents an important application of IVUS. Angiographic and IVUS studies after PTCA reveal a poor correlation of final lumen diameter. Since angiographically "normal" segments often have occult atherosclerosis,[1] this could lead to undersizing of devices by angiography. However, there are no prospective data to document a need for device sizing by IVUS, either to improve safety or reduce late cardiac events.

References:
1. Nissen SE, De Franco AC, Raymond RE, Franco I, et al. Angiographically unrecognized disease at "normal" reference sites: a risk factor for sub-optimal results after coronary interventions. Circulation 1993;88:I-412A.

472. Answer: b (false)

"Optimal" directional coronary atherectomy involves the use of atherectomy and adjunctive PTCA to achieve final diameter stenoses < 15%. Although the Optimal Atherectomy Restenosis Study (OARS) suggested that IVUS can be used to achieve optimal results, the Balloon vs. Optimal Atherectomy Trial (BOAT) demonstrated that similar results could be achieved without IVUS.

473. Answer: a, b

IVUS studies have demonstrated that despite excellent angiographic appearance, some stents are incompletely apposed to the vessel wall and/or asymmetrically expanded. A single-center, retrospective analysis suggested that the level of systemic anticoagulation may be safely reduced if optimal stenting is confirmed by IVUS; these IVUS observations have led to the routine use of high-pressure balloons to fully deploy stents. While IVUS-guidance can further enlarge lumen dimensions after routine high-pressure balloon inflations,[1] results from the AVID (Angiography vs. Intravascular ultrasound-Directed Stent Placement) trial have not shown a beneficial effect on 30-day clinical event rate (longterm results are pending).[2] Other randomized studies (STARS, Stent Anticoagulation Regimen Study) are in progress to determine the value of IVUS as an adjunct to stenting, and for identifying suitable patients for low-intensity anticoagulation regimens.

IVUS Criteria for Optimal Stent Deployment

Stent Result	Gap*	CSA Index**	Symmetry Index***
Inadequate	> 0.3 mm	< 0.6	< 0.5
Marginal	0.1 - 0.3 mm	0.6 - 0.8	0.5 - 0.7
Optimal	< 0.1 mm	≥ 0.8	> 0.7

*   Gap = Maximum distance between stent strut (or coil) and underlying wall
**   CSA Index = ratio of minimal cross-sectional area (CSA) of stent/CSA of normal reference vessel (average CSA proximal and distal to stent)
*** Symmetry Index = ratio of stent minor diameter/stent major diameter

References.
1. Russo RJ, Teirstein PS. Angiography versus intravascular ultrasound-directed stent placement. J Am Coll Cardiol 1996;27:306A.
2. Goldberg SL, Hall P, Nakamura S, et al. Is there a benefit from intravascular ultrasound when high-pressure stent expansion is routinely performed prior to ultrasound imaging? J Am Coll Cardiol 1996;27:306A.

474. Answer: c, e

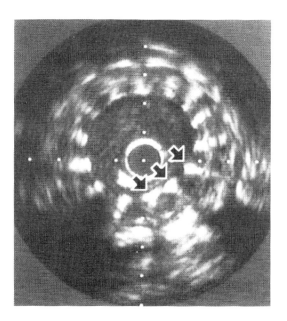

Suboptimal Stent Deployment

After deployment of a Palmaz-Schatz stent at 18 atmospheres, several stent struts are not opposed to the vessel wall (black arrows); subsequent inflations with a larger balloon resulted in optimal stent deployment.

475. Answer: c

476. Answer: b (false)

Anginal chest pain in the absence of significant epicardial coronary atherosclerosis may be due to Syndrome-X (microvascular disease), and is readily detected by evaluation of coronary blood flow using the Doppler Flowire.

477. Answer: b, c, d, e

Comparison of Imaging and Doppler Techniques

	Digital Angiography	Angioscopy	IVUS	Doppler Flowire
Vessel lumen detail	+	++++	++	-
Vessel wall detail	-	-	++++	-
Vessel dimensions	++	-	++++	-
Coronary flow	++	-	+	++++
Borderline lesions	+	++	+++	++++
Ostial lesions	+	-	+++	++
Detect diffuse disease	+	+++	++++	-
Suboptimal results	+	+++	+++	+++
Clot vs dissection	±	++++	+++	-
Continuous record	-	-	-	+++
Predict complications	+	Possible	Possible	+++
Predict restenosis	±	-	Possible	Possible
Microvascular disease	-	-	-	+++
Cause ischemia	-	+++	++	-

Abbreviation: IVUS = intravascular ultrasound
- = no value; ± = limited value; + - ++++ = increasing value

478. Answer: a (6); b (5); c (4); d (3); e (2); f (1)

479. Answer: b (false)

Ultrasound catheters may be used for ultrasound examination of coronary arteries and bypass grafts; the risk of no-reflow is probably similar to other devices.

480. Answer: a, b, c, d, e

Complications after IVUS are rare, but include arterial dissection, perforation, abrupt closure, death, unstable angina, myocardial infarction, ventricular fibrillation, and air embolism.

Peripheral Vascular Disease

481. Answer: a

It is helpful to consider peripheral vascular obstruction in three anatomic zones: The inflow tract, the outflow tract, and the runoff bed.

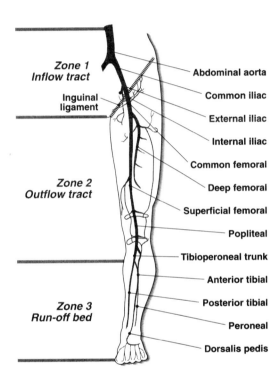

Arterial Circulation of the Lower Extremity

Zone 1: In-flow tract (abdominal aorta, common iliac artery, and external iliac artery)
Zone 2: Out-flow tract, extends from the inguinal ligament to the knee (common femoral artery, superficial femoral and popliteal artery)
Zone 3: Run-off bed (anterior tibial artery, posterior tibial artery, and peroneal artery)

482. Answer: b

The abdominal aorta and common and external iliac arteries make up the inflow tract to the lower extremities.

483. Answer: b

Diffuse atherosclerosis is often present throughout the infrarenal aorta; the most severe lesions are typically found at the aortic bifurcation involving the origin of the common iliac arteries, or at the iliac bifurcation involving the origin of the external and internal iliac arteries. Aorto-iliac disease usually causes claudication in the hips and buttocks, but may extend into the thighs and calves with further exertion. Femoral artery pulses may or may not be diminished, depending on the degree of proximal obstructive disease;[1] however, the quality of the femoral pluses does not correlate with stenosis severity.

References:
1. Glover JL, Bendick PJ, Dilley RS, et al. Efficacy of balloon catheter dilatation for lower extremity atherosclerosis. Surgery 1982;91:560-565.

484. Answer: b

The outflow tract extends from the inguinal ligament to just below the knee, and consists of the common femoral, superficial femoral, and popliteal arteries (the femoropopliteal system).

485. Answer: b, d

The common femoral artery and the mid segment of the popliteal artery are often spared; the superficial femoral artery may be involved throughout its length, and the most critical lesions frequently occur near the adductor hiatus. [1]

References:
1. Rutherford RB. Evaluation and selection of patients for vascular surgery. In Rutherford RB (Ed). Vascular Surgery, Third Edition. WB Saunders, Philadelphia, 1989;10-16.

486. Answer: a

The runoff bed consists of the anterior tibial artery, posterior tibial artery and peroneal artery (the trifurcation vessel system) in the lower leg.

487. Answer: a

The proximal segments of the tibioperoneal vessels are frequently diseased, limiting distal runoff to the foot.

488. Answer: a, b, c, d

Diabetic patients comprise a unique population: One-third of diabetics with peripheral atherosclerotic lesions have disease limited to the lower leg trifurcation vessels; one-third have disease limited to the aortoiliac or femoro-popliteal vessels; and one-third have multiple segmental disease involving the inflow, outflow and runoff systems. [1,2]

References:
1. Bendick PJ, Glover JL, Kuebler TJ, et al. Progression of atherosclerosis in diabetics. Surgery 1983;93:834-838.
2. Krajewski LP, Olin JW. Atherosclerosis of the aorta and lower extremity arteries, In Young JR, Graor RA, Olin JW, et al. Peripheral Vascular Diseases. Mosby, St Louis, 1991;179-200.

489. Answer: a

Isolated trifurcation vessel lesions in diabetic patients are often not amenable to surgical bypass; small diameter balloon catheters provide an alternative endovascular approach.

490. Answer: b

The clinical history will determine the likelihood of ischemia and the degree of functional impairment; the quality of pulses will help localize the site(s) of obstruction, but is unreliable for estimating disease severity. [1]

References:
1. Strandness DE Jr. Noninvasive vascular laboratory and vascular imaging. In Young JR, Graor RA, Olin JW, et al. Peripheral Vascular Diseases. Mosby, St Louis, 1991;39-69.

491. Answer: a, c

Objective data are provided by the ankle-brachial index (ABI), defined as the ratio of systolic pressure in the ankle to the upper arm. [1-3] Brachial systolic pressure should be measured in both arms; the higher value is used to calculate the right and left ABI. Ankle systolic pressures are measured with a standard adult blood pressure cuff (12 x 23 cm bladder) wrapped snugly around the ankle, with the lower edge of the cuff just above the malleoli. While using a Doppler pencil probe to monitor the signal from the posterior or anterior tibial artery, inflate the cuff to 30 mmHg above systolic pressure to temporarily occlude flow; as the cuff is slowly deflated (2 - 4 mmHg per second), the pressure at which a Doppler flow signal is heard is recorded as the ankle systolic pressure.

References:
1. Yao JST. Hemodynamic studies in peripheral arterial disease. Br J Surg 1970;57:761-770.
2. Bridges RA, Barnes RW. Segmental limb pressures. In Kempczinski RF, Yao JST (Eds). Practical Noninvasive Vascular Diagnosis, Second Edition. Year Book Medical Publishers, Chicago, 1987;112-126.
3. Binnington HB. Segmental limb pressures, doppler waveforms, and stress testing. In Hershey FB, Barnes RW, Sumner DS (Eds). Noninvasive Diagnosis of Vascular Disease. Appleton Davies, Pasadena, California, 1984;16-23.

492. Answer: a, b

Excellent noninvasive evaluation is provided by duplex ultrasound, which allows direct real-time ultrasound imaging of obstructive lesions and simultaneous assessment of hemodynamic significance by Doppler. The entire peripheral arterial tree from the abdominal aorta to the tibial arteries can be surveyed if necessary. The Doppler flow signals can be subjectively graded and stenosis severity can be estimated using Doppler velocity spectra. [1-4]

References:
1. Jager KA, Ricketts HJ, Strandness DE Jr. Duplex scanning for the evaluation of lower limb disease. In Bernstein EF (Ed). Noninvasive diagnostic techniques in vascular disease. Mosby, St Louis, 1985;619-631.
2. Kohler TR, Nance DR, Cramer M, et al. Duplex scanning for diagnosis of aortoiliac and femoropopliteal disease: a prospective study. Circulation 1987;76:1074-1080.
3. Strandness DE Jr. Duplex scanning in vascular disorders. Raven Press, New York,1990;121-145.
4. Bandyk DF. Postoperative surveillance of infrainguinal bypass. In Pearce WH, Yao JST (Eds). Surg Clin NA 1990;70:71-85.

493. Answer: b

The North American Symptomatic Carotid Endarterectomy Trial (NASCET) and Asymptomatic Carotid Artery Stenosis (ACAS) studies showed benefit for surgical management of symptomatic patients with carotid stenosis > 60% and asymptomatic patients with carotid stenosis > 70%.

494. Answer: a

At present, the most sensitive indicator is the absolute peak velocity at end-diastole at the site of stenosis; velocity >100 cm/sec suggests a high likelihood of severe stenosis, and further workup is warranted.

495. Answer: a (6); b (5); c (4); d (3); e (2); f (1)

Correlation of Ankle-Brachial Index (ABI) with Clinical Presentation and Severity of Obstructive Lesions

ABI	Symptoms	Disease Severity
> 1.30	Indeterminate	Medial wall calcification; nondiagnostic
0.90 - 1.25	Asymptomatic	No hemodynamically significant lesions
0.60 - 0.90	Claudication	Single segment stenosis or well-collateralized occlusion
0.30 - 0.60	Claudication	Multiple segment disease
0.15 - .030	Resting pain	Multiple segment total occlusions
< 0.15	Impending tissue loss	Multiple segment total occlusions, poor runoff

496. Answer: a, b, c, d

Qualitative Assessment of Doppler Flow Signals (Lower Extremity)

Flow Pattern	Characteristics	Significance
Normal	Multiphasic flow signal with a brisk, well-defined high pitched systolic peak; lower pitched signals during diastole; transient reversal of flow during early diastole.	No significant obstruction

497. Answer: b, c, d

Qualitative Assessment of Doppler Flow Signals (Lower Extremity)

Flow Pattern	Characteristics	Significance
Damped	Slow systolic upstroke with a poorly defined systolic peak; slowly diminishing flow from systole through diastole, with antegrade flow during the entire cardiac cycle.	Significant proximal obstruction

498. Answer: a

Qualitative Assessment of Doppler Flow Signals (Lower Extremity)

Flow Pattern	Characteristics	Significance
Absent	No flow signal	Total vessel occlusion; absent collateral reconstitution

499. Answer: b

Doppler Velocity Criteria for Grading Severity of Internal Carotid Artery Stenosis

Diameter Stenosis (%)	Spectrum Characteristics
< 20	No increase in V_p relative to proximal arterial segment; minimal spectral broadening.
20 - 49	>30% increase in V_p relative to proximal artery segment; V_p <125 cm/sec; spectral broadening throughout pulse cycle.
50 - 75	>100% increase in V_p relative to proximal arterial segment; V_p <125 cm/sec; spectral broadening throughout pulse cycle.
> 75	Spectrum similar to 50-75% diameter stenosis, with end-diastolic velocity > 100 cm/sec.

Abbreviations: V_p = Peak systolic velocity

500. Answer: b

The renal arteries, celiac axis and superior mesenteric artery (SMA) may all be evaluated at their origin from the abdominal aorta using duplex ultrasound techniques.[1]

References:
1.   Vascular Technology, vol ii of vascular registry review and vascular educational program, 1995. Society of Vascular Technology, Lanham, MD.

501. Answer: a, b, c

The Doppler flow signal from the aorta just above the renal artery is used as a reference signal to determine the Renal/Aortic Ratio (RAR); absolute velocities are used in the celiac trunk and SMA. Patients should be fasting for at least eight hours prior to an abdominal vascular examination.

502. Answer: b

Following a caloric challenge, (e.g., 16 oz. Ensure) vascular resistance in the gut decreases sharply, with an attendant increase in end diastolic flow velocity. In the normal mesenteric circulation, the SMA end diastolic velocity should at least double (compared to fasting) within 30 minutes of a caloric challenge.

503. Answer: b, d

A systolic pressure difference $\geq$ 20 mm Hg between the two arms suggests significant subclavian artery obstruction; reversal of flow in the ipsilateral vertebral artery is diagnostic for hemodynamically significant subclavian stenosis. Direct evaluation of the subclavian artery by duplex ultrasound will show post-stenotic turbulence for subtotal lesions, or a damped flow waveform indicative of collateral reconstitution.

504. Answer: b

Aspirin should be given at least 24 hours before PTA.

505. Answer: a

Nifedipine 10 mg SL and intra-arterial Nitroglycerin (NTG) 100-200 mcg are recommended before crossing target lesions in the renal artery and infrapopliteal vessels, to minimize spasm.

Answers

506. Answer: b

Duplex Ultrasound Diagnostic Criteria for the Carotid, Renal and Mesenteric System[1]

Arterial System	Duplex Criteria*
Carotid artery	Absolute Peak Velocity > 100 cm/sec at end-diastole at the lesion site.
Renal artery	Renal/Aortic Ratio (RAR) > 3.5, and Peak Systolic Velocity > 180 cm/sec.
Celiac trunk	Peak Systolic Velocity > 200 cm/sec.
Superior mesenteric artery (SMA)	Peak Systolic Velocity > 275 cm/sec; failure to increase post-prandial end-diastolic velocity by at least two-fold compared to fasting velocity (within 30 minutes).

* Significant stenosis is defined as renal artery stenosis > 60%; iliac or SMA stenosis > 70%

References:
1.   Vascular Technology, vol ii of vascular registry review and vascular educational program, 1995. Society of Vascular Technology, Lanham, MD.

507. Answer: a, b, d

Indications and Contraindications for Peripheral Vascular Intervention[1,2]

Target Vessel	Indications	Relative Contraindications	Absolute Contraindications
Aorta[20,21]	• Short stenoses of infrarenal aorta without other aortic disease • Buttock or lower extremity claudication or impotence	• Stenoses > 4 cm in infrarenal aorta • Stenoses resulting in blue-toe syndrome • Stenoses 2-4 cm in length associated with diffuse infrarenal atherosclerosis	• Total occlusion of aorta • Stenoses associated with abdominal aortic aneurysm

References:
1.   Standards of practice committee of the society of cardiovascular and interventional radiology. Guidelines for percutaneous transluminal angioplasty. Radiology 1990; 177: 619-626.
2.   Schwarten DE, Tadavarthy SM, Casta–eda-Zu–iga WR. Aortic, iliac, and peripheral arterial angioplasty. Castaneda-Zuniga WR. Tadavarthy SM (eds). Interventional Radiology. 2ed. Williams & Wilkins, Baltimore, 1992; 378-421.

508. Answer: a, b, c, d

Indications and Contraindications for Peripheral Vascular Intervention[1,2]

Target Vessel	Indications	Relative Contraindications	Absolute Contraindications
Peripheral Artery	• Intermittent claudication • Critical limb ischemic (rest pain, ulceration, gangrene, poor wound healing) • Improve inflow or outflow, before or after vascular bypass surgery • Bypass graft stenosis or anastomotic lesion • Impending amputation (to improve the level)	• Ulcerated plaque with atheroemboli • Long total occlusion (iliac > 4 cm, SFA > 10 cm), unless converted to shorter occlusions by thrombolysis • Long segment of infrapopliteal disease • Heavy, eccentric calcification • Lesion in or adjacent to an essential collateral	• Mild-moderate stenosis with no significant pressure gradient (>10 mm Hg, at rest, > 20 mm Hg after priscoline • Stenosis immediately adjacent to an aneurysm • Embolic occlusions

References:
1. Standards of practice committee of the society of cardiovascular and interventional radiology. Guidelines for percutaneous transluminal angioplasty. Radiology 1990; 177: 619-626.
2. Schwarten DE, Tadavarthy SM, Casta–eda-Zu–iga WR. Aortic, iliac, and peripheral arterial angioplasty. Castaneda-Zuniga WR. Tadavarthy SM (eds). Interventional Radiology. 2ed. Williams & Wilkins, Baltimore, 1992; 378-421.

509. Answer: a

Indications and Contraindications for Peripheral Vascular Intervention[1-13]

Target Vessel	Indications	Relative Contraindications	Absolute Contraindications
Renal Artery	• Renovascular Hypertension: correction of a stenosis > 50%, resting pressure gradient > 10 mm Hg or occlusion associated with refractory hypertension or documentation of renovascular hypertension • Renal Insufficiency: deterioration of renal function or asymmetric decrease in real size, and renal artery stenosis > 50% • Recurrent pulmonary edema: due to bilateral renal artery stenosis • Renal transplant arterial stenosis or bypass stenosis producing hypertension, azotemia, or both	• Long occlusion • Stenosis associated with renal artery aneurysm • Atherosclerotic stenoses involving ostia (some authors recommend initial angioplasty, others advocate primary stenting) • Stenosis in renal artery arising from severely diseased or aneurysmal aorta	• Irreversible renal dysfunction • Hemodynamically insignficiant stenosis • Medically unstable patient • Renal size < 6 cm

References:
1. Becker GJ, Katzen BT, Dake, MD. Noncoronary angioplasty. Radiology, 1989;170:921-940.
2. Pickering TG. Diagnosis and evaluation of renovascular hypertension: indications for therapy. Circulation 1991; 83: I-147--I-154.
3. Tegtmeyer Cj, Kellum CD, Ayers A. Percutaneous transluminal renal angioplasty of renal arteries: Results and long term follow-up. Radiol 1984; 153: 77-84
4. Sos TA, Pickering TG, Sniderman K, et al. Percutaneous transluminal renal angioplasty for renovascular hypertension due to atherosclerosis and fibromuscular dysplasia. N Engl J Med 1983; 309 274-279.

Answers

5. Gerlock AJ, MacDonnell RC Jr, Smith CW, et al. Renal transplant arterial stenosis: Percutaneous transluminal angioplasty. Am J Roentgen 1983; 140: 325-331.
6. Miller GA, Ford KK, Braun SD, et al. Percutaneous transluminal angioplasty vs. surgery for renovascular hypertension. Am J Roentgen 1985; 144: 447-450.
7. Kuhlman U, Greninger P, Gruntzig A, et al. Long term experience in percutaneous transluminal dilation of renal artery stenosis. Am J Med 1985; 79: 692-698.
8. Martin LG, Casarella WJ, Gaylord GM. Azotemia caused by renal artery stenosis: treatment by percutaneous angioplasty. Am J Roentgen 1988; 150: 839-844.
9. Pickering TG, Sos TA, Saddekni S, et al. Renal angioplasty in patients with azotemia and renovascular hypertension. J Hypertension 1986; 4: s667-s669.
10. Pickering TG, Sos Ta, Vaughan ED, Case DB, Sealey JE, Harshfield GA, Laragh JH. Predictive value and changes of renin secretion in hypertensive patients with unilateral renovascular disease undergoing successful renal angioplasty. Am J Med 1984; 76: 398-404.
11. Martin EC, Mattern RF, Baer L et al. Renal angioplasty for hypertension: predictive factors for long term success. Am J Roentgen 1981; 137:921-924.
12. Sos TA. Angioplasty for the treatment of azotemia and renovascular hypertension in atherosclerotic renal artery disease. Circulation 1991; 83: I-162--I-166.
13. Pickering TG, Devereux RB, James GD, et al. Recurrent pulmonary edema in hypertension due to bil;ateral renal artery stenosis: treatment by angioplasty or surgical revascularization. Lancet 1988; 9: 551-552.

510. Answer: a

Indications and Contraindications for Peripheral Vascular Intervention[1,2]

Target Vessel	Indications	Relative Contraindications
Visceral/Mesenteric	• Chronic mesenteric ischemia (unexplained weight loss with postprandial pain and chronic nausea, vomiting, diarrhea) with significant stenoses or occlusion of two or more visceral vessels or acute symptoms in a patient who is not a surgical candidate. At this time surgery remains the first line of treatment	• Stenoses > 3 cm or ostial lesions of the superior mesenteric or celiac arteries • Occlusion of visceral vessels • Acute mesenteric ischemia

References:
1. Sniderman, KW. Transluminal angioplasty in the management of chronic intestinal ischemia. In DE Strandness and A Van Breda (eds), vascular diseases: surgical and interventional therapy. New York: Churchill Livingstone, 1994. pp. 803-809.
2. Roberts L, Wertman DA, Mills SR, et al: Transluminal angioplasty of the superior mesenteric artery: an alternative to surgical revascularization. Am J Roentgen 141: 1039, 1983.

511. Answers: b, c, d

Arterial access should be achieved as close as possible to the target lesion. Retrograde punctures are made with Seldinger or single wall techniques; antegrade puncture is most commonly performed with a single wall technique. Axillary and brachial artery punctures are typically performed with a single wall technique using a Potts-Cournand needle; alternatively, a micropuncture set may cause less arterial spasm. Placement of an appropriate arterial sheath facilitates exchange of catheters and guidewires.

512. Answer: a

This contralateral route often provides a better angle for reaching iliac artery branches, for dilating distal iliac and proximal femoral artery lesions, for thrombolytic therapy of occluded femoro-popliteal grafts, and for gaining access to distal femoral artery branches when the ipsilateral antegrade approach is difficult. Catheterization is performed by retrograde puncture of the contralateral femoral artery, initially advancing a guidewire up the iliac, then using a Cobra catheter, Simmons sidewinder, or internal mammary artery catheter to direct the wire down the opposite iliac artery. A stiff teflon-coated guidewire (Amplatz or Rosen guidewire) may be used to further advance the catheter around the bifurcation; an alternative technique is to use a flow-directed balloon catheter.

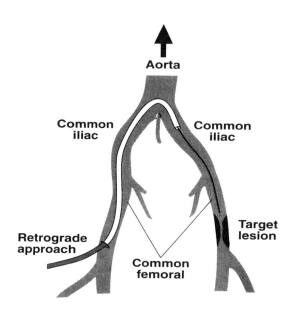

Peripheral Angioplasty: Contralateral Femoral Artery Approach

513. Answer: a

Site of Vascular Access for Peripheral Vascular Interventions

Arterial Approach	Target Lesion Location
Retrograde femoral*	Aorta, common iliac, proximal external iliac, renal, visceral
Antegrade femoral*	Superficial femoral, profunda femoral, popliteal, infrapopliteal
Contralateral femoral (retrograde)+*	Internal iliac and its branches, distal external iliac, common femoral; can be used for fem-pop vessels if antegrade approach is not feasible
Left brachial ++	Indicated if femoral access is not feasible
Left axillary +++	Indicated if all other routes are not available

   *   Arterial puncture is over the femoral head
   +   Internal mammary, Simmons sidewinder, or Cobra catheter may be used to hook the contralateral iliac artery
   ++ Nifedipine 10 mg SL may be given to prevent spasm
   +++ Puncture over the humeral head

514. Answer: a

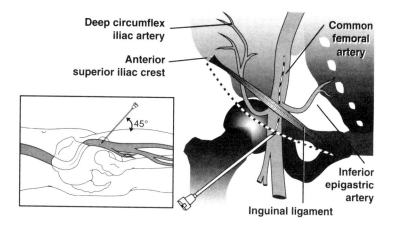

Common Femoral Artery: Retrograde Puncture

515. Answer: b

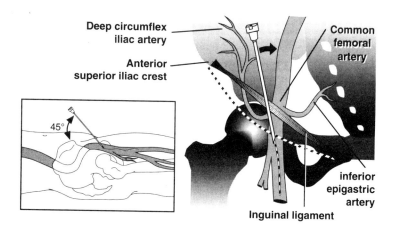

Common Femoral Artery: Antegrade Puncture

516. Answer: a

The axillary approach is used when there is no femoral artery access, and if there is no stenosis in the subclavian or axillary arteries. This approach may be useful for gaining access to sharply angulated lesions at the origin of the renal or mesenteric arteries.

517. Answer: b

Radiographic Views for Peripheral Angiography and Intervention[1]

Vessel	Radiology Film-Screen	Cine/DSA
Carotid bifurcation	Lateral and AP (with head turned to opposite extreme)	AP/oblique or lateral
Aortic arch (to open arch)	AP and RPO	AP and LAO
Aortic arch (for brachycephalic vessels)	45° RPO with head turned, chin raised, shoulders dropped down	45° LAO
Origins of mesenteric vessels	Lateral aorta	Lateral
Origin of renal arteries	Left: 15° RPO Right: 15° LPO	Left: 15° LAO* Right: 15° RAO*
Common iliac bifurcation	Ipsilateral posterior oblique	Right: 15-30° LAO* Left: 15-30° RAO*
Common femoral bifurcation	Contralateral posterior oblique	Right: 15-30° RAO* Left: 15-30° LAO*

Abbreviations: DSA = digital-subtraction angiography; AP = anteroposterior; RPO = right posterior oblique; LPO = left posterior oblique; LAO = left anterior oblique; RAO = right anterior oblique
* Varying degrees of cranial and caudal angulation may be necessary

References:
1. Kandarpa, K. Handbook of cardiovascular and interventional radiologic procedures, 1st ed. Little, Brown and Company, Boston, 1989.

518. Answer: a, b, c, e

Long-acting antihypertensive medications should be discontinued; short acting drugs should be substituted. Vascular surgery back-up is recommended for renal artery interventions. Guiding catheters (7-9F) facilitate selective angiography, wire manipulations, catheter exchanges, PTA, and stent placement, if necessary; high pressure polyethylene balloons are useful. Blood pressure and renal function must be closely monitored before, during, and after the procedure.

519. Answers: a

Renal angioplasty is technically more difficult than iliac or peripheral angioplasty; failures usually result from inability to cross the lesion or elastic recoil. Slightly oversized balloon may reduce the

Answers

incidence of restenosis.[1] Several large series[1-6] reported angiographic success in 79-96% and a favorable blood pressure response in 80-90%. If a good initial result is obtained, the renal arteries may remain patent in 70-93% of patients for up to 6 years. Procedural success and long-term results are dependent upon lesion location, morphology and underlying pathology: Fibromuscular dysplasia is associated with excellent initial and long-term results; atherosclerotic stenoses are associated with a higher incidence of restenosis.[1,7-12] Procedural success has been reported in 75-100% of non-ostial stenoses;[1,7-9,13-24] total occlusions or ostial stenoses have lower success rates, with success in 25% in one study.[25] Some interventionalists recommend primary stenting in ostial lesions,[26,27] but further study is needed. Restenosis occurs in approximately 15% of non-ostial lesions[27] these patients may be treated with repeat PTA, with similar initial and long-term results.

Results of Percutaneous Renal Artery Angioplasty

Series	No.	Initial Success (%)	Long-Term Patency (%)	Follow-up (months)
Tegtmeyer[1] (1984)	149	94	93*	72
Sos[2] (1983)	101	79	-	-
Colapinto[3] (1982)	68	85	81	36
Puijlaert[5] (1981)	54	96	70	-
Schwarten[6] (1981)	70	93	71	6
Katzen[4] (1979)	17	94	75	12

Abbreviation: - = not reported
* Includes successful redilatations

References:
1. Tegtmeyer CJ, Kellum CD, Ayers C. Percutaneous transluminal angioplasty of the renal artery: results and long-term follow-up. Radiol 1984;153:77
2. Sos TA, Pickering TG, Sniderman K, et al. Percutaneous transluminal renal angioplasty for renovascular hypertension due to atherosclerosis and fibromuscular dysplasia. N Engl J Med 1983; 309 274-279.
3. Colapinto RF, Stronell RD, Harries-Jones EP, et al. Percutaneous transluminal dilatation of the renal artery: follow-up studies on renovascular hypertension. Am J Roentgen 1982;139:727-732.
4. Katzen BT, Chang J, Knox WG. Percutaneous transluminal angioplasty with the gruntzig balloon catheter: a review of 70 cases. Arch Surg 1979;114:1389-1399.
5. Puijlaert CBAJ, Boomsma JHB, Ruijs JHJ, et al. Transluminal renal artery dilatation in hypertension: technique, results and complications in 60 cases. Urol Radiol 1981;2:201-210.
6. Schwarten DE. Percutaneous transluminal renal angioplasty. Urol Radiol 1981;2:193-200.
7. Tegtmeyer Cj, Kellum CD, Ayers A. Percutaneous transluminal renal angioplasty of renal arteries: Results and long term follow-up. Radiol 1984; 153: 77-84.
8. Miller GA, Ford KK, Braun SD, et al. Percutaneous transluminal angioplasty vs. surgery for renovascular hypertension. Am J Roentgen 1985; 144: 447-450.
9. Sos TA. Angioplasty for the treatment of azotemia and renovascular hypertension in atherosclerotic renal artery disease. Circulation 1991; 83: I-162-- I-166.
10. Tegtmeyer CJ, Sos TA. Techniques of renal angioplasty. Radiol 1986; 161: 577-586.
11. Tegtmeyer CJ, Sos TA. Percutaneous transluminal angioplasty of the renal arteriea. In WR Castenada-Zuniga and SM Tadavarthy (eds), interventional radiology (2nd ed). Baltimore: Williams & Wilkins 1992.pp364-377.
12. Losinno, F, Zuccala, A; Busato, F: Zuccali. Renal artery angioplasty for renovascular hypertension and preservation of renal funtion: long-term angiographic and clinical follow-up. Am J Roentgen 1994;16.2:853-7.

13. Pickering TG, Sos TA, Saddekni S, et al. Renal angioplasty in patients with azotemia and renovascular hypertension. J Hypertension 1986; 4: s667-s669.
14. Pickering TG, Sos Ta, Vaughan ED, Case DB, Sealey JE, Harshfield GA, Laragh JH. Predictive value and changes of renin secretion in hypertensive patients with unilateral renovascular disease undergoing successful renal angioplasty. Am J Med 1984; 76: 398-404.
15. Martin EC, Mattern RF, Baer L et al. Renal angioplasty for hypertension: predictive factors for long term success. Am J Roentgen 1981; 137:921-924.
16. Pickering TG, Devereux RB, James GD, et al. Recurrent pulmonary edema in hypertension due to bil;ateral renal artery stenosis: treatment by angioplasty or surgical revascularization. Lancet 1988; 9: 551-552.
17. Sniderman, KW. Transluminal angioplasty in the management of chronic intestinal ischemia. In DE Strandness and A Van Breda (eds), vascular diseases: surgical and interventional therapy. New York: Churchill Livingstone, 1994. pp. 803-809.
18. Roberts L, Wertman DA, Mills SR, et al: Transluminal angioplasty of the superior mesenteric artery: an alternative to surgical revascularization. Am J Roentgen 141: 1039, 1983.
19. Kaufman SL, Barth KH, Kadir S. et al. Hemodynamics measurements in the evaluation and follow-up of transluminal angioplasty of the iliac and femoral arteries. Radiol 1982; 142: 329-336.
20. Becker GJ. Femoropopliteal angioplasty, atherectomy, stents. Second international symposium on cardiovascular and ind interventional radiology. Harvard Medical School/Brigham and Women's Hospital, Vol. 1, 1994: 53-65.
21. Johnston KW. Femoral and popliteal arteries: reanalysis of results of balloon angioplasty. Radiol 1992; 183: 767-771.
22. Gardiner GA, Meyerovitz MF, Stokes KR, Clouse ME, Harrington DP, Bettmann MA. Complications of transluminal angioplasty. Radiol. 1986; 159: 201-208.
23. Werbull H, et al. Complications after percutaneous transluminal angioplasty in the iliac, femoral and popliteal arteries. J Vasc Surg, 5: 681-686, 1987.
24. Plecha FR, et al. The early results of vascular surgery in patients 75 years of age and older: an analysis of 3259 cases. J Vasc Surg, 2: 767-774, 1985.
25. Sos TA, Pickering TG, Sniderman K, et al. Percutaneous transluminal renal angioplasty for renovascular hypertension due to atherosclerosis and fibromuscular dysplasia. N Engl J Med 1983; 309 274-279..
26. Thomson, KR. Longterm results of renal artery stenting: the Australian experience. Harvard Medical School/Brigham and Women's Hospital second international symposium on cardiovascular and interventional radiology. 1994, Vol I, 892-6.
27. Sos, Thomas. Renal angioplasty: optimal techniques, long-term results. Harvard Medical School/Brigham and Women's Hospital second international symposium on cardiovascular and interventional radiology. 1994, Vol. I, 75-75N.

520. Answer: b

Long-term Outcome After Renal Artery Angioplasty for Renovascular Hypertension

Series	Follow-up (months)	Etiology	Outcome (%)		
			Cured	Improved	No Response
Sos[2,4]	16	Fibromuscular Dysplasia	59	33	8
		Atherosclerotic	27	60	13
Tegtmeyer[1,5,6]	39	Fibromuscular Dysplasia	37	63	0
		Atherosclerotic	25	55	20
Miller[3]	6	Fibromuscular Dysplasia	85	15	0
		Atherosclerotic	25	58	17
Lossino[7]	60	Fibromuscular Dysplasia	57	21	21
		Atherosclerotic	12	51	37

References:
1. Tegtmeyer Cj, Kellum CD, Ayers A. Percutaneous transluminal renal angioplasty of renal arteries: Results and long term follow-up. Radiol 1984; 153: 77-84
2. Sos TA, Pickering TG, Sniderman K, et al. Percutaneous transluminal renal angioplasty for renovascular hypertension due to atherosclerosis and fibromuscular dysplasia. N Engl J Med 1983; 309 274-279.
3. Miller GA, Ford KK, Braun SD, et al. Percutaneous transluminal angioplasty vs. surgery for renovascular hypertension. Am J Roentgen 1985; 144: 447-

450.

4. Sos TA. Angioplasty for the treatment of azotemia and renovascular hypertension in atherosclerotic renal artery disease. Circulation 1991; 83: I-162--I-166.
5. Tegtmeyer CJ, Sos TA. Techniques of renal angioplasty. Radiol 1986; 161: 577-586.
6. Tegtmeyer CJ, Selby JB. Percutaneous transluminal angioplasty of the renal arteria. In WR Castenada-Zuniga and SM Tadavarthy (eds), interventional radiology (2nd ed). Baltimore: Williams & Wilkins 1992.pp364-377.
7. Losinno, F, Zuccala, A; Busato, F: Zuccali. Renal artery angioplasty for renovascular hypertension and preservation of renal funtion: long-term angiographic and clinical follow-up. Am J Roentgen 1994;16.2:853-7.

521. Answer: a

PTA of the aorta an iliac arteries has high success rates and a lower incidence of restenosis;[1-3] initial procedural success rates are 83-100% in the aorta and 73-100% in iliac arteries. Long-term patency at 5 years is 70-92% and 32-92%, respectively.

Results of Aortoiliac Angioplasty[1-3]

Target Vessel	Success (%)	Long-Term Patency (%)		
		1-year	2-year	3-year
Aorta	83 - 100	83 - 100	83 - 96	70 - 92
Iliac artery	73 - 100	63 - 100	58 - 95	32 - 92

References:
1. Capek P, Mclean GK, Berkowitz HD. Femoropopliteal angioplasty: Factors influencing long-term success. Circulation 1991; 83: I-70-I-80.
2. Rholl KS and von Breda A, percutaneous intervention for aortoiliac disease. In: Vascular Diseases: Surgical and Interventional Therapy. 1994, Churchill Livingston, New York.
3. Gallino A, Mahler F, Probst P, Nachbur B. Percutaneous transluminal angioplasty of the arteries of the lower limbs: a 5-year follow-up. Circulation 1984; 70: 619-623.

522. Answer: a, b, c

Results are best in the ilio-femoral system, with initial success in 90-95% and 3-year patency of 75-80%.[1-6] For focal subtotal stenoses of the common iliac artery in patients with claudication, 3-year patency is 90%.[2] Total iliac occlusions and stenoses > 10 cm in length lead to poor technical results and are not suitable for PTA.[3,6]

References:
1. Becker GJ, Katzen BT, Dake, MD. Noncoronary angioplasty. Radiology, 1989;170:921-940.
2. van Andel GJ, van Erp WF, Krepel VM et al. Percutaneous transluminal dilatation of the iliac artery: long-term results. Radiol 1985;156:321-323.
3. Johnston KW, Rae M, Hogg S, et al. 5-year results of a prospective study of percutaneous transluminal angioplasty. Ann Surg 1987;206:403-413.
4. Wilson SE, Wolf GL, Cross AP. Percutaneous transluminal angioplasty versus operation for peripheral arteriosclerosis: report of a prospective randomized trial in a selected group of patients. J Vasc Surg 1989;9:1-9.
5. Rutherford RB, Durham J. Percutaneous balloon angioplasty for arteriosclerosis obliterans: long-term results. In Yao JST, Pearce WH (Eds). Technologies in vascular surgery. W.B. Saunders, Philadelphia, 1992;329-345.
6. Colapinto RF, Stronell RD, Johnston KW. Transluminal angioplasty of complete iliac obstructions. Am J Roentgen 1986;146:859-862.

523. Answer: a, b, c, d

Results in the common femoral and popliteal arteries are consistently worse than in the aortoiliac arteries, with higher rates of early failure and restenosis. For femoro-popliteal disease, initial success is achieved in 85%; 3-year patency is approximately 60%.[1-5] The best results are in focal stenoses or total occlusions <3 cm in length with good distal runoff; 3-year patency for this group is 75%.[5,6] In contrast, PTA of occlusions ≥ 9 cm in length with poor distal run off is associated with 3-year patency of 20-25%.[6,7] Although long-term patency is significantly decreased when PTA is performed for limb salvage as opposed to claudication, PTA alone will provide adequate inflow for limb salvage in 34%; PTA combined with bypass surgery may result in limb salvage in 71% of patients. Factors favorably influencing long-term outcome include proximal, focal stenoses in patients with claudication; adverse factors include distal lesions, total occlusion, poor distal run-off, and symptoms of critical ischemia.[1,8-11] Long-term success is most influenced by distal run-off.

References:
1. Schwarten DE, Tadavarthy SM, Casta–eda-Zu–iga WR. Aortic, iliac, and peripheral arterial angioplasty. Castaneda-Zuniga WR. Tadavarthy SM (eds). Interventional Radiology. 2ed. Williams & Wilkins, Baltimore, 1992; 378-421.
2. Johnston KW, Rae M, Hogg S, et al. 5-year results of a prospective study of percutaneous transluminal angioplasty. Ann Surg 1987;206:403-413.
3. Rutherford RB, Durham J. Percutaneous balloon angioplasty for arteriosclerosis obliterans: long-term results. In Yao JST, Pearce WH (Eds). Technologies in vascular surgery. W.B. Saunders, Philadelphia, 1992;329-345.
4. Schwarten DE. Clinical anatomical considerations for non-operative therapy in tibial disease and the results of angioplasty. First international symposium on cardiovascular and interventional radiology. Harvard Medical School/Brigham and Women's Hospital , 1992: pp 196-205.
5. Berkowitz HD, Spence RK, Frieman DB, et al. Long-term results of transluminal angioplasty of the femoral arteries. In Dotter CT, Gruntzig A, Schoop W, et al. (Eds). Percutaneous transluminal angioplasty. Springer-Verlag, Berlin 1983;207-214.
6. Jeans WD, Armstrong S, Cole SE, et al. Fate of patients undergoing transluminal angioplasty for lower limb ischemia. Radiol 1990;177;559-564.
7. Rutherford RB, Patt A, Kumpe DA. The current role of percutaneous transluminal angioplasty. In Greenhalgh KM, Jamieson CW, Nicolaides AN (Eds). Vascular surgery: issues in current practice. Grune & Stratton, London, 1986;229-244.
8. Johnston KW. Femoral and popleteal arteries: reanalysis of results of balloon angioplasty. Radiol 1992; 183: 767-771.
9. Capek P, Mclean GK, Berkowitz HD. Femoropopliteal angioplasty: Factors influencing long-term success. Circulation 1991; 83: I-70-I-80.
10. Rholl KS and von Breda A, percutaneous intervention for aortoiliac disease. In: Vascular Diseases: Surgical and Interventional Therapy. 1994, Churchill Livingston, New York.
11. Gallino A, Mahler F, Probst P, Nachbur B. Percutaneous transluminal angioplasty of the arteries of the lower limbs: a 5-year follow-up. Circulation 1984; 70: 619-623.

524. Answers: b, c

Until recently, PTA at or below the popliteal trifurcation has been reserved for patients with critical ischemia (rest pain or tissue necrosis) or for patients with disabling claudication who were poor surgical candidates.[1-4] This reluctance to perform infrapopliteal PTA was based on early reports, which showed a high incidence of serious complications, and the belief that such complications frequently resulted in amputation of the affected limb. However, improvements in guidewire and balloon catheter technology, combined with better use of adjunctive medication has limited the frequency of serious complications. Technical success is approximately 95%; 1-year patency is 75-80%. In selected cases, PTA may be a useful adjunct for salvaging critically ischemic limbs.[5] There are limited data on the long term success of PTA in the infrapopliteal trifurcation vessels; the availability of modified coronary angioplasty catheters has increased the utilization of this technique.[6,7]

Results of Infrapopliteal Angioplasty

Series	No.	Success (%)			Complications (%)	
		Technical	Early	Late	Major	Minor
Bull[4] (1992)	168	83	77	67	11	8
Brown[2] (1988)	12	75	66	50	17	-
Schwarten[3] (1988)	98	97	88	86	2	1

Abbreviation: - = not reported

References:

1. Adar R, Critchfield GC, Eddy DM. A confidence profile analysis of the results of femoro-popliteal percutaneous transluminal angioplasty in the treatment of lower-extremity ischemia. J Vasc Surg 1989;10:57-67.
2. Brown KT, Schoenberg NY, Moore, ED, Saddekni S. Percutaneous transluminal angioplasty of infrapopliteal vessels: preliminary results and technical considerations. Radiol 1988; 169: 78-78.
3. Schwarten DE Cutcliff WB. Arterial occlusive disease below the knee: treatment with percutaneous transluminal angioplasty performed with low profile catheters and steerable guide wires. Radiol 1988; 169: 71-74.
4. Bull PG, Mendel H, Hold M, Schlegl A, Denck H, Distal popliteal and tibioperoneal tibioperoneal transluminal angioplasty: long-term follow-up. J Vasc Interv Radiol 1992; 3: 15-53.
5. Schwarten DE. Clinical and anatomical considerations for nonoperative therapy in tibial disease and the results of angioplasty. Circulation 1991;83:86-90.
6. Horvath W, Oertl M, Haidinger D. Percutaneous transluminal angioplasty of crural arteries. Radiol 1990;177:565-569.
7. Tamura S, Sniderman KW, Beinart C, et al. Percutaneous transluminal angioplasty of the popliteal artery and its branches. Radiol 1982;143:645-648.

525. **Answer: a**

Suboptimal results after PTA are due to elastic recoil and/or extensive dissection. Stents approved by the FDA in the iliac arteries are the Palmaz Stent (Johnson & Johnson, Warren, NJ) and the Schneider Wallstent (Schneider Stent Division, Pfizer, Minneapolis, MN).

526. **Answer: a, b, c, d**

Possible indications for stenting include eccentric lesions or total occlusions in the renal or iliac arteries; ostial renal artery stenoses; residual gradient > 10 mm Hg or stenosis > 30% post PTA; renal artery stenosis; and dissection or restenosis after PTA.[1-7]

References:

1. Thomson, KR. Long-term results of renal artery stenting: the Australian experience. Harvard Medical School/Brigham and Women's Hospital second international symposium on cardiovascular and interventional radiology. 1994, Vol I, 892-6.
2. Rutherford RB, Becker GJ. Standards for evaluating and reporting the results of surgical and percutaneous therapy for peripheral arterial disease. Radiol 1991; 181: 277-281.
3. Saeed M. Aortoiliac and Renal Artery Stenting. In: Kandarpa K and Aruny J, (eds). Handbook of interventional radiologic procedures, 2nd edition. Boston: Little Brown, 1996. pp. 103-114.
4. Richter GM, Roeren T, Brado M, Noeldge G. Renal artery stents: Long-term results of a European trial. Society of Cardiovascular and Interventional Radiology Meeting Abstracts, J. Vasc Interv Radiol, 4: 47, 1993.
5. Becker GJ, Palmaz JC, Rees CR, et al. Angioplasty-induced dissections in human iliac arteries: management with Palmaz balloon-expandable intaluminal stents. Radiol 1990; 176:31-38.
6. Rees CT, Palmaz JC, Garcia O, et al. Angioplasty and stenting of completely occluded iliac arteries. Radiol 1989; 172:953-959.
7. Williams JB, Watts PW, Nguyen VA, Peterson CL. Balloon angioplasty with intraluminal stenting vs the initial treatment modality in aortoiliac occlusive disease. Am J Surg 1994; 168:202-204.

527. Answer: a, b, c, d

Coexisting aneurysmal disease requiring surgical intervention; heavily calcified stenoses; nondilatable lesions; and extravasation of contrast following PTA are contraindications to peripheral stenting. Specific contraindications to renal artery stenting include non-functional kidney or size < 6 cm; diffuse intrarenal vascular disease; renal artery diameter <4 mm.[1]

References:
1. Saeed M. Aortoiliac and Renal Artery Stenting. In: Kandarpa K and Aruny J, (eds). Handbook of interventional radiologic procedures, 2nd edition. Boston: Little Brown, 1996. pp. 103-114.

528. Answer: a, c, d

Procedural success in the iliac and renal arteries is > 95%;[1-5] iliac artery patency at 5-years is 93% with stents and 70% for PTA.[1] The incidence of complications is approximately 5-10%, including renal failure; hematoma or pseudoaneurysm at the puncture site; systemic or intracranial hemorrhage due to anticoagulation; and branch artery occlusion.[6] There are now several small studies of stenting innominate, subclavian, and carotid arteries with angiographic success rates > 90% and a low incidence of complications;[7-9] longterm follow-up is pending.

Stents for Peripheral Vascular Disease

Series	Target	No.	Stent	Success (%)	Comments
Henry[3] (1995)	Femoral, Popliteal	126	PS	99.6	RS 13%; 4-year patency 88% for upper SFA, 44% for lower SFA and popliteal; 4-year patency 39% for total occlusions
White[4] (1995)	Renal	98	BE	99	SAT 1.4%; RF 2.7%; Vasc 2.7%; ARS 28%
Bacharach[5] (1995)	Renal	116	-	-	DUS patency 79% (9.5m); AP = 70% (9m)
Sullivan[7] (1995)	Subclavian, Innominate	33	PS	94	DE 6%; VAO 3%; Vasc 12%
Yadav[10]	Carotid	96	PS+GR	99	SAT 0%; no MI, or death; minor stroke 5%; RS 4.5%
Iyer[8] (1995)	Carotid	55	BE	100	SAT 0%
Dietrich[9] (1995)	Carotid	55	PS	94.5	Death 1.8%; TIA 3.6%; Vasc 18%; direct carotid puncture technique in 44%
Dietrich[11] (1995)	SFA	47	PS-ELG	98	Graft migration 4.3%; thrombosis 12.8%; Vasc 4.3%; 10 month patency 75%

Abbreviations: PS = Palmaz stent; GR = Gianturco-Roubin stent; BE = balloon expandable stent; PS-ELG = Palmaz stent-endoluminal graft (PTFE); DE = distal embolization ; VAO = vertebral artery occlusion; Vasc = vascular injury; SAT = subacute thrombosis; RF = renal failure; ARS = angiographic restenosis; DUS = duplex ultrasound; AP = angiographic patency; - = not reported

Answers

References:
1. Richter GM, Noeldge, G, Roeren, T et al. Further analysis of the randomized trial: Primary iliac stenting vs. PTA. Harvard Medical School (BWH 2nd Intl'l Symposium of CVIR. 1994, vol 1, 52-52 L.
2. Palmaz JC, Laborde JC, Rivera FJ, et al. Stenting of the iliac arteries with the Palmaz stent: experience from a multicenter trial. Cardiovasc Interven Radiol 1992; 15:291-297.
3. Henry M, Amor M, Henry I, Ethevenot G, et al. Placement of Palmaz-Schatz in femoropopliteal arteries: A 6-year experience. Factors influencing restenosis and longterm results. Circulation 1995;92:I-58.
4. White CJ, Ramee SR, Collins TJ, Jenkins JS, et al. Stent placement for unfavorable renal artery stenosis. Circulation 1995;92:I-129.
5. Bacharach JM, Olin JW, Sullivan TM, Childs MB, Piedmonte M. Renal artery stents: Early patency and clinical followup. Circulation 1995;92:I-128.
6. Saeed M. Aortoiliac and Renal Artery Stenting. In: Kandarpa K and Aruny J, (eds). Handbook of interventional radiologic procedures, 2nd edition. Boston: Little Brown, 1996. pp. 103-114.
7. Sullivan TM, Bacharach JM, Childs MB. PTA and primary stenting of the subclavian and innominate arteries. Circulation 1995;92:I-383.
8. Iyer SS, Yadav S, Vitek J, Wadlington V, et al. Technical approaches to angioplasty and stenting of the extracranial carotid arteries. Circulation 1995;92:I-383.
9. Diethrich EB, Lopez JR, Galarza L. Stents for vascular reconstruction in the carotid artereis. Circulation 1995;92:I-383.
10. Yadav S, Roubin G, Iyver S, et al. Immediate and late outcome after carotid angioplasty (PTA) and stenting. J Am Coll Cardiol 1996;27:277A.
11. Diethrich EB, Papazoglou CO, Lopez JR, Lopez-Galarza L. Endoluminal grafts for aneurysm exclusion and intraluminal bypass in the superficial femoral arteries. Circulation 1995;92:I-377.

529. Answer: a

Peripheral Intra-Arterial Thrombolysis (PIAT) consists of direct intra-arterial infusion of fibrinolytic agents to restore blood flow to an ischemic limb due to thrombotic or embolic occlusion. Adjunctive thrombolytic therapy can convert a long occlusion to a short occlusion or discrete stenosis, thus limiting the extent of surgical revascularization or making the lesion more amenable to percutaneous intervention. Although no thrombolytic agent has received FDA approval for peripheral vascular use, Urokinase is currently the most commonly used agent for PIAT because it offers distinct advantages over Streptokinase (shorter infusion time, fewer complications)[1,2] and tissue plasminogen activator (lower cost, fewer hemorrhagic complications). [3,4]

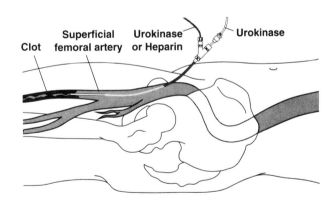

Peripheral Intra-Arterial Thrombolysis (PIAT)

References:
1. Belkin M, Belkin B, Buckman CA, et al. Intra-arterial fibrinolytic therapy: efficacy of streptokinase vs urokinase. Arch Surg 1986; 121: 769-773.
2. Van Breda A, Groar RA, Katzen BT, et al. Relative cost-effectiveness of urokinase versus streptokinase in the treatment of peripheral vascular disease. J Vasc Interv Radiol 1991; 2: 77-87.
3. Graor RA, Olin J,Bartholomew JR, et al. Efficacy and safety of intraarterial local infusion of streptokinase, urokinase and tissue plasminogen activator for peripheral arterial occlusion: a retrospective review. J Vasc Med Biol;1990:310-5.

4. Meyerovitz MF, Goldhaber SZ, Reagan K, et al., recombinant tissue-type plasminogen activator versus urokinase in peripheral arterial and graft occlusions: a randomized trial. Radiol 1990; 175:75-78.

530. Answer: b

Mechanical atherectomy is undergoing extensive evaluation; [1-6] 4 devices have received FDA approval in the peripheral vessels: DCA, TEC, the Kensey catheter, and Rotablator. With the exception of the Kensey catheter, all depend on the ability to pass a guidewire through the lesion. Initial success after directional atherectomy is 95% for femoro-popliteal stenoses in patients with claudication; 2-year patency is only 45% and major complications occur in 5%. Directional atherectomy is not useful for distal vessels, long total occlusions or for limb salvage. Despite early enthusiasm for directional atherectomy, several large series suggest worse results compared to PTA.[7-10] However, it may be useful for specific indications, such as ulcerated atheromas causing "Blue-toe syndrome"; extensive dissections which are not amenable to intravascular stents; and stenoses in vein grafts.[11,12] The rotational atherectomy devices have achieved initial success rates of 80%, with 6-month patency of 40% and 2--year patency of only 15%; 8% of patients require urgent surgery for perforation or distal embolization. Similar to all other angioplasty techniques, the worst results are observed in long occlusions in the femoro-popliteal system for limb salvage.

References:
1. Queral LA, Criado FJ, Patten P et al. Long-term results of simpson atherectomy. In Yao JST, Pearce WH (Eds). Technologies in Vascular Surgery. W.B. Saunders, Philadelphia, 1992;366-372.
2. Simpson JB, Selmon MR, Robertson GC et al. Transluminal atherectomy for occlusive peripheral vascular disease. Am J Cardiol 1988;61:96G-101G.
3. Ahn SS, Eton D, Mehigan JT. Preliminary clinical results of rotary atherectomy. In Yao JST, Pearce WH (Eds). Technologies in Vascular Surgery. W.B. Saunders, Philadelphia, 1992;388-401.
4. Snyder SO, Wheeler JR, Gregory RT et al. Kensey Catheter: early results with a transluminal endarterectomy tool. J Vasc Surg 1988;8:541-543.
5. Wholey MH, Smith JAM, Godlewski BS, et al. Recanalization of total arterial occlusions with the kensey dynamic angioplasty catheter. Radiol 1989;172:95-98.
6. Ahn SS, Auth D, Marcus D, et al. Removal of focal atheromatous lesions by angioscopically guided high-speed rotary atherectomy: preliminary experimental observations. J Vasc Surg 1988;7:292-300.
7. Becker GJ. Femoropopliteal angioplasty, atherectomy, stents. Second international symposium on cardiovascular and ind interventional radiology. Harvard Medical School/Brigham and Women's Hospital, Vol. 1, 1994: 53-65.
8. Dorros G, Lewin RF, Sachdev N, et al: Percutaneous atherectomy of occlusive peripheral vascular disease: Stenoses and/or occlusions. Cathet Cardiovasc Diagn 1989 18:1-6.
9. McLean GK. Percutaneous peripheral atherectomy. J Vasc Interv Radiol1993; 4:465-480.
10. Johnson DE, Hinohara T, Selmon MR, et al: Primary peripheral arterial stenoses and restenoses excised by transluminal atherectomy: A histopathological study. J Am Coll Cardiol 1990 15:410-425.
11. Dolmatch BL, Rholl KS, Moskowitz LB, et al. Blue toe syndrome: Treatment with percutaneous Atherectomy. Radiol 1989; 172:799-804.
12. Katzen BT, Becker GJ, Benenati JF, et al. Long-term follow-up of directional atherectomy in the femoral and popliteal arteries. (abstr). J Vasc Interv Radiol 1992; 3:38-39.

531. Answer: a

Hot-tip laser assisted balloon angioplasty and excimer laser angioplasty are rarely used; immediate results and long-term patency are worse than PTA.[1-8]

References:
1. Rosenthal D. Hot-tip Laser Angioplasty: a three year follow-up study. In Yao JST, Pearce WH (Eds). Technologies in Vascular Surgery. W.B. Saunders, Philadelphia, 1992, pg. 357-365.
2. Rosenthal D, Pesa FA, Gottsegen WL, et al. Thermal laser balloon angioplasty of the superficial femoral artery: a multicenter review of 602 cases. J Vasc Surg 1989;14:152-159.
3. White RA, Grundfest WS. Lasers in cardiovascular disease. Year Book Medical Publishers, Chicago, 1987.
4. Choy DSJ. History of Lasers in Medicine. Thorac Cardiovasc Surg 1988;36:114-117.
5. Litvack F, Grundfest WS, Adler L, et al. Percutaneous excimer-laser and excimer-laser-assisted angioplasty of the lower extremities: results of initial clinical

trial. Radiol 1989;172:231-235.

6. McCarthy WJ, Vogelzang RL, Nemcek AA Jr et al. Excimer laser-assisted femoral angioplasty: early results. J Vasc Surg 1991;13:607-614.

7. McCarthy WJ, Vogelzang RL, Pearce WH et al. Excimer laser treatment of femoral artery atherosclerosis. In Yao JST, Pearce WH (Eds). Technologies in Vascular Surgery. W.B. Saunders, Philadelphia, 1992;346-356.

8. Perler BA, Osterman FA, White RI et al. Percutaneous laser probe femoropopliteal angioplasty: a preliminary experience. J Vasc Surg 1989;10:352-357.

Balloon Valvuloplasty

532. Answer: a

Closed surgical commissurotomy and PBMV increase orifice diameter and leaflet mobility by separating fused commissures and fracturing calcified nodules.[1-4] In contrast to open surgical commissurotomy (i.e., performed under direct vision using circulatory arrest and cardiopulmonary bypass), PBMV and closed commissurotomy have little or no impact on subvalvular thickening or chordal involvement.

References:

1. McKay RG, Lock JE, Safian RD, et al. Balloon dilation of mitral stenosis in adult patients: post morterm and percutaneous mitral valvuloplasty studies. J Am Coll Cardiol 1987;9:723-731.

2. Block PC, Palaeios IF, Jacobs ML, et al. Mechanism of percutaneous mitral valvotomy. Am J Cardiol 1987;59:178-179.

3.. Kaplan JD, Isner JM, Karas RH, et al. In vitro analysis of mechanisms of balloon valvuloplasty of stenotic mitral valves. Am J Cardiol 1987;59:318-323.

4.. Hogan K, Ramaswamy K, Losordo DW, et al. Pathology at mitral commissurotomy performed with the Inoue catheter: implication for mechanisms and complications. Cathet Cardiovasc Diagn 1994;32(Suppl 2):42-51.

533. Answer: a

Once the diagnosis of mitral stenosis is established, 2-D and transesophageal echocardiography (TEE) are recommended to assess the extent of mitral valve thickening, calcification, leaflet mobility, subchordal disease, and mitral regurgitation. Findings by 2-D echocardiography can be used to generate an "echo score," which has important prognostic impact on the immediate and longterm results after PBMV.[1] TEE is particularly useful in evaluating left atrial thrombus, especially in patients with atrial fibrillation: Patients with cavitary thrombus should be treated with anticoagulants for 2 - 3 months prior to valvuloplasty (due to the risk of systemic embolization). Persistent thrombus is a contraindication to PBMV, although small numbers of patients with thrombus limited to the left atrial appendage have undergone PBMV with TEE guidance.[2-5] A prior history of embolism in the absence of thrombus on TEE is not a contraindication to PBMV.[6-8]

References:

1. Palacios IF, Block PC, Wilkins GT, et al. Follow-up of patients undergoing percutaneous mitral balloon valvotomy. Analysis of factors determining restenosis. Circulation 1989;79:573-579.

2. Yeh K-H, Hung J-S, Wu C-J, Fu M. Safety of inoue balloon mitral commissurotomy in patients with left atrial appendage thrombi. Am J Cardiol 1995;75:302-304.

3. Hung J. Mitral stenosis with left atrial thrombi: Inoue balloon catheter technique. New York: Igakushoin Medical, 1992:280-293.

4. Fu M, Hung J-S, Lee C-B, Cherng W-J. Coronary neovascularization as a specific sign for left atrial appendage thrombus in mitral stenosis. Am J Cardiol 1991;67:1158-1160.

5. Chen WJ, Chen MF, Liau CS, Chung C. Safety of percutaneous transvenous balloon mitral commissurotomy in patients with mitral stenosis and thrombus in the left atrial appendage. Am J Cardiol 1992;70:117-119.

6. Chow WH, Chow TS, Yip A, Cheung KL. Percutaneous balloon mitral valvotomy in patients with history of embolism. Am J Cardiol 1993;71:1243-1244.

7. Kamalesh M, Burger AJ, Shubrooks SJ. The use of transesophageal echocardiography to avoid left atrial thrombus during percutaneous mitral valvuloplasty. Cathet Cardiovasc Diagn 1993;28:320-322.

8. Vahanian A, Acar J. Mitral valvuloplasty: The French Experience. In: Topol EJ, Editor. Textbook of Interventional Cardiology; Philadelphia, WB Saunders, 1994.

534. Answer: a, b, c, d

Mitral Valve Echo Score Based on Morphologic Features *

Grade	Definition
	Leaflet Mobility
1	Highly mobile valve; only leaflet tips restricted
2	Normal mobility (mid portion and base of leaflet)
3	Valve moves forward in diastole, mainly from the base
4	No forward movement of leaflets in diastole
	Leaflet Thickening
1	Leaflets normal in thickness (4-5mm)
2	Mid portion of leaflets normal; thickening of margins (5-8mm)
3	Moderate thickening of entire leaflet (5-8mm)
4	Marked thickening of leaflet (>8 mm)
	Subvalvular Disease
1	Minimal thickening just below mitral leaflets
2	Thickening of chordal structures extending up to one-third of the chordal length
3	Thickening extends to distal third of the chords
4	Extensive thickening and shortening of all chordal structures to papillary muscles
	Calcification
1	Single area of increased echo brightness
2	Scattered areas of brightness confined to leaflet margins
3	Brightness extends into mid portion of leaflets
4	Extensive brightness throughout the leaflets

* Echo score is determined by adding the individual scores for leaflet mobility, leaflet thickening, subvalvular disease, and calcification

535. Answer: b

The two general approaches to PBMV are the antegrade tansvenous approach and the retrograde transarterial approach.

536. Answer: a, c, d

The technique of transseptal left heart catheterization is as follows: An 8F sheath is introduced into the right femoral vein and exchanged for a modified 8F Mullins sheath and dilator, which is advanced over a 0.032-inch J-guidewire into the superior vena cava. The guidewire is removed, a Brockenbrough needle is advanced to within a few mm of the tip of the dilator, and the needle is then flushed and connected to a transducer for continuous pressure monitoring. There are several techniques for crossing the interatrial septum; the easiest is to orient the arrow on the Brockenbrough handle to 5 o'clock while monitoring the position of the needle in the AP projection. In this position, as the sheath, dilator, and needle are withdrawn along the shadow of the spine, the needle tip will descend over the top of the aortic knob, and then drop into the fossa ovalis. Further slight pullback and then gentle re-advancement of the Mullins sheath and dilator will usually produce a "catching" sensation, indicating that the tip is in the fossa ovalis. This position can be confirmed by further imaging in a standard 30° RAO projection, which should demonstrate that the needle is directed toward the atrial side of the AV groove. Similarly, fluoroscopy can be employed in the lateral projection. In some cases, a high left atrial pressure may result in flattening and posterior displacement of the fossa ovalis. If the fossa cannot be easily identified as described above, the needle can be oriented more posteriorly by turning the arrow to 6 o'clock. In some cases, it may be necessary to repeat the entire approach after adding an extra bend to the tip of the Brockenbrough needle. In particularly difficult cases, transesophageal echo may be useful for identifying the fossa ovalis. Once proper position is achieved, the Mullins sheath and dilator are gently advanced into the fossa (which may result in transient pressure damping), and the Brockenbrough needle is advanced across the atrial septum to the left atrium, which is usually associated with a slight "popping" sensation. In general, the AP and RAO projection result in mild foreshortening of the atrial septum and left atrium; it is therefore preferable to advance the needle into the left atrium in a 60°-90° LAO projection. Transseptal catheterization described above is safe: Perforation leading to tamponade has been reported in 1.3%; mortality is less than 0.1%.[1]

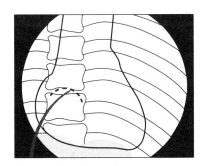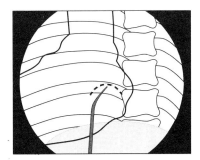

Transseptal Puncture

Orientation of needle in antero-posterior (A) and left lateral (B) view. The dotted line represents the limbus of the fossa ovalis.

References:
1. Roelke M, Smith AJ, Palacios IF. The technique and safety of transseptal left heart catheterization: the Massachusetts General Hospital experience with 1279 procedures. Cathet Cardiovasc Diagn 1994;32:332-339.

537. Answer: a

PBMV produces immediate improvement in hemodynamic and clinical status in the majority of patients.[1-19] In general, there is a 50-70% decrease in transmitral gradient and a 50-100% increase in mitral valve area. Approximately 10% of patients have persistent mitral valve area $< 1.0 \text{ cm}^2$.

Immediate Results of PBMV

Series	Technique	N (pts)	MVA (cm²)		MVG (mm Hg)	
			Pre	Post	Pre	Post
Fawzy[19] (1996)	I	220	0.7	1.7	15	6
Chen[6] (1995)	I	4832	1.1	2.1	18	5
Arora[9] (1994)	2,I	600	0.8	2.2	27	4
Block[10] (1994)	1,2	570	0.9	2.0	16	6
Vahanian[8] (1994)	2,I	790	1.1	2.1	15	6
Stephandis[1] (1994)	R	154	1.0	2.2	16	6
Feldman[12] (1993)	I	260	1.0	1.8	14	6
Pan[13] (1993)	2,I	350	1.0	2.1	18	7
NHLBI[2] (1992)	1,2	738	1.0	2.0	14	6
Cohen[3] (1992)	1,2	146	1.0	2.1	14	6
Abascal[4] (1992)	1,2	130	0.9	1.8	16	6
Stephanadis[7] (1992)	R	86	0.9	2.1	16	5
Hung[14] (1991)	I	219	1.0	2.0	13	6
Ruiz[15] (1990)	2	276	0.9	2.4	16	5

Abbreviations: MVA = mitral valve area; MVG = transmitral valve gradient; I = Inoue technique; 1 = single balloon technique; 2 = double balloon technique; R = retrograde (transarterial) technique

Answers

References:
1. Vahanian A, Michel PL, Cormier B, et al. Results of percutaneous mitral commissurotomy in 200 patients. Am J Cardiol 1989;63:847-852.
2. The National Heart, Lung, and Blood Institute Balloon Valvuloplasty Registry Participants Multicenter Experience with Balloon Mitral Commissurotomy: NHLBI Balloon Valvuloplasty Registry report on immediate and 30-day follow-up results. Circulation 1992;85:448-461.
3. Cohen DT, Kuntz RE Gorday SP, et al. Predictors of Longterm outcome after percutaneous balloon mitral valvuloplasty. N Engl J Med 1992;327:1329-1335.
4. Abascal VM, Wilkins GT, O'Shea JP, et al. Prediction of successful outcome in 130 patients undergoing percutaneous mitral valvotomy. Circulation 1990;82:448-456.
5. Nobuyoshi M, Hameishi N, Dimura T, et al. Indications, complications, and short-term clinical out-come of percutaneous transvenous mitral commissurotomy. Circulation 1989;80:782-792.
6. Chen CR, Cheng TO. Percutaneous balloon mitral valvuloplasty by the Inoue technique. A multicenter study of 4832 patients in China. Am Heart J 1995;129:1197-1203.
7. Stefanadis C, Stratos C, Pitsaves C, et al. Retrograde nontransseptal balloon mitral valvuloplasty immediate results and Longterm follow-up. Circulation 1992;85:1760-1767.
8. Vahanian A, Acar J. Mitral valvuloplasty: The French Experience. In: Topol EJ, Editor. Textbook of Interventional Cardiology; Philadelphia, WB Saunders, 1994.
9. Arora R, Kalra G, Murty G, et al. Percutaneous transatrial mitral commissurotomy: Immediate and intermediate results. J Am Coll Cardiol 1994;23:1327-32.
10. Block PC, Palacies IF. Aortic and mitral balloon valvuloplasty. The US Experience. In: Topol EJ, Editor. Textbook of Interventional Cardiology; Philadelphia, WB Saunders, 1994.
11. Stephanadis, Toutouzas P. Retrograde nontransseptal mitral valvuloplasty. In: Topol EJ, Editor. Textbook of Interventional Cardiology; Philadelphia, WB Saunders, 1994.
12. Feldman T, Carroll JD, Herrmann HC, Holmes DR. Effect of balloon size and stepwise inflation technique on the acute results of inoue mitral commissurotomy. Cathet Cardiovasc Diagn 1993;28:199-205.
13. Pan M, Medina A, deLexo JS, Hernandez E. Factors determining late success after mitral balloon valvulotomy. Am J Cardiol 1993;71:1181-1185.
14. Hung J, Chern M, Wu J, Fu M. Short and longterm results of catheter balloon percutaneous transvenous mitral commissurotomy. Am J Cardiol 1991;67:854-862.
15. Ruiz CE, Allen J, Lau F. Percutaneous double balloon valvotomy for severe rheumatic mitral stenosis. Am J Cardiol 1990;65:473-477.
16. Park SJ, Kim JJ, Park SW, et al. Immediate and one-year results of PBMV using Inoue and double-balloon techniques. Am J Cardiol 1993;71:938-943.
17. Ribeiro PA, Fawzy ME, Arafat MA, Dunn B. Comparison of mitral valve area results of balloon mitral valvotomy using the inoue and double balloon techniques. Am J Cardiol 1991;68:687-688.
18. Bassand J, Schiele F, Bernard Y, Anguenot T. The double-balloon and inoue techniques in percutaneous mitral valvuloplasty: comparative results in a series of 232 cases. J Am Coll Cardiol 1991;18:982-989
19. Fawzy ME, Mimish L, Sivanandam V, et al. Advantage of Inoue balloon catheter in mitral balloon valvotomy: Experience with 220 consecutive patients. Cathet Cardiovasc Diagn 1996;38:9-14.

538. Answer: a

Valve areas are smaller after PBMV with single balloons than double balloons, and results with the Inoue balloon are similar to the double balloon technique.[1-4]

Immediate Results and Technique of PBMV

| Series | N (pts) | Technique | MVA (cm²) | | MVG (mmHg) | |
			Pre	Post	Pre	Post
Park[1]	59	I	0.9	1.9	-	-
(1993)	61	2	0.9	2.0	-	-
Ribeiro[2]	9	I	0.8	1.8	-	-
(1993)	9	2	0.8	1.9	-	-
NHLBI[3]	114	1	0.9	1.7	14	7
(1992)	591	2	1.0	2.0	14	6
Bassand[4]	161	2	1.0	2.0	13	5
(1991)	60	I	1.1	2.0	12	5

Abbreviations: MVA = mitral valve area; MVG = transmitral valve gradient; I = Inoue technique; 1 = single balloon technique; 2 = double balloon technique; R = retrograde (transarterial) technique; - = not reported

References:
1. Park SJ, Kim JJ, Park SW, et al. Immediate and one-year results of PBMV using Inoue and double-balloon techniques. Am J Cardiol 1993;71:938-943.
2. Ribeiro PA, Fawzy ME, Arafat MA, Dunn B. Comparison of mitral valve area results of balloon mitral valvotomy using the inoue and double balloon techniques. Am J Cardiol 1991;68:687-688.
3. Bassand J, Schiele F, Bernard Y, Anguenot T. The double-balloon and inoue techniques in percutaneous mitral valvuloplasty: comparative results in a series of 232 cases. J Am Coll Cardiol 1991;18:982-989.
4. The National Heart, Lung, and Blood Institute Balloon Valvuloplasty Registry Participants Multicenter Experience with Balloon Mitral Commissurotomy: NHLBI Balloon Valvuloplasty Registry report on immediate and 30-day follow-up results. Circulation

539. Answer: b

Several reports confirm the effectiveness of PBMV after previous surgical commissurotomy[1-4] (although symptom recurrence is more frequent at 6 months),[1-3] and for pregnant women with mitral stenosis.[5-10]

References:
1. Davidson CT, Bashere TM, Mickel M, et al. Balloon mitral commissurotomy after previous surgical commissurotomy. The NHLBI balloon valvuloplasty registry participants. Circulation 1992;86:91-99.
2. Jang I-K, Block P, Newell J, Tuzcu M, Palacios I. Percutaneous mitral balloon valvotomy for recurrent mitral stenosis after surgical commissurotomy. Am J Cardiol 1995;75:601-605.
3. Serra A, Bonan R, Lefevre T, Barraud P. Balloon mitral commissurotomy for mitral restenosis after surgical commissurotomy. Am J Cardiol 1993;71:1311-1315.
4. Rediker D, Block P, Abascal V. Mitral balloon valvuloplasty for mitral restenosis after surgical commissurotomy. J Am Coll Cardiol 1988;11:252-256.
5. Vahanian A, Acar J. Mitral valvuloplasty: The French Experience. In: Topol EJ, Editor. Textbook of Interventional Cardiology; Philadelphia, WB Saunders, 1994.
6. Glantz JC, Pomerantz RM, Cunningham MJ, et al. Percutaneous balloon valvuloplasty for severe mitral stenosis during pregnancy: a review of therapeutic options. Obstet Gyn Surg 1993;48:503-508.
7. Kalra G, Arora R, Kahn J, Nigam M. Percutaneous mitral commissurotomy for severe mitral stenosis during pregnancy. Cathet Cardiovasc Diagn 1994;33:28-30.
8. Lung B, Cormier B, Elias J, Michel P. Usefulness of percutaneous balloon commissurotomy for mitral stenosis during pregnancy. Am J Cardiol 1994;73:398-400.
9. Safian R, Berman A, Sachs B, et al. Percutaneous balloon mitral valvuloplasty in a pregnant woman with mitral stenosis. Cathet Cardiovasc Diagn 1988;15:103-108.
10. Esteves CA, Ramos AIO. Effectiveness of percutaneous balloon mitral valvotomy during pregnancy. Am J Cardiol 1991;68:930-934.

540. Answer: a, b, c, d, e

Serious complications include death (0-1.6%), thromboembolic events (0-6.5%), and severe mitral regurgitation requiring valve replacement (0.9%-3%); transient heart block and pericardial tamponade occur infrequently (<5%) with the transseptal techniques.[1] While a left-to-right shunt is detected in 20% of patients immediately after transseptal PBMV, the shunt ratio is usually < 1.5 and decreases over the next 6 months in the majority of cases.[2-5]

Complications of PBMV

Series	N (pts)	Death (%)	Emb/CVA (%)	Perf/Tamp (%)	MR (%)
Fawzy[6] (1996)	220	0	0	0.9	1.4
Chen[7] (1995)	4832	0.1	0.5	0.8	0.4

Answers

Series	N (pts)	Death (%)	Emb/CVA (%)	Perf/Tamp (%)	MR (%)
Arora[8] (1994)	600	1.0	0.5	1.3	1.0
Block[9] (1994)	570	0.5	1.0	1.0	1.4
Vahanian[10] (1994)	810	0.5	3.6	0.9	3.5
Stephanadis[11] (1994)	155	0.6	0	0	1.3
Feldman[12] (1993)	260	1.1	0.7	0.7	2.7
NHLBI[13] (1992)	737	1.6	1.7	0.4	-
Cohen[14] (1992)	146	1.0	2.0	4.0	2.7
Stephanadis[15] (1992)	86	0	0	0	1.2
Bassand[16] (1991)	232	0	6.5	2.6	-
Ruiz[17] (1990)	285	0.7	1.4	4.9	-
Hung[18] (1991)	219	0.5	1.4	0	6
Vahanian[19] (1989)	200	0	4	-	-
Noboyoshi[20] (1989)	106	0	0	2	4

Abbreviations: Emb/CVA = embolic event or stroke; Perf/Tamp = cardiac perforation or tamponade; MR = severe mitral regurgitation; - = not reported

References:
1. Roelke M, Smith AJ, Palacios IF. The technique and safety of transseptal left heart catheterization: the Massachusetts General Hospital experience with 1279 procedures. Cathet Cardiovasc Diagn 1994;32:332-339.
2. Thomas MR, Monaghan MJ, Metealfe JM, et al. Residual atrial septal defects following balloon mitral valvuloplasty using different techniques. A transthoracic and transesophageal study demonstrating an advantage of the Inoue balloon. Eur Heart J 1992;13:496-502.
3. Arora R, Jolly N, Kalra GS, et al. Atrial septal defect after balloon mitral valvuloplasty: a transesophageal echocardiographic study. Angiology 1993;44:217-221.
4. Cequier A, Bonan R, Serra A, et al. Left to right shunting after percutaneous mitral valvuloplasty. Incidence and longterm hemodynamic follow-up. Circulation 1990;81:1190-1197.
5. Casale P, Block PC, O'Shea JP, et al. Atrial septal defect after percutaneous mitral balloon valvuloplasty: Immediate results and follow-up. J Am Coll Cardiol 1990;15:1300-1304.
6. Fawzy ME, Mimish L, Sivanandam V, et al. Advantage of Inoue balloon catheter in mitral balloon valvotomy: Experience with 220 consecutive patients. Cathet Cardiovasc Diagn 1996;38:9-14.
7. Chen CR, Cheng TO. Percutaneous balloon mitral valvuloplasty by the Inoue technique. A multicenter study of 4832 patients in China. Am Heart J 1995;129:1197-1203.

8. Arora R, Kalra G, Murty G, et al. Percutaneous transatrial mitral commissurotomy: Immediate and intermediate results. J Am Coll Cardiol 1994;23:1327-32.
9. Block PC, Palacies IF. Aortic and mitral balloon valvuloplasty. The US Experience. In: Topol EJ, Editor. Textbook of Interventional Cardiology; Philadelphia, WB Saunders, 1994.
10. Vahanian A, Acar J. Mitral valvuloplasty: The French Experience. In: Topol EJ, Editor. Textbook of Interventional Cardiology; Philadelphia, WB Saunders, 1994.
11. Stephanadis, Toutouzas P. Retrograde nontransseptal mitral valvuloplasty. In: Topol EJ, Editor. Textbook of Interventional Cardiology; Philadelphia, WB Saunders, 1994.
12. Feldman T, Carroll JD, Herrmann HC, Holmes DR. Effect of balloon size and stepwise inflation technique on the acute results of inoue mitral commissurotomy. Cathet Cardiovasc Diagn 1993;28:199-205.
13. The National Heart, Lung, and Blood Institute Balloon Valvuloplasty Registry Participants Multicenter Experience with Balloon Mitral Commissurotomy: NHLBI Balloon Valvuloplasty Registry report on immediate and 30-day follow-up results. Circulation 1992;85:448-461.
14. Cohen DT, Kuntz RE Gorday SP, et al. Predictors of Longterm outcome after percutaneous balloon mitral valvuloplasty. N Engl J Med 1992;327:1329-1335.
15. Stefanadis C, Stratos C, Pitsaves C, et al. Retrograde nontransseptal balloon mitral valvuloplasty immediate results and Longterm follow-up. Circulation 1992;85:1760-1767.
16. Bassand J, Schiele F, Bernard Y, Anguenot T. The double-balloon and inoue techniques in percutaneous mitral valvuloplasty: comparative results in a series of 232 cases. J Am Coll Cardiol 1991;18:982-989.
17. Ruiz CE, Allen J, Lau F. Percutaneous double balloon valvotomy for severe rheumatic mitral stenosis. Am J Cardiol 1990;65:473-477.
18. Hung J, Chern M, Wu J, Fu M. Short and longterm results of catheter balloon percutaneous transvenous mitral commissurotomy. Am J Cardiol 1991;67:854-862.
19. Vahanian A, Michel PL, Cormier B, et al. Results of percutaneous mitral commissurotomy in 200 patients. Am J Cardiol 1989;63:847-852.
20. Nobuyoshi M, Hameishi N, Dimura T, et al. Indications, complications, and short-term clinical out-come of percutaneous transvenous mitral commissurotomy. Circulation 1989;80:782-792.

541. Answer: b

In general, improvement in hemodynamic and clinical status persists in the majority of patients.[1-10] However, restenosis, defined as a loss of $\geq$ 50% of the original gain in mitral valve area, develops in 7-24% of patients within 5 years.

Clinical Follow-up After PBMV

Series	N (pts)	F/U (months)	Restenosis (%)	RePBMV (%)	MVR (%)	Death (%)
Chen[2] (1995)	4832	32	5.2	0.4	-	-
Arora[4] (1994)	600	37	1.7	0.3	0.2	-
Chan[8] (1994)	253	20	23.5	3.6	10.3	3.9
Pan[5] (1993)	350	38	11.7	0.6	5.1	1.7
Chen[9] (1992)	85	60	6.8	1.1	4.7	-
Cohen[1] (1992)	146	36	18	4.1	12.4	22.1
Stephanadis[3] (1992)	84	24	15.4	-	3.6	-

Abbreviations: F/U = follow-up interval; RePBMV = repeat PBMV; MVR = mitral valve replacement; - = not reported

Answers

Hemodynamic Follow-up after PBMV

Series	N (pts)	F/U (years)	Technique	MVA (cm^2)		
				Pre	Post	F/U
Chen[2] (1995)	-	2.6	I	1.1	2.1	1.8
Park[7] (1993)	-	1	I,2	0.9	1.9	1.7
Chen[9] (1992)	85	5	I	1.1	2.0	1.8
Block[10] (1992)	41	2	1,2	1.1	1.8	1.6
Stephanadi[3] (1992)	26	2	R	0.9	2.0	1.9

Abbreviations: F/U = follow-up interval; I = Inoue technique; 1 = single balloon technique; 2 = double balloon technique; R = retrograde (transarterial) technique; MVA = mitral valve area; - = not reported

References:
1. Cohen DT, Kuntz RE Gorday SP, et al. Predictors of Longterm outcome after percutaneous balloon mitral valvuloplasty. N Engl J Med 1992;327:1329-1335.
2. Chen CR, Cheng TO. Percutaneous balloon mitral valvuloplasty by the Inoue technique. A multicenter study of 4832 patients in China. Am Heart J 1995;129:1197-1203.
3. Stefanadis C, Stratos C, Pitsaves C, et al. Retrograde nontransseptal balloon mitral valvuloplasty immediate results and Longterm follow-up. Circulation 1992;85:1760-1767.
4. Arora R, Kalra G, Murty G, et al. Percutaneous transatrial mitral commissurotomy: Immediate and intermediate results. J Am Coll Cardiol 1994;23:1327-32.
5. Pan M, Medina A, deLexo JS, Hernandez E. Factors determining late success after mitral balloon valvotomy. Am J Cardiol 1993;71:1181-1185.
6. Hung J, Chern M, Wu J, Fu M. Short and longterm results of catheter balloon percutaneous transvenous mitral commissurotomy. Am J Cardiol 1991;67:854-862.
7. Park SJ, Kim JJ, Park SW, et al. Immediate and one-year results of PBMV using Inoue and double-balloon techniques. Am J Cardiol 1993;71:938-943.
8. Chan C, Berland J, Cribier A, Rocha P. Results of percutaneous transseptal mitral commissurotomy in patients 40 years and above with those under 40 years of age: Immediate and 5-year follow-up results. Cathet Cardiovasc Diagn 1994;32:223-230.
9. Chen CR, Cheng To, Chen JY, et al. Longterm results of percutaneous mitral valvuloplasty with the Inoue balloon catheter. Am J Cardiol 1992;70:1445-8.
10. Block PC, Palacios IF, Block EH, et al. Late (two-year) follow-up after percutaneous mitral balloon valvotomy. Am J Cardiol 1992;69:537-554.

542. Answer: a

Factors adversely affecting longterm outcome include high echo score, elevated left ventricular end diastolic pressure, and higher NYHA functional class; predicted 5-year event-free survival is 60-84% and 13-41% in patients with ≤ 1 risk factor and ≥ 2 risk factors, respectively.[1] Total survival and event-free survival at 2 years were 98% and 79% for patients with an echo score ≤ 8, and 72% and 39% for patients with echo score > 8. In another study, independent predictors of event-free survival at 2 years were echo score, change in valve gradient, and change in left ventricular end-diastolic pressure.[2]

References:
1. Palacios IF, Block PC, Wilkins GT, et al. Follow-up of patients undergoing percutaneous mitral balloon valvotomy. Analysis of factors determining restenosis. Circulation 1989;79:573-579.
2. Pavlides GS, Hauser AM, Dudlets PI, et al. The value of transesophageal echocardiography in predicting immediate and Long-term outcome in balloon mitral valvuloplasty. Comparison with transthoracic echocardiography. J Interven Cardiol 1994;7:401-408.

543. Answer: a, b, c, d, e

Clinical, echocardiographic, hemodynamic and procedural factors associated with a less successful immediate outcome include:[1-12] Advanced age (only 50% of patients > 65 years achieve a final valve area > 1.5 cm²); rhythm other than sinus; high echo score (although some patients with high scores have good results); mitral valve calcification (mitral valve area after PBMV was smaller in calcified than noncalcified valves and treatment with smaller balloons.

References:
1. Palacios IF, Block PC, Wilkins GT, et al. Follow-up of patients undergoing percutaneous mitral balloon valvotomy. Analysis of factors determining restenosis. Circulation 1989;79:573-579.
2. The National Heart, Lung, and Blood Institute Balloon Valvuloplasty Registry Participants Multicenter Experience with Balloon Mitral Commissurotomy: NHLBI Balloon Valvuloplasty Registry report on immediate and 30-day follow-up results. Circulation 1992;85:448-461.
3. Cohen DT, Kuntz RE Gorday SP, et al. Predictors of Longterm outcome after percutaneous balloon mitral valvuloplasty. N Engl J Med 1992;327:1329-1335.
4. Abascal VM, Wilkins GT, O'Shea JP, et al. Prediction of successful outcome in 130 patients undergoing percutaneous mitral valvotomy. Circulation 1990;82:448-456.
5. Pan M, Medina A, deLexo JS, Hernandez E. Factors determining late success after mitral balloon valvotomy. Am J Cardiol 1993;71:1181-1185.
6. Wilkins GT, Weyman AE, Abascal VM, et al. Percutaneous mitral valvotomy: An analysis of echocardiographic variables related to outcome and the mechanism of dilation. Br Heart J 1988;60:299-308.
7. Herrmann HE, Wilkins GT, Abascal VM, et al. Percutaneous balloon mitral valvotomy for patients with mitral stenosis. Analysis of factors influencing early results. J Thorac Cardiovasc Surg 1988;96:33-38.
8. Abascal VM, Wilkins GT, Choong CY, et al. Mitral regurgitation after percutaneous balloon mitral valvuloplasty in adults: Evaluation by pulsed Doppler echocardiography. J Am Cardiol 1988;11:257-263.
9. Come PC, Riley MF, Diver DJ, et al. Noninvasive assessment of mitral stenosis before and after percutaneous balloon mitral valvuloplasty. Am J Coll Cardiol 1988;61:817-825.
10. Reid CL, Chandraratna AN, Kawamishi DT, et al. Influence of mitral valve morphology on double-balloon catheter balloon valvuloplasty in patients with mitral stenosis. Analysis of factors predicting immediate and 3-month results. Circulation 1989;80:515-524.
11. Reid CL, Otto CM, Davis KB, et al. Influence of mitral valve morphology on mitral balloon commissurotomy: Immediate and six-month results from the NHLBI Balloon Valvuloplasty Registry. Am Heart J 1992;124:657-665.
12. Complications and mortality of percutaneous balloon mitral commissurotomy. A report from the National Heart, Lung, and Blood Institute Balloon Valvuloplasty Registry. Circulation 1992;85:2014-2024.

544. Answer: b

Selection of the technique for mitral valvuloplasty is based primarily on personal experience and available equipment. In appropriate hands, all techniques are effective and safe.[1-9] In studies comparing double balloons to the Inoue technique, final valve area was slightly larger after double balloons (2.0-2.2 cm² vs. 1.7-2.0 cm²), but the degree of mitral regurgitation and intracardiac shunting were similar. (There are no studies that directly compare transarterial and transseptal techniques.) PBMV and surgical techniques (closed[10-12] and open commissurotomy[12]) have been shown to achieve similar early results, although in one report, mitral valve area at 3 years was greater in patients treated with PBMV (2.4 vs. 1.8 cm²).[12]

References:
1. The National Heart, Lung, and Blood Institute Balloon Valvuloplasty Registry Participants Multicenter Experience with Balloon Mitral Commissurotomy: NHLBI Balloon Valvuloplasty Registry report on immediate and 30-day follow-up results. Circulation 1992;85:448-461.
2. Park SJ, Kim JJ, Park SW, et al. Immediate and one-year results of PBMV using Inoue and double-balloon techniques. Am J Cardiol 1993;71:938-943.
3. Ribeiro PA, Fawzy ME, Arafat MA, Dunn B. Comparison of mitral valve area results of balloon mitral valvotomy using the inoue and double balloon techniques. Am J Cardiol 1991;68:687-688.
4. Bassand J, Schiele F, Bernard Y, Anguenot T. The double-balloon and inoue techniques in percutaneous mitral valvuloplasty: comparative results in a series of 232 cases. J Am Coll Cardiol 1991;18:982-989.
5. Kasper W, Wollschlager H, Gerbel A, et al. Percutaneous mitral balloon valvuloplasty: a comparative evaluation of two transatrial techniques. Am Heart J 1992;124:1562-6.
6. Abdullah M, Halim M, Rajedran V. Comparison between single (Inoue) and double balloon mitral valvuloplasty. Immediate and short-term results. Am Heart J 1992;123:1581-1588.
7. Rihal CS, Nishimura RA, Reeder GS, et al. Percutaneous balloon mitral valvuloplasty: Comparison of double and single (Inoue) techniques. Cathet Cardiovasc

Answers

Diagn 1993;29:183-190.

8. Manga P, Landless P, Gebka M. Comparative results of PBMV using the Trefoil/Biofoil and Inoue balloon techniques. Int J Cardiol 1994;43:21-25.

9. Zhang HP, Gamra H, Allen J, Lau F, Ruiz C. Comparison of late outcome between inoue balloon and double-balloon techniques for percutaneous mitral valvotomy in a matched study. Am Heart J 1995;130:340-4

10. Shrivastava S, Mathur A, Der V, et al. Comparison of immediate hemodynamic response to closed mitral commissurotomy, single balloon and double balloon mitral valvuloplasty in rheumatic mitral stenosis. J Thorac Cardiovasc Surg 1992;104:1262-7.

11. Turi ZG, Reyes VP, Raju BS, et al. Percutaneous balloon versus surgical closed commissurotomy for mitral stenosis: a prospective randomized trial. Circulation 1991;83:1179-1185.

12. Reyes VP, Raju BS, Wynne J, et al. Percutaneous balloon valvuloplasty compared with open surgical commissurotomy for mitral stenosis. N Engl J Med 1994;331:961-967.

545. Answer: b

Aortic stenosis (AS) in adults is most commonly caused by degenerative calcification of a congenital bicuspid valve. Characterized by a long latent period during which progressive stenosis and left ventricular hypertrophy occur, patients with severe AS may remain asymptomatic for years. However, once symptoms develop, prognosis is poor: Life-expectancy for those with angina, syncope, and heart failure is 5-, 3-, and 2-years, respectively.

546. Answer: b

Percutaneous balloon aortic valvuloplasty (PBAV) was first performed in children and adults with aortic stenosis,[1] and later applied to adults with degenerative calcific aortic stenosis.[2,3] Although PBMV has become a viable alternative to surgical commissurotomy for select patients with mitral stenosis, PBAV has not become a viable alternative to aortic valve replacement in adults.

References:

1. Lababidi Z, Wu JR, Walls JT. Percutaneous balloon aortic valvuloplasty. Results in 23 patients. Am J Cardiol 1984;53:194-197.

2. Cribier A, Saoudi N, Berland J, et al. Percutaneous transluminal valvuloplasty of acquired aortic stenosis in elderly patients: An alternative to valve replacement? Lancet 1986;1:63-67.

3. Lombard JT, Selzer A. Valvular aortic stenosis. A clinical and hemodynamic profile of patients. Ann Int Med 1987;106:292-298.

547. Answer: a, c

AVR is the standard treatment for adults with symptomatic aortic stenosis and is typically associated with marked hemodynamic improvement, regression of LV hypertrophy, enhanced LV performance, and increased survival;[1,2] perioperative mortality rates are 1.5-5% but may be as high as 15-40% for emergency operations or in patients with severe LV dysfunction and shock.[3] The impact of advanced age per se is somewhat controversial; some studies of AVR in patients > 70 years reported perioperative mortality rates of 12-33%,[4,5] but contemporary studies report perioperative mortality rates < 10%.[6,7] Actuarial 1- and 5-year survival rates are 83% and 67% for octogenarians treated with isolated AVR for aortic stenosis, which is similar to the actuarial survival of octogenarians without aortic stenosis.[6]

References:

1. Smith N, McAnulty J, Rahimtoola S. Severe aortic stenosis with impaired left ventricular function and clinical heart failure: Results of valve replacement. Circulation 1978;58:255-264.

2. Pantely G, Morton M, Rahimtoola S. Effects of successful, uncomplicated valve replacement on ventricular hypertrophy, volume and performance in aortic stenosis and in aortic incompetence. J Thorac Surg 1978;75:383-391

.3. Magovern J, Pennock J, Campbell D, Pae W. Aortic valve replacement and combined aortic valve replacement and coronary artery bypass grafting: Predicting high risk groups. J Am Coll Cardiol 1987;9:38-43.

4. Copeland J, Griepp R, Stinson E, Shumway N. Isolated aortic valve replacement in patients older than 65 years. JAMA 1977;237:1578-1581.

5. Edmunds H, Stephenson L, Edie R, Ratcliffe M. Open-heart surgery in octogenarians. N Engl J Med 1988;319:131-136.

6. Levinson JR, Akins CW, Buckley MJ, et al. Octogenarians with aortic stenosis: outcome after aortic valve replacement. Circulation 1989;80:I-49-I-56

7. Fremes S, Goldman B, Ivanov J, Weisel R. Valvular surgery in the elderly. Circulation 1989;80:I77-90.

548. Answer: a

Post-mortem and intraoperative studies indicate that the mechanisms of PBAV include fracture of calcified nodules, separation of fused commissures (rheumatic aortic stenosis), and simple stretching of valve leaflets. Although leaflet mobility and orifice dimensions improve, valve leaflets remain severely deformed, calcified, and stenotic.[1]

References:

1. Safian RD, Mandell VS, Thurer RE, et a. Postmortem and intraoperative balloon valvuloplasty of calcific aortic stenosis in elderly patients: Mechanisms of successful dilatation. J Am Coll Cardiol 1987;9:655-660.

549. Answer: a

Adults with clinical evidence of aortic stenosis should undergo 2-D echocardiography to evaluate valve function and morphology, and left ventricular performance. Right and left heart catheterization, coronary angiography, and aortography are recommended to assess the extent of coronary artery disease and aortic insufficiency.

550. Answer: b

The two potential approaches for PBAV are the retrograde arterial approach and the antegrade transvenous approach.

551. Answer: a

The most common approach to PBAV is the retrograde femoral arterial approach. A retrograde brachial approach may also be used if femoral arterial access cannot be achieved.

552. Answer: b

The antegrade transvenous approach requires transseptal left heart catheterization, as described for balloon mitral valvuloplasty. This techniques should be reserved for operators experienced in transseptal techniques and in circumstances where retrograde crossing of the aortic valve is impossible.

553. Answer: b

PBAV may be performed using single or multiple balloons; multiple balloon techniques seem to achieve slightly larger valve areas, but no difference in late outcome. In most patients, the simplest approach is the single balloon technique using a 20 mm balloon; if necessary, larger or multiple balloons may be used.[1]

References:
1. Safian RD, Kuntz RE, Berman AD. Aortic valvuloplasty. Cardiol Clin 1991;9:289-299.

554. Answer: b

PBAV results in a 50-70% decrease in aortic valve gradient, and a 40-60% increase in aortic valve area. Despite these results, all patients still have severe AS. The hemodynamic results are similar for retrograde or antegrade approaches, and for single or multiple balloons.[1-8]

Immediate Hemodynamic Results of PBAV

Series	N (pts)	Approach	AVA (cm^2)		AVG (mm Hg)	
			Pre	Post	Pre	Post
Block[2] (1994)	375	All	0.50	0.90	61	27
Letac[3] (1993)	406	S,R	0.55	0.97	72	29
Safian[1] (1991)	225	S,R	0.60	0.90	67	33
NHLBI[4] (1991)	674	All	0.5	0.8	65	31
McKay[5] (1991)	492	All	0.50	0.82	60	30
Lewin[6] (1989)	125	M,R	0.60	1.00	87	32

Abbreviations: S = single balloon; M = multiple balloons; R = retrograde approach; A = antegrade approach; AVA = aortic valve area; AVG = transaortic valve gradient

References:
1. Safian RD, Kuntz RE, Berman AD. Aortic valvuloplasty. Cardiol Clin 1991;9:289-299..
2. Block P, IF P. Aortic and mitral balloon valvuloplasty: The United States experience. In: Topol EJ, Editor. Textbook of Interventional Cardiology; Philadelphia, WB Saunders, 1994.
3. Letac B, Cribier A. Aortic balloon dilatation as a treatment of aortic stenosis: what are the indications? J Interven Cardiol 1993;6:1-6.
4. NHLBI Balloon Valvuloplasty Registry Participants. Percutaneous balloon aortic valvuloplasty. Acute and 30-day follow-up results in 674 patients from the NHLBI Balloon Valvuloplasty Registry. Circulation 1991;84:2383-2397.
5. McKay RG for the Mansfield Scientific Aortic Valvuloplasty Registry Investigators. Overview of acute hemodynamic results and procedural complications. J Am Coll Cardiol 1991;17:485-491.
6. Lewin R, Dorros G, King J, Mathiak L. Percutaneous transluminal aortic valvuloplasty: acute outcome and follow-up of 125 patients. J Am Coll Cardiol 1989;14:1210-1217.
7. Isner JM, Salem DN, Desnoyers MR, Fields CD. Dual balloon technique for valvuloplasty of aortic stenosis in adults. Am J Cardiol 1988;61:583-589.

8.   Block PC, Palacios IF. Comparison of hemodynamic results of anterograde versus retrograde percutaneous balloon aortic valvuloplasty. Am J Cardiol 1987;60:659-662.

555.   Answer: a, b, c, d, e

Major clinical complications after PBAV are not infrequent and include death (2.6-10.4%), cerebrovascular events (0.4-4.6%), cardiac perforation (0-1.8%), myocardial infarction (0.3-1.6%), severe aortic insufficiency (0-1.6%), and vascular injury requiring blood transfusion and/or vascular repair (7.5-27%).[1-7]

Complications of PBAV

Series	N (pts)	Death (%)	CVA (%)	Perf (%)	MI (%)	AI (%)	Vasc (%)
Block[2] (1994)	308	5	2	0.3	0.5	0	9
Safian[1] (1991)	225	3.1	0.4	1.2	0.5	0.8	7.5
Isner[7] (1991)	492	2.6	-	1.8	-	0.8	-
NHLBI[3] (1991)	672	3	4.6	1	1	1	27
McKay[4] (1991)	492	7.5	2.2	1.8	0.2	1	11
Cribier[6] (1990)	334	4.5	1.4	0.6	0.3	0	13.1
Lewin[5] (1989)	125	10.4	3.2	0	1.6	1.6	9.6

Abbreviations: CVA = stroke; Perf = cardiac perforation; MI = myocardial infarction; AI = severe aortic insufficiency; Vasc = vascular injury requiring surgical repair or blood transfusion; - = not reported

References:
1.   Safian RD, Kuntz RE, Berman AD. Aortic valvuloplasty. Cardiol Clin 1991;9:289-299.
2.   Block P, IF P. Aortic and mitral balloon valvuloplasty: The United States experience. In: Topol EJ, Editor. Textbook of Interventional Cardiology; Philadelphia, WB Saunders, 1994.
3.   NHLBI Balloon Valvuloplasty Registry Participants. Percutaneous balloon aortic valvuloplasty. Acute and 30-day follow-up results in 674 patients from the NHLBI Balloon Valvuloplasty Registry. Circulation 1991;84:2383-2397.
4.   McKay RG for the Mansfield Scientific Aortic Valvuloplasty Registry Investigators. Overview of acute hemodynamic results and procedural complications. J Am Coll Cardiol 1991;17:485-491.
5.   Lewin R, Dorros G, King J, Mathiak L. Percutaneous transluminal aortic valvuloplasty: acute outcome and follow-up of 125 patients. J Am Coll Cardiol 1989;14:1210-1217.
6.   Cribier A, Gerber L, Letac B. Percutaneous Balloon Aortic Valvuloplasty: The French Experience,. Philadelphia: WB Saunders, 1990. (Eds) Topol,E. Textbook of Interventional Cardiology; vol p.849).
7.   Isner JM. Acute catastrophic complications of balloon aortic valvuloplasty. J Am Coll Cardiol 1991;17:1436-1444.

Answers

556. Answer: a

557. Answer: a

Sudden hemodynamic collapse during the procedure is usually due to cardiac tamponade or aortic valve disruption,[1-4] while worsening congestive heart failure immediately after PBAV is usually due to aortic insufficiency.[5,6]

References:
1. Lewin RF, Dorros G, King JF, Seifert PE. Aortic annular tear after valvuloplasty: The role of aortic annulus echocardiographic measurement. Cathet Cardiovasc Diagn 1989;16:123-129.
2. Seifert PE, Auer JE. Surgical repair of annular disruption following percutaneous balloon aortic valvuloplasty. Ann Thorac Surg 1988;46:242-243.
3. Vrolix M, Piessens J, Moerman P, Vanhaecke J, De Geest H. Fatal aortic rupture: An unusual complication of percutaneous balloon valvuloplasty for acquired valvular aortic stenosis. Cathet Cardiovasc Diagn 1989;16:119-122.
4. Lembo NJ, King SB, Roubin GS, Hammami A. Fatal aortic rupture during percutaneous balloon valvuloplasty for valvular aortic stenosis. Am J Cardiol 1987;60:733-736.
5. Dean LS, Chandler JW, Saenz CB, Baxley WA. Severe aortic regurgitation complicating percutaneous aortic valve valvuloplasty. Cathet Cardiovasc Diagn 1989;16:130-132.
6. Sadaniantz A, Malhotra R, Korr KS. Transient acute severe aortic regurgitation complicating balloon aortic valvuloplasty. Cathet Cardiovas Diagn 1989;17:186-189.

558. Answer: b

In contrast to balloon mitral valvuloplasty, the longterm results of PBAV are poor. Available studies of 1-3 year follow-up report a high incidence of late cardiac events, including death in 30-60%, aortic valve replacement in 7-27%, and repeat balloon valvuloplasty in 4-22%.[1-4] Acute and longterm results of repeat PBAV are similar to initial PBAV.[5-7]

Clinical Follow-up After PBAV

Series	N (pts)	F/U (months)	Death (%)	AVR (%)	reBAV (%)
Safian[1] (1991)	225	24	40	27	22
NHLBI[2] (1991)	648	36	60	13	4
Cribier[4] (1990)	300	16	30	19	17
Lewin[3] (1989)	125	12	42	7	8

Abbreviations: F/U = follow-up interval (months); AVR = aortic valve replacement; reBAV = repeat BAV

References:
1. Safian RD, Kuntz RE, Berman AD. Aortic valvuloplasty. Cardiol Clin 1991;9:289-299.
2. NHLBI Balloon Valvuloplasty Registry Participants. Percutaneous balloon aortic valvuloplasty. Acute and 30-day follow-up results in 674 patients from the NHLBI Balloon Valvuloplasty Registry. Circulation 1991;84:2383-2397.
3. Lewin R, Dorros G, King J, Mathiak L. Percutaneous transluminal aortic valvuloplasty: acute outcome and follow-up of 125 patients. J Am Coll Cardiol 1989;14:1210-1217.
4. Cribier A, Gerber L, Letac B. Percutaneous Balloon Aortic Valvuloplasty: The French Experience,. Philadelphia: WB Saunders, 1990. (Eds) Topol,E.

Textbook of Interventional Cardiology; vol p.849).

5. Ferguson J, Garza R. Efficacy of multiple balloon aortic valvuloplasty procedures. J Am Coll Cardiol 1991;17:1430-1435.
6. Kuntz R, Tosteson, Anna, Maitland L, Gordon P. Immediate results and Longterm follow-up after repeat balloon aortic valvuloplasty. Cathet Cardiovasc Diagn 1992;25:4-9.
7. Koning R, Cribier A, Asselin C, Mouton-Schleifer D, Derumeaux G, Letac B. Repeat balloon aortic valvuloplasty. Cathet Cardiovasc Diagn 1992;26:249-254.

559. Answer: a, b, c, d

The poor longterm results of PBAV are secondary to several factors, including persistent severe aortic stenosis despite successful dilation, a high incidence (30-60%) of early restenosis, the presence of concomitant severe coronary artery disease, and associated noncardiac comorbid diseases.

560. Answer: b

The most important determinants of event-free survival are those associated with baseline LV performance,[1-6] not improvement in valve area. In a study of 205 valvuloplasty patients, event-free survival correlated with baseline LV ejection fraction, LV systolic pressure, aortic systolic pressure, and percent reduction in valve gradient; baseline pulmonary wedge pressure was inversely related to outcome.[6] Although overall event-free survival at 2-years was 25%, it was only 4% in patients with all 3 baseline adverse predictors. Patients with severe LV dysfunction who underwent PBAV had longterm results similar to those of untreated aortic stenosis.[6]

References:

1. Kuntz RE, Tosteson AN, Berman AD, et al. Predictors of event-free survival after balloon aortic valvuloplasty. N Engl J Med 1991;325:17-23.
2. Otto K, Mickel M, Kennedy W, et al. Three-year outcome after balloon aortic valvuloplasty: Insights into prognosis of valvular aortic stenosis. Circulation 1994;89:642-650.
3. O'Neill WW. Predictors of Longterm survival after percutaneous aortic valvuloplasty: report of the Mansfield Scientific Balloon Aortic Valvuloplasty Registry. J Am Coll Cardiol 1991;17:193-198.
4. Holmes D, Nichimura R, Reeder G. In-hospital mortality after balloon aortic valvuloplasty: frequency and associated factors. J Am Coll Cardiol 1991;17:189-192.
5. Legrand V, Beckers J, Fastrez M, et al. Longterm follow-up of elderly patients with severe aortic stenosis treated by balloon aortic valvuloplasty. Importance of hemodynamic parameters before and after dilatation. Eur Heart J 1991;12:451-457.
6. Davidson C, Harrison K, Pieper K, Harding M. Determinants of one-year outcome from balloon aortic valvuloplasty. Am J Cardiol 1991;68:75-80.

561. Answer: b

There are no prospective randomized studies of PBAV and AVR. However, a single center observational study reported the superiority of AVR in octogenarians with symptomatic aortic stenosis: In-hospital mortality rates were similar, but event-free survival at 22 months was 78% in AVR patients but only 6.5% in PBAV patients.[1]

Answers

Comparison of PBAV and AVR[1]

	PBAV (n=46)	AVR (n=23)
Age (yrs)	80	78
Preop AVG (mm Hg) *	105	107
In-hospital death (%)	6.5	8.7
Follow-up** (%)		
Death	52	13
AVR	35	0.00
EFS	6.5	78
Total survival		
1 yr.	75	83
2 yr.	47	83
3 yr.	33	75

Abbreviations: AVR = aortic valve replacement; AVG = transaortic valve gradient; EFS = event free survival
* Doppler gradient
** Follow-up at 22 months

References:
1. Bernard Y, Etievent J, Mourand J, et al. Longterm results of percutaneous aortic valvuloplasty compared with aortic valve replacement in patients more than 75 years old. J Am Coll Cardiol 1992;20:796-801.

562. Answer: b

Available data are compelling: Aortic valve replacement is the preferred treatment for virtually all adults with symptomatic aortic stenosis. Octogenarians with aortic stenosis should not be denied the opportunity for valve replacement based on age alone.

563. Answer: a, b, c

Selected patients may be considered for PBAV: Some adult patients with aortic stenosis have severely depressed ejection (EF < 25%), but LV dysfunction may be explained by one or more factors such as critical aortic stenosis and afterload mismatch, previous myocardial infarction, coexisting hypertensive heart disease, advanced mitral regurgitation, or an undefined cardiomyopathy. Although patients with left ventricular dysfunction due to critical aortic stenosis and afterload mismatch will improve after aortic valve replacement, it is difficult to identify these patients using standard clinical criteria. In contrast, patients with aortic stenosis and left ventricular dysfunction secondary to causes other than afterload mismatch may not have improvement in left ventricular performance after aortic valve replacement. In patients with aortic stenosis and severe LV dysfunction, PBAV may be used to identify a subgroup of patients who are likely to improve after AVR. In such patients, significant improvement in LV ejection fraction is observed in 40-50% of patients 3 months after PBAV;[1] however, PBAV should not be considered definitive treatment since the late clinical outcome of these patient is poor.[2,3] However, patients who demonstrate improvement in LV ejection fraction after PBAV should be considered for AVR, to improve survival. The role of PBAV in improving mitral regurgitation associated with aortic stenosis is controversial; some studies suggest a benefit,[4] but others do not.[5] Some patients with symptomatic aortic stenosis, a low cardiac output, and a low transaortic valve gradient are at high risk for AVR and have a poor longterm prognosis. In these patients, PBAV may identify a subgroup of patients with hemodynamic and clinical improvement, who might then be considered for AVR.[6] PBAV may be a life-saving procedure in select patients with aortic stenosis and cardiogenic shock. However, because in-hospital mortality is high and longterm prognosis is poor, patients who survive hospitalization should be strongly considered for AVR, or rarely cardiac transplantation.[7-13]

References:
1. Safian R, Warren S, Berman A, et al. Improvement in symptoms and left ventricular performance after balloon aortic valvuloplasty in patients with aortic stenosis and depressed left ventricular ejection fraction. Circulation 1988;78:1181-1191.
2. Berland J, Cribier A, Savin T, Lefebvre E, Koning R, Letac B. Percutaneous balloon valvuloplasty in patients with severe aortic stenosis and low ejection fraction: Immediate results and 1-year follow-up. Circulation 1989;79:1189-1196.
3. Davidson CJ, Harrison K, Leithe M, Kisslo K. Failure of balloon aortic valvuloplasty to result in sustained clinical improvement in patients with depressed left ventricular function. Am J Cardiol 1990;65:72-77.
4. Come P, Riley M, Berman A, Safian R, Waksmonski C, McKay R. Serial assessment of mitral regurgitation by pulsed doppler echocardiography in patients undergoing balloon aortic valvuloplasty. J Am Coll Cardiol 1989;14:677-682.
5. Adams P, Otto C. Lack of improvement in coexisting mitral regurgitation after relief of valvular aortic stenosis. Am J Cardiol 1990;66:105-107.
6. Nishimura R, Holmes D, Michela M. Follow-up of patients with low output, low gradient hemodynamics after percutaneous balloon aortic valvuloplasty: the Mansfield Scientific Aortic Valvuloplasty Registry. J Am Coll Cardiol 1991;17:828-833.
7. Moreno P, Jank I-K, Newell J. The role of percutaneous aortic balloon valvuloplasty in patients with cardiogenic shock and critical aortic stenosis. J Am Coll Cardiol 1994;23:1071-1075.
8. Smedira NG, Ports TA Merrick SH, et al. Balloon aortic valvuloplasty as a bridge to aortic valve replacement in critically ill patients. Ann Thorac Surg 1993;55:914-916.
9. Friedman H, Cragg D, O'Neill W. Cardiac resuscitation using emergency aortic balloon valvuloplasty. Am J Cardiol 1989;63:387-8.
10. Desnoyers M, Salem D, Rosenfield K, Mackey W, O'Donnell T, Isner J. Treatment of cardiogenic shock by emergency aortic balloon valvuloplasty. Ann Int Med 1988;108:833-5.
11. Losordo D, Ramaswamy K, Rosenfield K, Isner J. Use of emergency balloon dilation to reverse acute hemodynamic decompensation developing during diagnostic cardiac catheterization for aortic stenosis (bailout valvuloplasty). Am J Cardiol 1989;63:388-9.
12. Brady S, Davis C, Kussmaul W, Laskey W. Percutaneous aortic balloon valvuloplasty in octogenarians: Morbidity and mortality. Ann Int Med. 1989;110:761-766.
13. Cribier A, Remadi F, Koning R, Rath P, Stix G, Letac B. Emergency balloon valvuloplasty as initial treatment of patients with aortic stenosis and cardiogenic shock. N Engl J Med 1992;326:646.

564. Answer: b

PBAV may be considered in some patients with aortic stenosis who require urgent noncardiac surgery.[1-3] In these patients, PBAV results is significant hemodynamic improvement, similar to that observed in other patients treated with PBAV. In spite of this hemodynamic improvement, there are no data to suggest that routine PBAV will improve the perioperative risks of noncardiac surgery. In fact, in one study of 48 patients with severe aortic stenosis, careful monitoring of anesthesia resulted in no major complications, despite the need for vascular, orthopedic, abdominal, and other forms of surgery without preoperative PBAV.[4] We empirically proceed with valvuloplasty in patients with overt heart failure or systolic blood pressures < 100 mmHg, who require urgent noncardiac surgery.

Answers

References:
1. Levine MJ, Berman AD, Safian RD, Diver DJ. Palliation of valvular aortic stenosis by balloon valvuloplasty as preoperative preparation for noncardiac surgery. Am J Cardiol 1988;62:1309-1310.
2. Roth R, Palacios I, Block P. Percutaneous aortic balloon valvuloplasty: Its role in the management of patients with aortic stenosis requiring major noncardiac surgery. J Am Coll Cardiol 1989;13:1039-1041.
3. Hayes SN, Holmes DR, Nishimura RA, Reeder GS. Palliative percutaneous aortic balloon valvuloplasty before noncardiac operations and invasive diagnostic procedures. Mayo Clin Proc 1989;64:753-757.
4. O'Keefe JH, Shub C, Rettke SR. Risk of noncardiac surgical procedures in-patients with aortic stenosis. Mayo Clin Proc 1989;64:400-405.

Case Studies

565. Answer: b, c, d

Occasionally, conventional PTCA fails because lesion rigidity prevents full balloon expansion. Although this scenario creates considerable frustration and anxiety for the operator, there are a number of approaches that can be used to salvage these "nondilatable" lesions. One approach is to deliver higher pressures using one of several balloons capable of > 20 ATM without rupture. A second approach is to use "force-focused" angioplasty. This technique requires placement of a second 0.012-0.018-inch guidewire parallel to the original wire, followed by balloon inflation over the original wire using a noncompliant balloon. The parallel wire outside the inflated balloon can "score" the plaque, increasing lesion compliance and facilitating balloon inflation. A third technique relies on the cutting (Barath) balloon, which uses razor-sharp microtomes on a conventional balloon to score the plaque and facilitate balloon expansion. A fourth approach is to use the Rotablator, which is extremely effective and virtually always successful in nondilatable lesions. However, the risk of extending an inapparent dissection after PTCA must be weighed against the advantage of successful revascularization. However, if gross angiographic dissection is apparent after PTCA, Rotablator is contraindicated. Stent implantation should not be considered unless full balloon expansion is achieved.

566. Answer: b, c

The general considerations and approaches to nondilatable lesions in vein grafts are similar to those in native coronary arteries (see previous question). An important exception is the use of Rotablator in the body of vein grafts, which has been considered an absolute contraindication because of the risk of distal embolization and no-reflow. Personally, we have no experience with Rotablator in the body of vein grafts, but if performed, it is probably best to use the smallest burr possible to unroof the plaque while minimizing distal embolization. In many cases such as this, even slight unroofing of the rigid cap can favorably impact lesion compliance; directional atherectomy can be used for this purpose, followed by stenting, if necessary.

567.   Answer: a, b, e

This case represents an example of a nondilatable lesion due to elastic recoil (rather than lesion rigidity or calcification). Prolonged balloon inflations (with or without a perfusion balloon), higher inflation pressures, and oversize balloons may be of value, but the results are unpredictable and often associated with complications. Directional atherectomy is particularly well-suited for elastic, eccentric lesions in large vessels; other atherectomy devices are less useful unless there is associated thrombus (TEC) or calcification (Rotablator). Finally, stenting is a reasonable approach to such lesions, because of its predictability and reliability in eliminating elastic recoil.

568.   Answer: b, c, d

"Watermelon-seeding" is a fairly common source of operator frustration. Generally, this problem arises when low-profile coated balloons are used to dilate rigid lesions. There are several approaches to this problem: One approach is to gently retract the balloon during slow inflation, to see if the balloon will "seat" across the lesion. Unfortunately, this maneuver often results in "watermelon-seeding" proximal to the stenosis. Another approach is to redilate the lesion with a long (30-40 mm) balloon, which generally works nicely; shorter balloons exacerbate the problem. Since these lesions are frequently rigid, it is a good idea to use a noncompliant balloon, in case higher pressures are needed to achieve full balloon expansion. A third approach is to use Rotablator or directional atherectomy to "unroof" the rigid cap on the lesion and facilitate subsequent lumen enlargement. Although stenting could be considered, we would be concerned about the ability to seat the stent in the lesion, and would not recommend stenting until the lesion can be fully expanded with a balloon.

569.   Answer: a, b, d, e

Before the availability of stents, this type of angiographic result would have been considered a "success," even though the risk of angiographic restenosis (diameter stenosis > 50% at 6-months) is ~ 50% and the need for repeat intervention is ~ 30%. For operators who perform only PTCA, one option is to terminate the procedure and follow the patient clinically. A second option is to insert a perfusion balloon and perform a 5-30 minute inflation, with the hope that a better result will be achieved. A third option is to use higher pressures or larger balloons, but neither has been shown to improve results. In fact, oversize balloons (balloon/artery ratio > 1.1) may increase the risk of dissection and major complications. Finally, this patient could be referred to a center where stents are available. Unfortunately, the "right" answer is unknown. In most contemporary interventional practices, this lesion would be treated by stenting, because of the predictability of this approach and the expectation of a lower restenosis rate. If the Doppler guidewire is available, this is a perfect case for its use, since coronary flow reserve ≥ 2.0 predicts an excellent clinical outcome without further intervention.

570. Answer: a, b, c, d

In situations where atherectomy results in a mild persistent residual stenosis, the next course of action is to either perform additional atherectomy with the same AtheroCath at higher pressures, increase the size of the AtheroCath, or use adjunctive PTCA with a balloon/artery ratio ~ 1.0-1.1. Stenting is certainly feasible, and could have been employed as the original intervention without antecedent atherectomy. If the goal is to achieve "optimal atherectomy", this result is "suboptimal".

571. Answer: a, c, d, e

Intraluminal haziness is a common, relatively nonspecific angiographic finding after conventional PTCA. Although some operators equate intraluminal haziness with thrombus, the most common causes are intimal dissection and residual plaque.[1] The following approach to the hazy result may be useful: First, confirm that the ACT is ≥ 300 seconds. Because of the lack of specificity of intraluminal haziness for thrombus, intracoronary lytic therapy is not recommended. Second, attempt to achieve optimal PTCA results using a full-size balloon (balloon/artery ratio ~ 1.0) for at least 2 minutes at nominal inflation pressure. If inflations are not tolerated or if longer inflations are desired, a perfusion balloon can be used. Third, consider use of IVUS (to help identify residual plaque and dissection) or angioscopy (the most sensitive tool for distinguishing thrombus, dissection, and residual plaque). Although these techniques are not mandatory, they can be useful in individual cases to help assess the results and guide further intervention, if necessary. Finally, a practical solution to this problem is to simply implant a stent, because of the reliability and predictability of this approach.

References:
1. Ziada KM, Tuzcu E, deFranco AC, et al. Intravascular ultrasound assessment of the prevalence and causes of angiographic "haziness" following high-pressure coronary stenting. Am J Cardiol 1997;80:116-121.

572. Answers: c

This lesion has a disturbing angiographic appearance after PTCA, and angiography alone cannot accurately distinguish the relative contributions of dissection, thrombus, and plaque separation. Although angioscopy can be used to make these distinctions, most operators do not use it, and the future of angioscopy is questionable (at least from a marketing standpoint). The most important aspect of treating this patient is to stabilize the lesion and prevent abrupt closure; this is best accomplished by intracoronary stenting. The choice of stents is wide, but virtually all balloon-expandable (e.g., Palmaz biliary stent and all coronary stents) and self-expanding (e.g., the Wallstent) stents would work nicely. Directional atherectomy is a reasonable technique, but would require exchange of vascular sheaths and guiding catheters, and could add considerable complexity to the procedure. Although ReoPro might be a useful adjunct, it is doubtful that ReoPro alone would have much impact on stabilizing this awful result. Intracoronary lytic therapy has not been shown to be useful in this setting.

573. Answer: f

This is a fairly typical result after conventional PTCA. If the operator has little experience with new devices, there are a number of alternatives to treat this fairly typical result after PTCA. First, in spite of the minor dissection (which is how PTCA works), this result may remain stable, and the procedure could be terminated at this point. If the operator is reluctant to pursue further intervention, it would be prudent to observe the patient in the catheterization laboratory for 15 minutes, and repeat the angiogram in multiple projections to be certain the result is stable. A second approach is to gather additional information about the lesion, using any one of a number of different techniques. The easiest technique is to advance the balloon catheter into the distal vessel and measure a translesional gradient. Although routine pressure gradient measurements have fallen out of favor, identification of a pressure gradient < 15 mm Hg may be reassuring, whereas a gradient > 30 mm Hg suggests that the result is unsatisfactory (a gradient of 15-30 mm Hg is in the "gray zone"). Intravascular ultrasound can provide additional information about the nature and extent of dissection and more precise quantitation of lumen geometry. Measurement of coronary flow reserve with the Doppler Flowire is quick and easy, and offers important physiologic information that correlates with outcome; coronary flow reserve > 2 would argue against the need for further intervention. Another advantage of the Doppler Flowire is the potential for following trends in blood flow velocity over 15 minutes, which can be used to predict complications. Of all imaging modalities, angioscopy is probably the least useful, since it will simply corroborate the presence of dissection, but offers no quantitative or physiologic data. A third approach is to perform a prolonged inflation with a perfusion balloon, which could potentially "tack-up" the dissection flap and improve the angiographic result; before the availability of stents, this would have been considered "standard fare" for this lesion. Any of the above recommendations could be employed with ReoPro, although further studies using this potent antiplatelet agent are required before firm recommendations can be offered. Data suggest that prolonged postprocedural heparin not only fails to prevent ischemic complications, but may increase bleeding and vascular injury. Finally, this lesion could be easily and successfully treated with virtually any stent. Directional atherectomy should be avoided since the presence of an extraluminal cap suggests medial dissection, which is associated with a higher risk of vessel perforation.

574. Answer: a, d

After primary PTCA, the risk of recurrent ischemia before discharge is approximately 10-15%; it is likely that many of these events are associated with the type of angiographic result observed in this patient. All of the considerations discussed in the previous case also apply to this patient, with the exception of the utility of the Doppler Flowire, since abnormal coronary flow reserve is difficult to interpret during acute myocardial infarction. The main issue surrounding this case is whether stents can be safely implanted during acute myocardial infarction. Data from our own institution and others suggest that stents should not be withheld from patients with failed primary PTCA, since the risk of stent thrombosis in this setting is no higher than for bailout stenting without acute myocardial infarction. When stenting is performed, contemporary studies suggest that Coumadin may be associated with a higher incidence of bleeding and ischemic complications than combined antiplatelet therapy with aspirin and Ticlopidine. The use of ReoPro is unproven, but not unreasonable.

575. Answer: e

This focal but severe dissection is best treated by stenting — virtually any stent would work nicely. Directional atherectomy is a reasonable alternative, since the dissection is focal and does not involve the deep layers of the arterial wall. For operators who perform only PTCA, prolonged balloon inflations with a perfusion balloon may reverse abrupt closure. Since flow impairment appears to be caused by dissection and/or plaque separation, rather than thrombus, it is doubtful that ReoPro alone would be beneficial.

576. Answer: b, c

From an angiographic standpoint, this stent result is perfect. However, it is important to resist the temptation to do nothing. At this point, the operator should either perform IVUS to confirm optimal stent deployment, or dilate the stent at high-pressure (16-20 ATM) with or without IVUS guidance. This patient underwent adjunctive PTCA with a 3.0 x 20 mm high-pressure balloon at 16 ATM, which resulted in extensive distal dissection requiring emergency bypass surgery. It is important to limit high-pressure inflations to the stented segment; a 3.0 x 9-15 mm balloon would have been a better choice.

577. Answer: b

Operators who perform percutaneous interventions on saphenous vein grafts should always anticipate the possibility of no-reflow, keeping a consistent treatment strategy in mind. It is of paramount importance to clearly distinguish no-reflow from abrupt closure of the target vessel, since treatment strategies are totally different. There are no prospective randomized trials comparing treatments of no-reflow, although several observational studies permit reasonable recommendations. First and foremost is the observation that many cases of no-reflow can be reversed by intracoronary calcium antagonists. Most experience is with verapamil (100-250 mcg bolus every 2-4 minutes up to 2 mg as needed), but Diltiazem is also effective (1-2 mg bolus every 2-4 minutes, not to exceed 10 mg). The key point is to ensure drug delivery to the distal capillary bed: If there is TIMI flow ≤ 1, drug administered through the guiding catheter (particularly those with sideholes) will never reach the distal capillary bed. In these circumstances, it is best to advance a deflated balloon catheter, infusion catheter, or any suitable transfer catheter into the distal vessel, and administer an intracoronary calcium antagonist through the central lumen. A very nice catheter for this purpose is the Ultrafuse-X, which is a double lumen catheter that allows distal drug delivery without relinquishing guidewire access. If there is "slow-flow" (TIMI flow = 2), a calcium antagonist can be delivered through the guiding catheter. The second point is that intracoronary nitroglycerin has not been shown to effectively reverse no-reflow, and should not be used as sole therapy. However, since it is not deleterious, may reverse associated epicardial spasm, and is not associated with any delays, intracoronary nitroglycerin is a reasonable adjunct. Third, while intracoronary lytics are potentially useful for distal embolization of thrombus to epicardial vessels, they are not useful for the distal microembolization characteristic of no-reflow; in our experience, intracoronary urokinase restores flow in < 10% of no-reflow cases, and increases the risk of bleeding and femoral vascular injury. Fourth, the value of intraaortic balloon pump counterpulsation is a matter of debate; it is clearly useful when there is hemodynamic compromise, possibly useful in milder degrees of "slow-flow," and probably not useful for true no-reflow. Fifth, limited anecdotal experience with ReoPro is positive, but further study is needed. Finally, conventional approaches to abrupt closure (prolonged balloon inflations, stents, emergency bypass surgery) have no role in the treatment of no-reflow.

578. Answer: d

This rare but catastrophic complication is more common after lasers and atherectomy than after PTCA. Regardless of the cause of perforation, immediate attention must be devoted to hemodynamic stabilization — ischemia is a secondary issue. An inflated balloon should be immediately positioned at the site of perforation. If the exact location of the perforation cannot be ascertained, a long (30-40 mm) balloon should be inserted to ensure coverage. A properly positioned balloon will prevent any further extravasation into the pericardium, and afford the operator more time to resuscitate the patient. Subsequent preparation and insertion of a perfusion balloon can follow, if appropriate. If there is hemodynamic collapse, the operator should do 4 more things at the same time: Protect the airway, initiate CPR, notify the surgeons, and perform immediate pericardiocentesis, leaving the pericardial drainage catheter in place. If there is any more than a moments delay in retrieving the pericardiocentesis tray, intravenous pressors and fluids should be administered to support the blood pressure. Heparin-induced anticoagulation should be reversed slowly (e.g., protamine 5-10 mg IV every 5 minutes, aiming for an ACT of 150-180 seconds). Although percutaneous CPS can be lifesaving, it can rarely be primed and instituted within minutes, and efforts are better directed at evacuating the pericardium, even by emergency pericardial window. If the patient is not in hemodynamic collapse initially, or once the patient is successfully resuscitated, further attention can be devoted to the coronary artery. Approximately two-thirds of perforations can be managed without emergency surgery, but the need for surgery is higher after free perforations caused by laser and atherectomy devices compared to those caused by PTCA. Indications for surgery include persistent (or recurrent) extravasation of contrast despite prolonged balloon inflations, and severe ischemia from vessel injury or as a consequence of balloon inflations. If the patient can be stabilized without surgical intervention, continuous monitoring of right heart filling pressures, observation in the coronary care unit, continuous pericardial drainage, and serial echocardiograms are recommended. There are a few investigational approaches to perforation, including implantation of stents covered with autologous veins or synthetic materials such as PTFE (Teflon), and coil embolization of perforated vessels that supply small areas of viable myocardium.

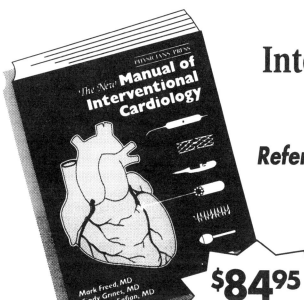
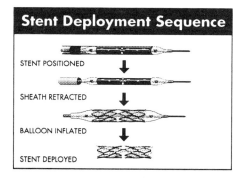
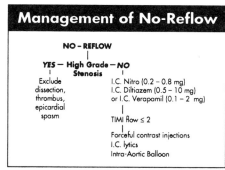

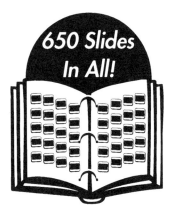
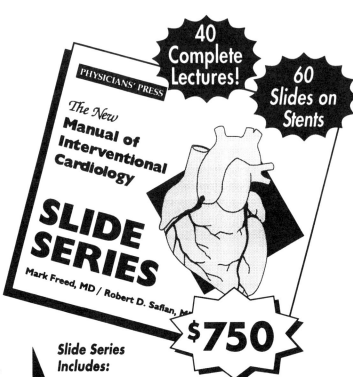
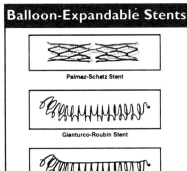
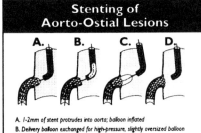

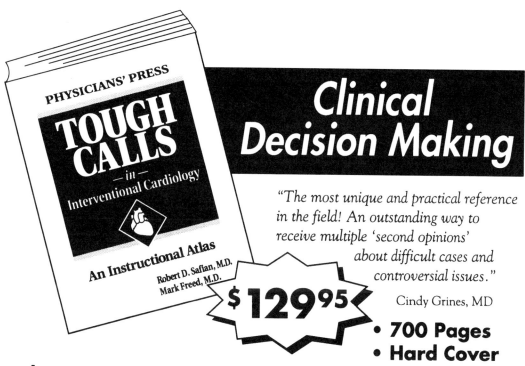
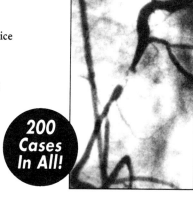

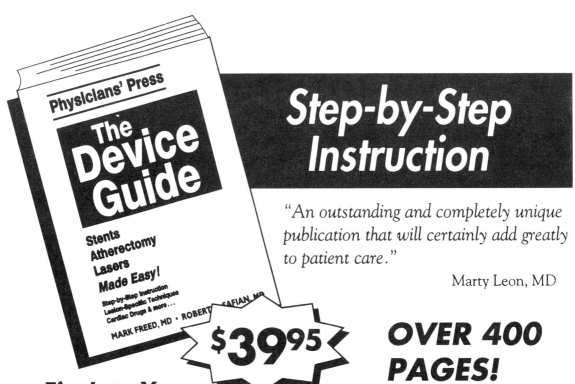
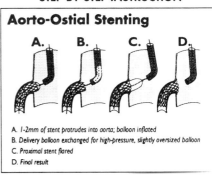
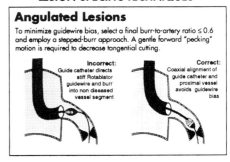

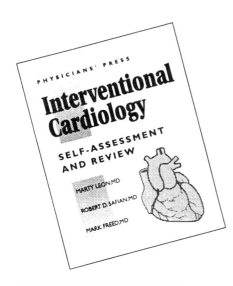

INTERVENTIONAL CARDIOLOGY:
Self–Assessment & Review

by Marty Leon, MD, Robert D. Safian, MD, and Mark Freed, MD

More than 500 questions and answers (*with literature references*) on simple and complex angioplasty; acute ischemic syndromes; lesion morphology and location, intraprocedural complications; adjunctive pharmacotherapy, imaging, and hemodynamic support; peripheral interventional, valvuloplasty; and more...

approx. 500 pages; 81/2 x 11; **$45.00**

The Stenter's Notebook

by Paul Phillips, MD, Morton Kern, MD, and Patrick Serruys, MD

A Lesion–Specific Approach to Intracoronary Stenting

Case studies, equipment selection, simple and advanced stenting techniques, adjunctive imaging and pharmacotherapy, and management of complications.

350 pages; 71/2 x 9; **$49.95**

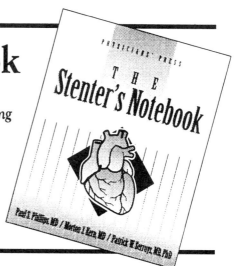

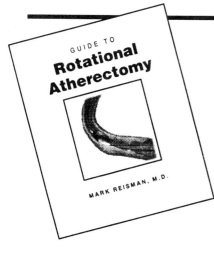

Guide to Rotational Atherectomy

by Mark Reisman, MD

A Lesion–Specific Approach to Rotational Atherectomy

Case studies, equipment selection, simple and advanced Rotablator techniques, adjunctive imaging and pharmacotherapy, and management of complications.

350 pages; 71/2" x 9"; all figures in color; **$59.95**

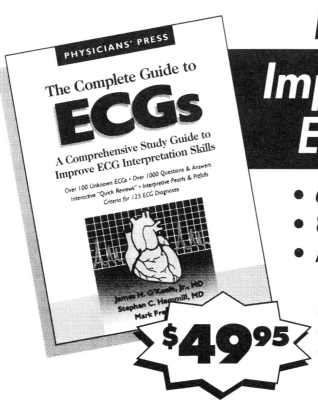

NEW!

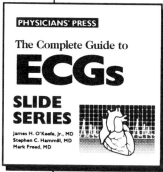

The Complete Guide to ECGs SLIDE SERIES

by James O'Keefe, Jr., MD, Stephen Hammill, MD, and Mark Freed, MD

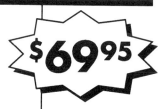

- Full color slides of all 103 ECGs from
  The Complete Guide to ECGs

- Ideal for ECG teaching conferences and study groups

- *Includes 3-ring binder,
  slide holders and paper copy of interpretations*

The ECG Criteria and ACLS Handbook

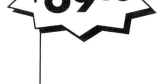

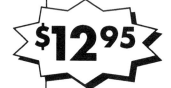

Fits a Shirt Pocket!

by James O'Keefe, Jr., MD, Stephen Hammill, MD,
Mark Freed, MD, and Steven Pogwizd, MD

Shirt-pocket companion to *The Complete Guide to ECGs*.
Provides ECG criteria and sample tracings (in color)
for 125 ECG diagnoses, including arrhythmias and
conduction disturbances; chamber enlargement and
hypertrophy; ischemic syndromes; pacemakers; and drug,
electrolyte and medical disorders. Also includes interpretive
pearls and pitfalls, and ACLS algorithms.
Approx. 160 pages; 4" x 6"

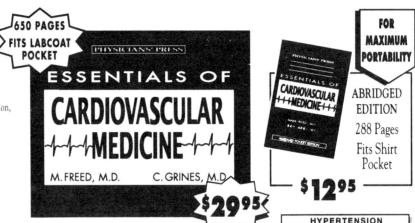
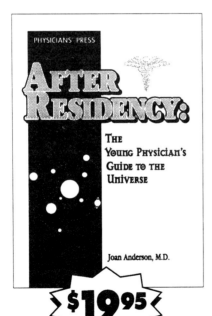

ORDERING INFORMATION
30 DAY MONEY-BACK GUARANTEE

ELECTROCARDIOGRAPHY

ITEM	DESCRIPTION	PRICE (US Dollars)
1	The Complete Guide to ECGs	$ 49.95
2	The Complete Guide to ECGs Slide Set (100 slides)	69.95
3	The ECG Criteria and ACLS Handbook	12.95

INTERVENTIONAL CARDIOLOGY

ITEM	DESCRIPTION	PRICE (US Dollars)
4	The New Manual of Interventional Cardiology	84.95
5	The New Manual of Interventional Cardiology Slide Series (650 slides)	750.00
6	Tough Calls in Interventional Cardiology	129.95
7	The Device Guide	39.95
8	Guide to Rotational Atherectomy	59.95
9	Interventional Cardiology: Self-Assessment and Review	45.00
10	The Stenter's Notebook	49.95

OTHER PUBLICATIONS

ITEM	DESCRIPTION	PRICE (US Dollars)
11a	Essentials of Cardiovascular Medicine (unabridged)	29.95
11b	Essentials of Cardiovascular Medicine (abridged)	12.95
11c	Essentials of Cardiovascular Medicine (bookset)	39.95
12	After Residency: The Young Physician's Guide to the Universe	19.95

DISCOUNT PACKAGES

ITEM	DESCRIPTION	PRICE (US Dollars)	
13	Interventional Package I: Items 4, 6, & 7	229.95	SAVE $25
14	Interventional Package II: Items 4, 5, 6, & 7	899.95	SAVE $105
15	Interventional Package III: All 6 Interventional Publications & Slides	1009.75	SAVE $150

5 Ways to Order:

Contact your local medical bookstore or:

By Phone:

(USA) (800) 642-5494

(Outside USA) (248) 645-6443

By Fax:

Fax order page to: (248) 642-4949

By Internet:

www.physicianspress.com

By Mail: Mail to:

Physicians' Press
555 S. Old Woodward
Suite 1409
Birmingham, Michigan
USA 48009-6679

§ Prices subject to change.

Sales Tax: Michigan residents add 6%; Canadian residents add 7% GST

Shipping & Handling Policy: Books & Slides are shipped immediately upon publication. It is possible to receive 2 or more shipments. **Overnight delivery available – call for charge.**

FAX/MAIL ORDER FORM

ITEM	QUANTITY	TOTAL COST (US Dollars)
_____	_____	_____
_____	_____	_____
_____	_____	_____
_____	_____	_____
_____	_____	_____

5 Ways to Order:

Contact your local medical bookstore or:

By Phone:

(USA) (800) 642-5494

(Outside USA)

(248) 645-6443

By Fax:

Fax order page to:
(248) 642-4949

By Internet:

www.physicianspress.com

By Mail: Mail to:

Physicians' Press
555 S. Old Woodward
Suite 1409
Birmingham, Michigan
USA 48009-6679

Sales Tax _____

(Michigan residents add 6%;
Canadian residents add 7% GST)

Shipping _____

(Compute shipping charge based on chart below)

TOTAL (U.S. DOLLARS) $ _____

TOTAL PURCHASE	USA UPS Ground; arrives 3–7 days	OUTSIDE USA*		
		US Postal Surface Arrives 6–8 weeks	**US Postal Air** Arrives 10-14 Days	**Express Air** UPS, FEDEX, DHL Arrives 2-5 Days
$1–35	Add $4	Add $10	Add $20	Add $30
$36–90	Add $7	Add $15	Add $30	Add $60
$91–150	Add $12	Add $20	Add $40	Add $75
$151–400	Add $14	Add $25	Add $50	Add $90
$401–750	Add $16	Add $30	Add $60	Add $120
$751+	Add $20	Add $35	Add $70	Add $150

* If shipping charges exceed those listed in the chart, you will be contacted for approval prior to shipment.

For shipping outside USA, check one: ☐ Express Air ☐ US Postal Air ☐ US Postal Surface

☐ Check Enclosed
(US Dollars from US Bank)

☐ Bill Me

☐ Credit Card: ☐ Visa ☐ MasterCard ☐ AMEX

☐ 3-Payment Plan: Orders over $300, bill my credit card each month for 3 consecutive months.

Card No.: _____

Exp. Date: _____

Signature: _____

Name: _____
(PLEASE PRINT)

Address: _____

_____

_____

Telephone (important): _____

FAX (important): _____

e-mail _____

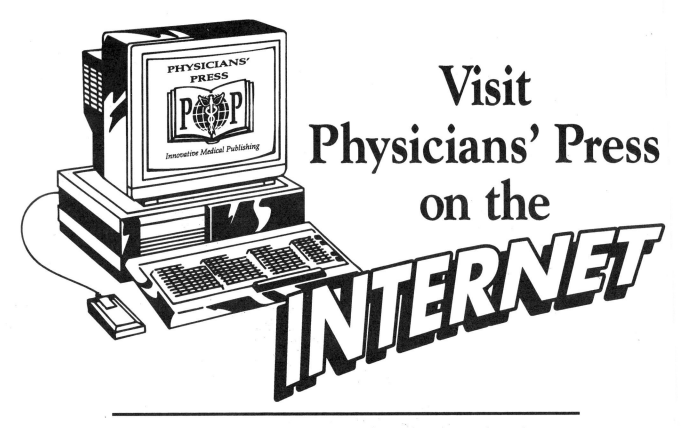